The Physiology of
BONE

The Physiology of
BONE

JANET VAUGHAN, DM, FRS

THIRD EDITION

CLARENDON PRESS · OXFORD
1981

Oxford University Press, Walton Street, Oxford OX2 6DP

London Glasgow New York Toronto
Delhi Bombay Calcutta Madras Karachi
Kuala Lumpur Singapore Hong Kong Tokyo
Nairobi Dar es Salaam Cape Town Salisbury
Melbourne Auckland

and associate companies in
Beirut Berlin Ibadan Mexico City

Published in the United States by
Oxford University Press, New York

FIRST EDITION 1970
SECOND EDITION 1975
THIRD EDITION 1981

British Library Cataloguing in Publication Data

Vaughan, Janet
 The physiology of bone. — 3rd ed.
 1. Bones
 I. Title
 612′.75 ~~QM101~~
 ISBN 0–19–857584–X

Filmset by Latimer Trend & Company Ltd, Plymouth
Printed in Great Britain
at the University Press, Oxford
by Eric Buckley
Printer to the University

Many shall run to and fro and knowledge shall be increased
The Book of Daniel 12:4

For Somerville College

Preface to Third edition

SINCE the first edition of this book in 1970 there has been increasing interest in the problems that are raised for many different disciplines in an attempt to understand the physiology of bone. The present volume is intended for readers who want a bird's-eye view of the subject and directions as to where they can find more detailed information on particular aspects. It does not attempt to give a complete account or even a full bibliography of the many exciting and often controversial questions that are covered by specialist journals and monographs. It can only hope to provide some signposts to both the past and the present, and perhaps the future.

Oxford   J.M.V.
May 1980

Preface to Second edition

CERTAIN aspects of the physiology of bone have advanced with amazing rapidity since the first edition of the book with this title appeared in 1970. This is particularly true of our understanding, still incomplete, of the behaviour of vitamin D and of the complicated story of the effects of parathyroid hormone and calcitonin on calcium homeostasis. An attempt is now made to bring our knowledge of the physiology of bone up-to-date without increasing the length of the book. This has necessitated a complete rewriting of some sections though others are little changed. The bibliography represents an attempt to include mainly references to papers and monographs that have appeared since 1969. On the other hand, mention is made of classical papers of an earlier date and in some cases knowledge is dependent on older work entirely. Again I must apologize to authors who have received inadequate mention. The bibliography is personal rather than complete.

It is hoped that this new edition will be useful to both medical students and their teachers.

Oxford   J.M.V.
May 1975

Preface to First edition

THE skeleton, for purposes of the present monograph, is taken to include both bone and the cartilage closely related to bone. The teeth are excluded. The anatomical structure and the supporting function of the skeleton is not discussed in any detail, nor is the haemopoetic marrow, a tissue which in some ways it is difficult to dissociate from consideration of bone. Emphasis is laid rather on the complex mechanisms involved in enabling the skeleton to play its essential role in mineral homeostasis.

Attention is given to the most recent work available, particularly that in journals and symposia. The bibliography does not attempt to be comprehensive. Certain questions are discussed at greater length than others for the reason that at the moment they are arousing lively interest and therefore new knowledge is available. No attempt is made to replace standard works such as *Mineral metabolism: an advanced treatise*, by Comar and Bronner, or *The biochemistry and physiology of bone*, edited by Bourne. It is certainly presumptious for one individual to attempt to survey a field which today occupies the attention of specialists from many different disciplines. However, it is hoped that a bird's-eye view of an exciting and expanding subject may be of use to medical students and their teachers.

Acknowledgements

I AM grateful to many people who have helped me in different ways in preparing this edition. My special thanks must go to John Loutit for exciting discussions and for having read the whole manuscript. I am also much indebted to Dr G. E. Harrison for his advice and help over Chapter 8. Once again I must take sole responsibility for the pattern of the book, the views expressed, and for the omission of many important references.

Thanks are due to the editors and publishers of the following journals, symposia, and books for permission to use new figures and tables. I regret that in two cases no permission has been obtained as I have not been able to trace the origin of the picture, which I had in my files: Fig. 2.3 and Fig. 1.14. *The biochemistry and physiology of bone* (2nd edn), Academic Press; *Histopathology of cartilage, bone and joints*, J. B. Lippincott Company; *Human growth*, Cassell Ltd; *Nature (London)*; *Calcified tissue Research*; *Annals of Human Biology*; *The New England Journal of Medicine*, Pergamon Press; *The Journal of Cell Biology*; *Proceedings of the Royal Society*; *Professional and Scientific Publications*, Springer Verlag.

I am also grateful to my photographer, Richard McAvoy, for his careful work. This revised edition has only been made possible because of the devoted work and patience of my secretary, Janet Judge.

Contents

1. Bone as a Tissue

BONE is a highly specialized form of connective tissue. It is distinguished from other forms of connective tissue by the fact that it is extremely hard, owing to the deposition within a relatively soft organic matrix of a complex mineral substance, largely composed of calcium, phosphate, and carbonate.

1. DEVELOPMENT

Bone is often described as developing by two different methods: intramembranous (in membrane), and endochondral (in cartilage). The fundamental process is, however, similar. An organic matrix, the osteoid, is laid down by cells, the osteoblasts. This becomes calcified with the deposition of amorphous and crystalline apatite. The bones of the calvarium of the skull are formed by intramembranous ossification, the basal bones of the skull and the majority of bones of the skeleton by endochondral ossification.

1.1. Intramembranous ossification

In early foetal life a condensation of mesenchyme cells occurs in the case of both membrane and endochondral bone formation. In the former a group of cells differentiate into osteoblasts, so forming centres of ossification (Ham 1974). These cells secrete osteoid and in so doing some of them become surrounded and become osteocytes lying in their lacunae. Others continue to form osteoid and surround ingrowing capillaries which will bring in the haemopoietic cells of the future marrow (Ham 1974), (Fig. 1.1). Spicules of bone are found radiating out from the ossification centre as a result of matrix formation by the osteoblasts lying on the surface of the condensation, thus creating a spongy type of bone. Calcification of the osteoid proceeds by the same process of vesicle formation as is seen in trabecular bone (see p. 37) (Bernard and Pease 1969). In early foetal life, in human or long gestation species, resorption and apposition begin to take place, so that the spongy or cancellous bone occupies the centre of the mass while a layer of compact bone is formed on each surface by the continuous addition of new sheets of bone by the active osteoblasts.

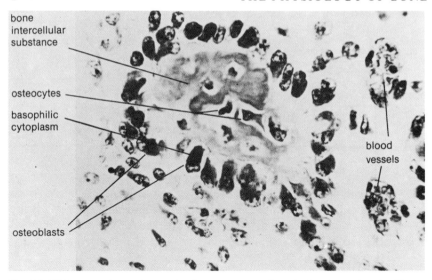

bone
intercellular
substance

osteocytes

basophilic
cytoplasm

blood
vessels

osteoblasts

FIG. 1.1. High-power photomicrograph of a transverse section of a forming trabecula of bone, in the developing skull of a pig embryo. Osteoblasts arranged around its periphery are laying down intercellular substance of bone. Some bone cells have entirely surrounded themselves with intercellular substance so as to become buried as osteocytes in it; these reside in lacunae. (From Ham and Cormack (1979) by courtesy of authors and publishers.)

1.2. Endochondral ossification

In an area of mesenchymal condensation, in the case of endochondral ossification, cells with oval or round nuclei appear packed together forming a model of the future bone (Fig. 1.2). These cells surround themselves with an intracellular matrix or ground substance which is largely composed of glycoproteins peculiar to cartilage (see p. 58). The cells at the periphery of the original condensation become orientated to form, which is described as a perichondrium. The inner layer of cells of this perichondrium differentiate and can be shown to contain alkaline phosphatase, the *sine qua non* of the osteoblast. These differentiated cells lay down a layer of osteoid, i.e. the matrix characteristic of bone. This immediately calcifies, so becoming a collar of periosteal bone directly in contact with the cartilaginous model. The cartilage cells in the centre of the model have in the meantime undergone degenerative changes which are associated with some calcification (Fig. 1.3). Capillaries from outside the perichondrium push through the perichondrium and the periosteal bone and invade the degenerating cartilage cells carrying with them stromal cells from the inner layers of the perichondrium which will form the marrow stroma (Jotereau and Le Douarin 1978) (Fig. 1.3). The vessels arborize and ultimately, together with their stromal cuff derived from

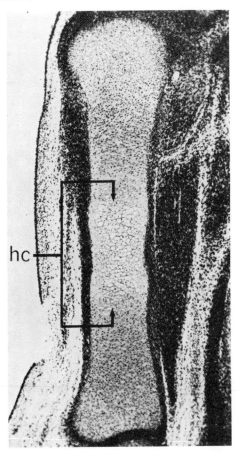

hc

F<small>IG</small>. 1.2. Low-power photomicrograph of part of a leg of a rabbit embryo. The future form of
the bone-to-be is well outlined. Note the hypertrophied chondrocytes (hc) in the mid-region of
the bone. (From Ham and Cormack (1979) by courtesy of authors and publishers.)

the perichondrium, replace the degenerating cartilage cells. The original
vascular endothelium forms the largely sinusoidal endothelium of the marrow, i.e. it is probably of haematogenous origin (Weiss 1976; Jotereau and
Le Douarin 1978). Within the capillaries are also the blood cells which leak
out either through gaps in the endothelial walls or as some observers think
through the endothelial cells themselves (Weiss 1973), to form the cells of
the haemopoietic marrow, the precursors of the erythrocytes, the lymphocytes, the megakaryocytes, the granulocytes, and the monocytes of the peripheral blood. From the monocyte, the macrophage and the osteoclast
differentiate (Van Furth and Cohn 1968; Van Furth, Cohn, Hirsch, Humphrey, Spector, and Langevoort 1972; Van Furth 1975; Van Furth, Lange-

Spaces in breaking-down calcified cartilage

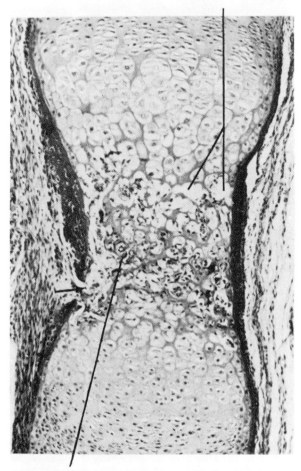

being invaded by blood vessels and osteoblasts of periosteal bud (arrow).

FIG. 1.3. Spaces in breaking-down calcified cartilage being invaded by blood vessels and osteoblasts of periosteal bud (arrow). (From Ham and Cormack (1979) by courtesy of authors and
publishers.)

voort, and Schaberg 1975; Owen 1978). These haemopoietic cells, carried
into the ossification centre within the invading capillaries, are derived from
a population of cells first appearing on the embryonic yolk sac (Moore and
Metcalf 1970; Metcalf and Moore 1971). They are carried from the yolk sac
by the blood to the liver, which they colonize, and then in turn to the marrow

cancellous bone
of epiphysis

articular
cartilage

epiphyseal
disk

trabeculae of
metaphysis

bone marrow
cavity of
diaphysis

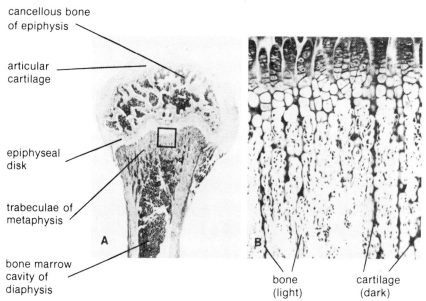

A

B

bone
(light)

cartilage
(dark)

FIG. 1.4. Low-power photomicrograph of one end of a growing long bone (rat). Osteogenesis has now spread from the epiphyseal centre of ossification so that only the articular cartilage above and the epiphyseal disc below remain cartilaginous. On the diaphyseal side of the epiphyseal plate (disc), metaphyseal trabeculae extend down into the diaphysis. (B) Medium-power photomicrograph of the area indicated in (A), showing trabeculae on the diaphyseal side of the epiphyseal plate (disc). These have cores of calcified cartilage on which bone has been deposited. The cartilaginous cores of the trabeculae were formerly partitions between columns of chondrocytes in the epiphyseal plate (disc). (From Ham and Cormack (1979) by courtesy of authors and publishers.)

which they also colonize. There are then in the bone marrow two distinct stem lines of different origin and potential, the osteogenic reticular cells, the mechanocytes (Friedenstein 1976), originating from the original mesenchyme cells of the perichondrium, and the haemopoietic stem cells originating from the yolk sac (Friedenstein 1976; Jotereau and Le Douarin 1978; Owen 1978). From the former, the osteoblast, the bone-forming cell is derived; from the latter, one or more bone-resorbing cells including the osteoclast (see p. 3). This view of the origin of both the osteoblast and the osteoclast is now generally accepted. The experimental evidence on which it is based is discussed in Chapter 2.

In the process of growth replacement of cartilage by marrow, the original area of condensation of cartilage cells extends centrifugally until a line of cartilage cells destined to form the epiphyseal cartilage is reached (Fig. 1.4). Here the process of endochondral ossification and growth takes place as discussed in Chapter 4.

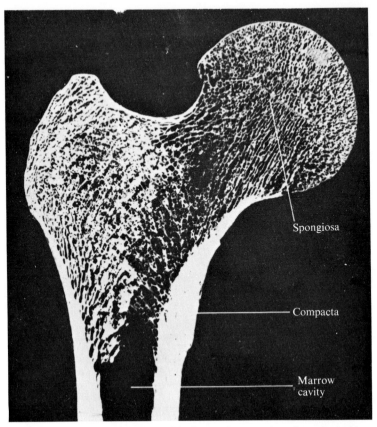

Fig. 1.5. Longitudinal section of the head of the human femur to show dense cortical bone, the compacta; spongiosa showing fine trabeculae; and marrow cavities between both the trabeculae and within the cortical bone. (From Moss (1966) by courtesy of author and publishers.)

2. STRUCTURE

Two types of bone structure are readily seen macroscopically in the mature skeleton:

    (a) spongy or cancellous bone, which is made up of a network of fine interlacing partitions, the trabeculae, enclosing cavities that contain either red or fatty marrow. Spongy bone is found in the vertebrae, in the majority of the flat bones, and in the ends of the long bones;

    (b) hard, compact cortical bone, found largely in the shafts of the long bones, which surround the marrow cavities.

Figure 1.5 is a photograph of a longitudinal section of the head of a human femur which shows both compact cortical and spongy, trabecular cancellous bone in relation to the marrow cavities.

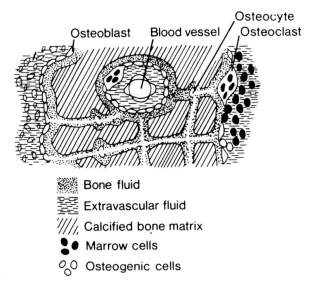

FIG. 1.6. Diagrammatic section of cortical bone — mid-shaft of femur of young rabbit.

2.1. Woven bone

The first bone to appear in embryonic development or in the repair of fractures differs from the mature types of bone just discussed. This immature bone is spoken of as woven bone or coarse bundled bone. It is usually more cellular, and the lacunae in which the osteocytes reside are not as flattened as they are in mature bone. The matrix often stains unevenly and may show a patchy basophilia. Immature bone is usually replaced, but some may persist, especially near tendon insertions and ligament attachments.

2.2. Trabecular bone

In spongy trabecular bone, remodelling takes place directly on the surface of the trabeculae and is more active than that in compact bone. This increased turnover of trabecular as compared to compact bone is important when considering the dosimetry of bone seeking radionuclides (Beddoe 1978).

2.3. Compact cortical bone

Figure 1.6 is a diagrammatic section of cortical bone which should be looked at together with microradiographs shown in Fig. 1.7 and 1.8, which indicate variations that occur in the mineralization of bone.

The three low-power microradiographs of cross sections from the mid-shaft of the femur from three normal individuals aged 15 years, 20 years, and

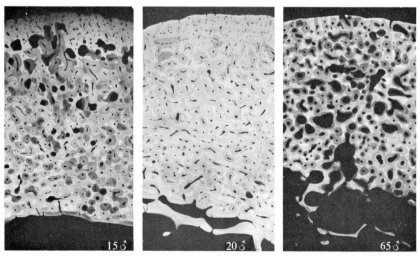

FIG. 1.7. Microradiographs of cross sections through the mid-shaft of the femur of normal individuals of different ages to show large number of Haversian systems, variations in the size of canals and in mineral density, also the change with age. (From Jowsey (1963) by courtesy of author and publishers.)

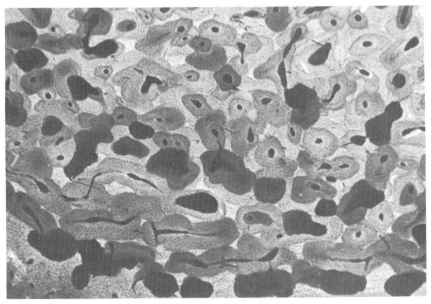

FIG. 1.8. Microradiograph of part of cross section through mid-shaft of the femur of normal man aged 25 years to show variation in size of Haversian systems, and in degree of mineralization in different osteons. Higher magnification than Fig. 1.3. (From Vaughan (1970) by courtesy of publishers.)

65 years, and a higher power view of a section from a man aged 25, indicate that the pattern of structure and mineralization varies with age and is extremely variable within a small area. The larger Haversian canals often have an irregular edge and are called resorption cavities. In such cavities active removal of both mineral and matrix may be occurring on one part of the surface while osteoid tissue is laid down on another. As osteoid tissue is laid down in an active Haversian system it becomes mineralized except in pathological conditions like rickets and osteomalacia.

Experimental results using radioactive calcium indicate that the process of mineralization in any osteon, i.e. the area of bone directly associated with a particular Haversian system, at first occurs rapidly so that about 70 per cent mineralization is completed within a matter of days; but complete mineralization occurs more slowly, requiring at least six weeks for completion and often longer (Frost 1967).

Why resorption or apposition should occur in any osteon at any point in time is not known. Many osteons remain quiescent for long periods. This constant remodelling accounts for the variable degrees of mineralization seen round Haversian canals. It is a process that goes on continuously throughout life within cortical bone. The degree and the rate at which it occurs is highly variable. In the microradiographs there can also be seen small areas of bone containing osteocytes and their lacunae between neighbouring Haversian systems. These are areas of mineralized matrix left by some earlier remodelling process. Such areas are well calcified. The diagram in Fig. 1.6 illustrates some further general structural points of cortical bone— which are now discussed.

3. BONE SURFACES

The term 'bone surface' is often used in a loose fashion to describe an extremely complex and physiologically important area of the skeleton (Vaughan 1972). It is anatomically extensive when the Haversian systems and Volkman's canals as well as the lining of all marrow cavities and the external surfaces of the bones are included. In man, the trabecular surface area in a vertebral body of approximately 40 cm³ is of the order of 1000 cm² and the periosteal area is 80 cm² (Dunnill, Anderson, and Whitehead 1967). The trabecular surface area of iliac bone is approximately 1600 cm² (Sissons, Holley, and Heighway 1967). The figure for cancellous bone in the head of the femur is of the same order (Dunnill, personal communication). In Table 1.1 is shown a summary of some published data on surface to volume ratios on normal human vertebrae (Lloyd and Hodges 1971), and in Table 1.2 some estimates of skeletal values of surface to volume ratios in four different species measured by Beddoe (1978). The constituents of any bone surface, excluding the walls of

TABLE 1.1
Surface to volume ratios of normal human vertebrae

	Percentage bone volume†	Sample thickness	Perimeter area (cm per cm²)	Surface area/volume bone mineral (cm² per cm³)	Surface area/volume bone tissue (cm² per cm³)
Dyson et al. (1970)	13·5 (1)	Surface only	165	207	28
Dunnill et al. (1967)	25 (30)	?	—	—	—
Amstutz and Sissons (1969)	25 (average 4 areas in 1 vert.)	27 μm	—	147	33
Atkinson (1967)	69 (calc.) (28)	2·5 mm	—	—	—
Bromley et al. (1966)	15 (7)	8 μm	100	127	19
Lloyd (1969)	27 (1)	100 μm	94	120	32

† Number of cases in parentheses.
From Lloyd and Hodges (1971) by courtesy of authors and publishers.

TABLE 1.2
Estimates of skeletal values of surface to volume in 4 species

Species	Skeletal surface to volume ratios cm²/cm³
1·7 years	220
9 years	225
Adult	190
Rhesus monkey	190
Beagle	185
Mini-pig	130

From Beddoe (1978) by courtesy of author and publisher.

the osteocyte lacunae are: (a) bone cells; (b) bone fluid; (c) osteoid tissue; (d) mineralized matrix (Fig. 1.6).

3.1. Bone cells

The character of the bone cells found on bone surfaces, those that form bone and those that resorb bone are discussed in the next chapter. It must be remembered that the bone-forming cells have a different origin from the cells responsible for resorbing bone. The former arise from stromal mesenchyme cells, the latter from cells of haemopoietic origin (Metcalf and Moore 1971).

The character of the cells on bone surfaces varies to some extent with the age of the animal from which the specimen is taken and the site in the skeleton under examination. Clearly an area of active resorption will differ from an area where apposition is active or an area where cellular activity is quiescent. In young actively growing bone the layer of tissue laying down bone is several cells thick (Fig. 1.9), p. 11. In older bone the layer is more often only one cell thick (p. 13). In the case of endosteal surfaces it may often be difficult to distinguish bone cells from closely adjacent haemopoietic cells. There is not present agreement among observers that all bone surfaces are completely covered by bone cells. Work by Vaughan and Sissons, published in 1973, concluded that such a cellular layer was continuous on all bone surfaces. They examined human adult bone by light microscopy and pointed out that, particularly on endosteal surfaces, for technical reasons it was often difficult to see the thin-layer of elongated resting osteoblasts, sometimes called lining cells, since the cells were apt either to separate from the mineral surface and remain attached to the marrow (see Figs 1.10, 1.11, and 1.12), or to be squeezed up against the mineral surface by marrow cells from which it was difficult to distinguish them.

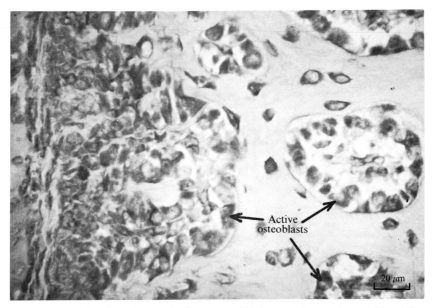

FIG. 1.9. Periosteal surface of the shaft of a young rabbit bone to show active osteoblasts lying adjacent to the mineral surface and within newly formed Haversian canals (methyl green–pyronin). (From Bingham (1968) by courtesy of the author.)

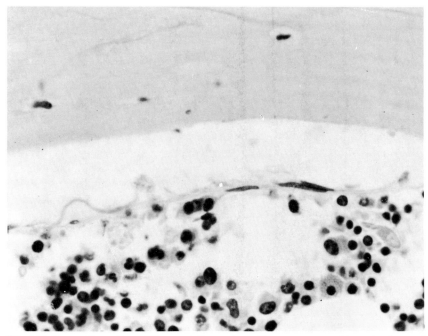

Fig. 1.10. 5μ paraffin section of iliac crest. Separation of bone marrow and investing layer of flattened cells from the bone surface (Sissons (1970) by courtesy of the author).

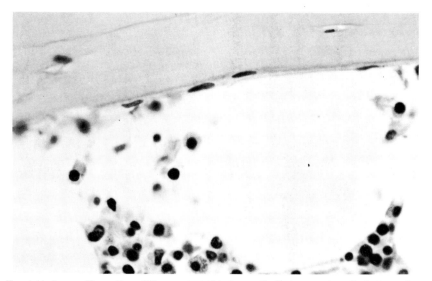

Fig. 1.11. 5μ paraffin section of iliac crest. A thin layer of cells is present on the bone surface separating the bone from fatty and haematopoietic bone marrow (Sissons (1970), by courtesy of the author).

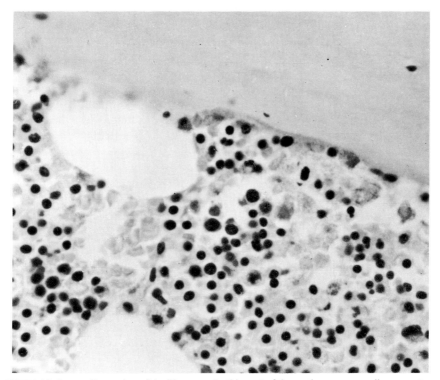

FIG. 1.12. 5μ paraffin section of the iliac crest. In this part of the section marrow cells appear to
be in contact with the bone surface (Sissons (1970), by courtesy of the author).

More recent electron micrographic studies of the cells on bone surfaces,
it is claimed, have confirmed that in normal trabecular bone, removed at
routine orthopaedic investigation in men and women aged 19–85, trabecular
surfaces were either covered with lining cells or there was sufficient evidence
to suggest that the uncovered surfaces had lost their cells during preparation
procedures (Matthews and Martin 1971; Woods, Earnshaw, and Kanis 1977;
Vander Wiel, Grubb, and Talmage 1978). Following elaborate studies by
Jee and his colleagues of the character of cells on bone surfaces (Kimmell and
Jee 1977, 1978a,b), the workers make no dogmatic statement as to whether
the entire surface is covered, but in describing certain types of cell they claim
they account for about 94 per cent of the surfaces examined.

Other workers (Loutit, personal communications), 1979, using both light
microscope and electron microscope techniques, while accepting that the
greater part of all bone surfaces are covered by cells, consider that gaps occur
and that bare areas of osteoid or fully mineralized bone are found, more
particularly on endosteal surfaces. It is, however, still open to question as to
whether such bare areas may be due to technical difficulties.

3.1.2. DOES A MEMBRANE EXIST SEPARATING BONE FLUID FROM EXTRAVASCULAR FLUID?

Is the layer of bone cell tissue continuous on bone surfaces and can it be regarded as the membrane first postulated by Howard (1956) and more recently by Neuman and his colleagues (Triffitt, Terepka, and Neuman 1968; Neuman 1969; Neuman and Ramp 1971) which separates extravascular tissue fluid from bone tissue fluid? This question was first raised when it was claimed by Neuman and his colleagues that bone fluid had a higher potassium content than extravascular fluid. Neuman himself having originally postulated the existence of a membrane between extravascular fluid and bone fluid does not necessarily accept this membrane as a cellular one, though he has at times postulated the existence of pumps in the osteogenic cells and has shown experimentally that there may be significant differences between bone fluid and extravascular fluid (Scarpace and Neuman 1976a,b; Neuman, Bromnage and Myers 1977). He has recently suggested that the zeta potential of hydroxyapatite may account for the different ionic concentration of potassium in bone fluid as opposed to extracellular fluid rather than a membrane (Bromnage and Neuman 1979). Brand and his colleagues (Brand, Cushing, and Hefley 1979) agree with Neuman that there is an excess of potassium in bone fluid while others (Morris, Day, Bassingthwaite, An, and Kelly 1979) consider the potassium is present in bone cells rather than in bone fluid. It is, however, generally accepted that there are gaps between the cells so large that macromolecules such as horse-radish peroxidase and thorium dioxide have been observed to penetrate the canalicular lacunar region when injected intravenously, presumably by means of bone fluid (Seliger 1970; Doty and Schofield 1972; Matthews and Martin 1971). Scherft (1972, 1978) has described a distinct area in the osteoid shown up by particular stains in decalcified bone, which outline what he considers the area where calcification begins, and which he calls 'The *Lamina Limitans*' which might serve as the barrier between extravascular and bone tissue fluid. He considers that 'the mineralized areas in bone and cartilage are bounded by a layer of more or less dense organic material, the *lamina limitans*, with the specific exception of the sites where the mineralization is extending, or resorption has taken place shortly before (Scherft 1972). Other workers have not been able to show this line in electron microscope studies of undecalcified bone (Vander Wiel, Grubb, and Talmage 1978).

3.2. Bone fluid

Whatever the character of the barrier, if it exists, that has been suggested as separating extracellular fluid from bone fluid, it is accepted that there are probably important differences between the two fluids.

Bone fluid is continuous throughout Haversian canals, on endosteal and periosteal surfaces and in the canaliculae and osteocyte lacunae as can be seen in Fig. 1.6. The passage of fluid through cortical bone is in the same net direction as the blood, mainly from the endosteal to the periosteal surface (Owen, Howlett, and Triffitt 1977). Owen and her colleagues speculate that it may vary in composition in different sites. This composition has never been directly examined since it has not yet proved possible to obtain samples.

3.2.1. MINERAL CONTENT

The question of the mineral content of bone fluid is still unsolved (see p. 14). Some observers consider it has a high potassium content, others that this high potassium can be accounted for by the cellular content. The concentration of ionic calcium is much lower than that in plasma, 0·5 mM compared with 1·5 mM (Neuman 1969).

3.2.2. PROTEIN CONTENT

Recently it has been shown that albumin which is immunologically identical to serum albumin is present throughout the bone fluid region. The greater part of extravascular albumin in kidney, intestine, skin, and muscle is exchangeable with plasma albumin whereas in bone only the proportion which is in bone fluid is exchangeable; the remaining fraction in calcified matrix is more permanently fixed. About 27 per cent of the albumin in young bone is in bone fluid, 57 per cent is in calcified matrix, and about 16 per cent is intravascular. The total amount of extravascular albumin per unit mass of bone is similar to that found in soft tissue. The rate of clearance of the albumin from tissue fluid in bone is approximately once every hour. This is more rapid than in skin and muscle, comparable with intestine, and less rapid than in kidney. The amount of albumin incorporated into calcified matrix of bone per day is calculated to be less than 0·5 per cent of the total albumin passing through the tissues of bone per day (Owen, Triffitt, and Melick 1973; Owen and Triffitt 1976). Other plasma proteins found in bone (see p. 75) presumably circulate in the bone fluid before being incorporated into the matrix or becoming associated with the mineral element. On the other hand it has been shown that macromolecules which are without metabolic significance such as polyvinylpyrrolidone, (PVP) a polymer of average molecular weight 35 000, may also circulate through bone fluid, following intravenous injection, without being incorporated into the matrix or held in any way (Owen, Howlett, and Triffitt 1977).

3.3. Osteoid matrix

The chemical character of osteoid or bone matrix is discussed in Chapter 3. It is laid down and removed by bone cells as described in Chapter 2. The

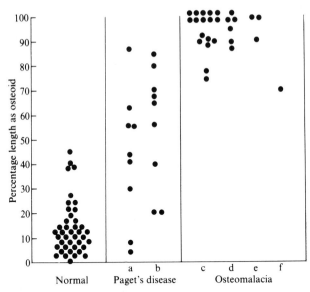

Fig. 1.13. Percentage of trabecular length covered by osteoid. (From Paterson *et al.* (1968) by courtesy of authors and publishers.)

rapidity with which it becomes mineralized is variable — in an ordinary light microscope examination it may appear at times that there is no uncalcified osteoid layer in a section of normal bone, while in other areas one or more layers of unmineralized osteoid may be apparent. It is probable that except when active resorption is in progress there is always an extremely thin layer of osteoid. In Fig. 1.13 is shown the percentage of trabecular length covered by observable osteoid in the normal adult ilium and in two pathological conditions, Paget's disease and osteomalacia (Paterson, Woods, and Morgan 1968). Chalmers and his colleagues (Chalmers, Barclay, Davison, MacLeod, and Williams 1969) estimate from biopsy studies that 6 per cent of osteoid relative to total bone matrix is the upper limit of normal. In electron microscope pictures of osteoblasts close to the bone surface the uncalcified osteoid border is well seen (Fig. 1.14). There is usually a well-defined interface between calcified matrix and uncalcified osteoid which is referred to as the calcification front. It stains intensely with certain lipid stains (Irving 1965) and with a variety of other staining procedures. This zone probably has an important physiological function which cannot, however, at present be explained. The possible part that the glycoproteins, found characteristically in the osteoid, may play in the binding of calcium ions, is discussed in Chapters 3 and 6.

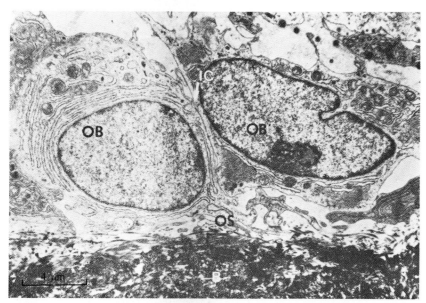

FIG. 1.14. Electron micrograph showing osteoblast layer (OB), osteoid (OS), and mineralized bone (B). Processes extend into canaliculi separated from mineralized walls by narrow channels containing some collagenous fibrils. Bone extracellular fluid occupies this and interstitial spaces of osteoid and intercellular channels (IC).

3.4. Mineralized matrix

The chemistry of bone mineral and the mechanism of calcification are discussed in Chapters 5 and 6.

4. PATTERNS OF GROWTH

Until adult stature is reached, growth in length of the long bones is achieved by a process of growth of cartilage at the end plates, with subsequent calcification, and growth in diameter by apposition of new bone on an existing bone surface. This apposition on the periosteal surface is accompanied by resorption on the endosteal surface, so in the case of a long bone the original shape is retained but the three dimensions of its geometry are increased (Lacroix 1971), (Fig. 1.15).

4.1. Endochondral ossification

A photograph of a longitudinal section of the cartilage plate of the femur of a young rabbit is shown in Fig. 1.4, A, and B with the zone of proliferating cells, zones of maturing chondrocytes, hypertrophic chondrocytes, and the invading capillaries that carry osteogenic tissue with them.

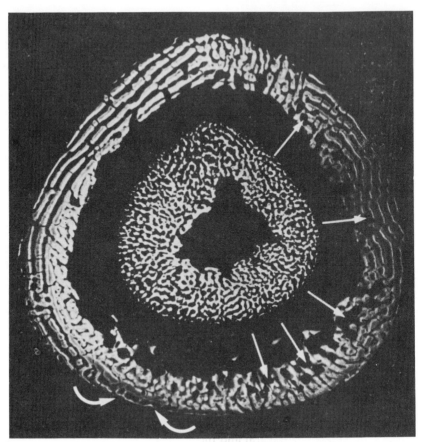

Fig. 1.15. This combined microradiographic illustration represents at the same scale (× 17) two transverse sections of the tibial diaphysis of the dog, the smaller from a newborn, the larger from a 7-week-old animal. At birth there is no internal remodelling. The 7-week stage catches the installation of the process: five thin arrows point to resorption cavities which will be filled with concentric lamellae. The two curved arrows indicate the regions where ostenonic structures are being added at the periphery of the diaphysis by periosteal bone formation. These addition osteons are an aspect of the external remodelling and should be clearly distinguished from the osteons which are the result of the internal remodelling of compact bone and those which are replacement osteons. (From Lacroix (1971), by courtesy of author and publishers.)

Though there is considerable confusion in the names given to the cartilage cells at different levels in the plate, there is agreement about their function. The cells in the zone of calcification enlarge; they lose their transverse walls, and their longitudinal walls calcify, while capillaries carrying osteogenic cells, particularly osteoblasts, but also osteoclasts and other bone resorbing cells (Loutit and Nisbet 1979), push up and invade the dying cells. The osteoblasts lay down osteoid on the calcified spicules of cartilage. This subsequently becomes calcified while further erosion is caused by the bone resorbing cells. In the meantime the dying hypertrophic cartilage cells are replaced by proliferation and maturation of the cells of the upper end of the plate, and the whole process is repeated continuously until the growth in length of the bone is complete. The detailed mechanism of cartilage calcification is discussed in Chapter 4.

4.2. Apposition

Bone grows in diameter by apposition, i.e. bone matrix is laid down by osteoblasts on an already existing bone surface and this subsequently becomes mineralized. The process of mineralization is extremely rapid on the periosteal surface, so that it is often difficult to demonstrate the line of underlying osteoid tissue. Mineralization of osteoid is less rapid in Haversian systems that are laying down bone, and here the use of radioactive isotopes has made it possible to demonstrate how first osteoid is laid down and then how this is subsequently calcified. If $^{35}SO_4$ is administered it can be shown by appropriate autoradiographic techniques immediately after injection in the outer edge of the osteoid borders of Haversian systems that are laying down bone. Within 24 hours it is found on the edge of the osteoid nearest to the mineralized surface. Experimental evidence suggests that it is incorporated into chondroitin sulphate (Kent, Jowsey, Steddon, Oliver, and Vaughan 1956; Lea and Vaughan 1957). ^{47}Ca is found immediately after injection behind the osteoid border.

5. THE BLOOD SUPPLY OF BONE

This is not the place for a detailed description of the blood-supply of bone. There are, however, certain facts that are essential for an understanding of bone physiology. Recent reviews with many references are available (Brookes 1971; Rhinelander 1972).

Blood flow through bone is mainly centrifugal. In certain regions in long bones where the muscle fascia are firmly attached some of the blood supply to the outer cortex may originate from the periosteal side (Rhinelander 1972; Owen, Howlett, and Triffitt 1977).

5.1. The afferent vascular system

A long bone has three basic blood supplies: (a) the nutrient artery; (b) the metaphyseal combined with the epiphyseal arteries after closure of the growth plate; (c) the periosteal arterioles.

5.1.1. THE NUTRIENT ARTERY

The nutrient artery varies in number according to the bone. It arises directly from an artery of the systemic circulation. It enters the diaphysis diagonally through a distinct foramen and branches into ascending and descending medullary arteries when it reaches the marrow cavity. The ascending and descending arteries, having reached the marrow, then divide further into arterioles which penetrate the endosteal surface to supply the diaphyseal cortex, spreading out into what Brookes has called an irregular arborization. He considers that the fine arterial twigs both in cortex and marrow are probably end arteries.

5.1.2. THE METAPHYSEAL AND EPIPHYSEAL VESSELS

The pattern of the blood-supply to the metaphysis and epiphysis of a long bone varies with age. During the period of growth the circulatory arrangements at the end of the long bones differs from that of the diaphysis because of the special circulation to the epiphyseal growth plate. When growth is complete the epiphyseal plate disappears and the cancellous bone circulation therefore changes.

5.1.3. THE PERIOSTEAL VESSELS

The question of a periosteal blood supply to bone is controversial. Brooks argues that though the periosteum itself has a rich supply of vessels the bone is supplied by nutrient endosteal vessels only. Rhinelander (1972) on the basis of much experimental work considers that periosteal arterioles supply the outer third or quarter of the compactum only in localized areas (related to fascial attachments) and that these become more important when the medullary supply is blocked.

5.2. The efferent vascular system

The components of the efferent vascular system are: (1) the large emissary veins and vena comitans of the principal nutrient artery; (2) the cortical venous channels and (3) the periosteal capillaries (Rhinelander 1972).

6. THE HAEMODYNAMICS OF BONE CIRCULATION

Only too little is known about what might be called the haemodynamics of the bone circulation. Brookes (1971) has collected some information for the rat femoral circulation which is shown in Table 1.3. Having reviewed all the available data he concludes that in standard man at rest about one-quarter of the cardiac output passes to the skeleton and the blood-flow rate in human bone is about 19 ml per 100 g per min—a figure which agrees well with rat-tissue flow rates. In the cortical vascular lattice the circulation is brisk, being 18 ml per 100 g per min in the rat femur, against 21 ml per 100 g per min

TABLE 1.3

Haemodynamic data for the rat femoral circulation

	Superior metaphysis	Marrow	Cortex	Inferior metaphysis	Inferior epiphysis
Red cell volume V (ml per 100 g)	1·2	1·6	0·9	1·9	1·1
Red cell flow rate					
$\quad F$ (ml per cent per min)	10	13	7·5	15	9
Transit time T (s)	7	9·2	9·2	7	6
Red cell velocity					
$S \propto \dfrac{\sqrt[3]{V}}{T^3\sqrt{100}}$ (mm s^{-1})	0·327	0·274	0·226	0·381	0·371
Haematocrit h	0·39	0·60	0·42	0·50	0·31
Plasma flow rate P	16	8	10	15	20
Whole blood flow rate Q	26	21	18	30	29
Rate of flow per unit vascular space Qh/V	8·4	7·9	8·4	7·9	7·9
Data as percentage of $\quad S$	86	72	59	100	97
inferior metaphyseal $\quad Q$	86	72	60	100	97
value (= 100 per cent) $\quad V$	64	85	50	100	60
$\qquad\qquad\qquad\qquad F$	64	85	50	100	60

Brookes (1971) by courtesy of author and publisher.

for diaphyseal marrow. Brookes believes that the intravascular pressure is high at the endosteal surface, about 60 mm Hg, but low at the periosteal surface, around 15 mm Hg (Brookes 1971).

Wootton (1974) has shown that in the rabbit 41 per cent of afferent blood to the femur flowed through a capillary bed in the marrow before reaching bone mineral and 28 per cent of tibial afferent blood flowed through the marrow. Epiphyseal and metaphyseal trabecular bone have approximately twofold higher blood flow rates than diaphyseal cortical bone (Whiteside, Simmons, and Lesker 1977). In man Wootton and his colleagues consider the values obtained for normal volunteers were found to have the smallest variation when flows were expressed as a fraction of blood volume per unit of time. The range in 8 normal young males was 4·4–5·9 per cent of blood volume per min. They (Wootton, Reeve, and Veall 1977) have found a close correlation between skeletal blood flow and the 24 h ^{47}Ca space, and that this relation can be used to estimate SBF in subjects for whom only ^{47}Ca data was available. They find SBF increased in Paget's disease, progressive diaphyseal dysplasia and myelomatosis by direct measurement. Using the ^{47}Ca extrapolation it appears raised in osteopetrosing osteitis fibrosa, and some untreated cases of osteomalacia. It appears normal in most cases of hyperparathyroidism, osteoporosis, thyroid dysfunction, and malignant hypercalcaemia. The latter is odd in view of the fact they found it raised in myelomatosis.

The mechanisms controlling the osseous circulation are as yet almost entirely unknown. Adrenaline reduces the flow rate (Weiss and Root 1959) while acetylcholine enhances it (Shim and Patterson 1967). Pituitrin possibly constricts skeletal arterioles independently of systemic arterial pressure (Stein, Morgan, and Porras 1958).

7. THE LYMPHATICS OF BONE

Brookes (1971) quotes Anderson (1960) for his categorical statement that there are no lymphatics in bone cortex and marrow. Owen (Owen *et al.* 1973), discussing the presence of albumin in bone tissue fluid, assumes that it may drain away into the lymph without explaining where the lymphatics are situated.

8. FUNCTION

Bone has many different functions. First, it constitutes the rigid skeleton of the body, yet by the muscle attachments of different bones mobility is made possible. Secondly, it provides protection for vital organs, like the brain, the lungs and the heart. Thirdly, through its high content of mineral ions it plays a crucial role in maintaining mineral homeostasis, i.e. a constant level of certain essential ions in plasma and tissue fluid. Further, there are extremely important interactions between bone and bone marrow (Patt 1976; Patt and Maloney 1975).

Growth and maintenance of the skeleton which are essential for the performance of bone's first two functions may be considered under the heading of skeletal homeostasis. The factors controlling both skeletal homeostasis and mineral homeostasis are complex. The mechanisms by which they act are at present far from completely understood. It is, however, recognized that to some extent these factors are interrelated. For convenience in later chapters they have been discussed separately but such a division is somewhat arbitrary. Many of these factors are hormones carried in the plasma to their target organs, others are more local, like osteoclast stimulating factor and the prostaglandins (see p. 51).

8.1. Skeletal homeostasis

During the first two decades of life there is general overall growth in the skeleton. The long bones for instance increase in length and diameter while maintaining their overall three dimensional geometry. After the adult skeletal pattern has been achieved continual remodelling occurs. It has been estimated that at any given time in an adult 3·5 per cent of the total skeleton is being remodelled (Rasmussen 1968).

8.1.1. HORMONAL CONTROL

There are many hormones which affect skeletal growth, in different and subtle ways. Lack of thyroid hormones results in the most severe form of dwarfism seen. Excess of pituitary hormone results in acromegaly. The growth spurt seen in boys and girls at puberty is dependent on the sex hormones, testosterone and oestrogen (Short 1980) and growth hormone (Aynsley-Green et al. 1976).

Factors affecting skeletal maintenance. The hormones indeed have an effect on skeletal maintenance but other external factors are involved, notably mechanical stress and pressure.

8.1.2. MECHANICAL STRESS AND PRESSURE

One of the external factors involved in maintaining skeletal homeostasis is mechanical stress and pressure. It has long been known that confinement to bed may result in a dramatic loss in bone mass (Minaire, Meunier, Edonard, Bernard, Courpron, and Bourret 1974). This will occur with ordinary illness: most marked is the *osteoporosis* that occurs particularly in young adults suddenly immobilized by paralytic poliomyelitis. Astronauts are subjected to weightlessness and therefore to little bone stress (Mack, Lachance, Vose, and Vogt 1967; Pyke, Mack, Hoffman, Gilchrist, Hood, and George 1968). From careful comparative metabolic studies on 3 astronauts who exercised regularly (Skylab 4) and three young quadriplegic patients, it would appear that mineral loss and increased loss of collagen degradation products (a measure of bone resorption) occur concomitantly in the quadriplegic patients (Minaire et al. 1974). It is of interest that analysis of the collagen degradation products indicated that skin as well as bone collagen was involved. In the astronauts during flight there was some loss of calcium (as evidenced by hypercalciuria) which corresponded with the loss of mineral seen radiographically in the calcaneus, but no increased excretion of collagen degradation products. The biochemical mechanisms responsible for the degradation of skeletal and cutaneous collagen in the quadriplegics is not clear. In the astronauts it is possible that the calcium loss was also associated with some matrix loss too small to be detected and that enhanced collagen degradation products were catabolized, but the fact that the calciuria stopped on re-entry makes it likely that there was a normal organic matrix ready to be recalcified (Claus-Walker, Singh, Leach, Hatton, Hubert, and Ferrante 1977).

8.1.3. PIEZOELECTRICITY

In 1964 Bassett and his colleagues (Becker, Bassett, and Bachman 1964) first emphasized the important part that biophysical events may play in bone remodelling. Having accepted the evidence from tissue culture experiments for the basic importance of genetic factors in determining the shape of any bone (Fell 1956) Bassett claims that 'from data now available the stimulus for bone formation and destruction involved in bone remodelling appears to be largely electrical in nature' (Bassett 1971). He suggests that control of remodelling is largely dependent on an indirect effect when mechanical energy is transduced to electrical energy by the bone matrix and vasculature, i.e. a deforming force produces stress which is converted to a proportional electric command signal. This signal tells the bone cells when, how, and in what orientation to function in order to adjust the mechanical properties of bone to the need. He mentions three possible deformation-based sources in the extracellular matrix of bone—piezo-electric, solid state (p-n junction), and streaming potentials—but suggests that the sum of all electric events occurring in bone, not only those dependent upon deformation, must be considered. He would include streaming potentials generated in vessels both by cardiac and skeletal muscle pumps, electric flow in the peripheral nervous system, electrical activity in the adjacent muscles, the total fixed charge and orientated dipole moment of collagen (and possibly protein–polysaccharide), and the electrical properties of cells.

During the last 15 years a variety of biological systems have been found capable of transducing mechanical to electrical energy. This behaviour has been attributed to piezoelectric properties of long chain polymers many of which are found in bone, collagen protein–polysaccharides and nucleic acids among others. Though there is an absence of hard data there are many physiological processes that hypothetically could be affected, such as replication of DNA and protein synthesis, the availability of unbound anions and cations, membrane permeability, adhesiveness and mobility, the function of contractile proteins (including microtubules) and cell communication (Bassett, Pawluk, and Pilla 1974). At present there is active interest in the possibility that electrical stimulation may be of value in the treatment of fractures through an observed effect on osteogenesis (Bassett, Pawluk, and Pilla 1974; Brighton 1977).

8.2. Mineral homeostasis

Calcium, magnesium, and phosphate ions particularly, in an appropriate and steady concentration, are essential for a proper working of many of the most delicate cellular mechanisms throughout the body (Rasmussen 1972). Of these calcium is probably the most important. It is essential that the concentration of these ions should remain constant in plasma, in extracellular and intercellular fluids. This mineral homeostasis is maintained by a complex system of controlling factors acting both on the skeleton, on the processes of absorption from the gastro intestinal tract, and excretion from the blood stream by the kidney. The importance of the skeleton in this system has been questioned by some workers (Peacock and Nordin 1973; Reynolds 1974). The former have stated that 'although bone may contribute to short-term regulation, it cannot in the long run contribute to the normal plasma concentration of young adults and does not seem to be the major factor behind most types of hypercalcaemia. We do not of course deny that bone is the ultimate reservoir for calcium and that in states of calcium deficiency and possibly during the early morning, calcium is mobilized from the skeleton to maintain the plasma calcium concentration'. Nordin admits, however, that the kidney can maintain the plasma calcium concentration only if there is an adequate input of calcium—as soon as the diet is low in calcium, bone must be involved as it must be during the night. 'When the nutritional status is normal, the gut and kidney are in control. The bone is in reserve.' The part played by the gut and kidney is discussed in Chapter 9. Here the part played by the skeleton is only briefly mentioned.

As already described, in the first 18–20 years of life, there is variable, but obvious constant growth and remodelling of the skeleton expressed by increase in size, but throughout life the process of apposition and resorption (i.e. bone-formation and bone-removal), though not obvious, are continuous. It is not now thought that such remodelling makes any significant contribution to mineral homeostasis.

There is, however, good evidence that the minute-to-minute regulation of blood calcium, phosphate and magnesium is mediated through the action of cells on all bone surfaces, particularly the osteoclasts and osteoblasts, as will be discussed in the next chapter and in Chapter 8 (Talmage 1969, 1970; Matthews and Martin 1971; Scarpace and Neuman 1976a,b; Neuman, Bromnage and Myers 1977; Talmage and Grubb 1977; Vander Wiel, Grubb, and Talmage 1978). This cellular action is to a large extent under the control of the parathyroid gland (see p. 151), vitamin D metabolites (see p. 139), and possibly calcitonin (see p. 163).

8.3. Bone–Bone marrow interaction

The importance of bone—marrow interactions has become increasingly appreciated over recent years. It is clear that there is still much to be learnt about the influence of the microenvironment provided by stromal elements close to mineralized bone upon differentiation and proliferation of both bone cells and blood cells (Patt and Maloney 1976; Trentin 1976). The close association between the development of haemopoietic marrow and bone is apparent in embryonic life (see pp. 2, 3). In adult life the association is also prominent. The formation of ectopic bone, irrespective of the initiating mechanism, generally leads to a new bone marrow even though there is no need for additional haemopoiesis (Patt 1976). The presumptive role of a bony

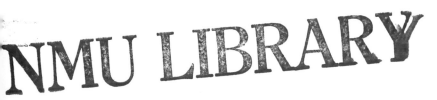

environment in creating haemopoietic marrow is further emphasized by experiments where marrow is removed either by perfusion or curetage from the shaft of a long bone *in vivo* (Patt and Maloney 1975). At first there is formation of granulation tissue which is followed by connective tissue, vasculature, and transient trabeculation of the medullary cavity as a prelude to the appearance of frankly haematopoietic tissue. As long as the bone is intact, haemopoietic marrow can be replaced. Further, if autologous implants of heterotopic marrow are made in subcutaneous tissues, for instance in the groin in normal rabbits, the probability of bone formation is greater than 90 per cent and the probability of bone-associated haemopoiesis exceeds 80 per cent (Patt and Maloney 1975). Implants of haematopoietic murine spleen are not osteogenic and do not generate the requisite environment for sustained haematopoiesis upon heterotopic implantation (Haley, Tjio, Smith, and Brecher 1975; Tavassoli, Ratzan, and Crosby 1973).

Evidence for the importance of both the stromal and haemopoietic elements in bone marrow in the origin and development of the bone cells, both the osteoblast and the osteoclast is discussed in Chapter 2.

2. Cellular Elements of the Skeleton

THERE are three groups of bone cells. First the osteoblasts, derived from stromal marrow cells, which lay down bone. Secondly, the osteocytes, 'imprisoned osteoblasts', which have an ill-defined role in maintaining both the mineral and matrix of bone, and thirdly the osteoclasts and associated mononuclear cells of haemopoietic origin, which resorb bone. Some consideration must also be given to the fibroblast.

The description of endochondral ossification in Chapter 1 indicated that in bone marrow there were two distinct stem cell lines of different origin and potential: first, the osteogenic reticular cells originating from the mesenchymal cells of the perichondrium which in due course formed the marrow stroma, and secondly, the haemopoietic stem cells originating from the yolk sac which reach the marrow via the liver and invading capillaries (Friedenstein 1976; Jotereau and Le Douarin 1978; Owen 1978). The stromal reticular cell is the stem cell of the bone forming osteoblast (Friedenstein 1976; Owen 1978). A multipotent haemopoietic stem cell: the precursor of the granulocyte, erythrocytes, the megakaryocytes, the lymphocytes and the monocytes, is at present thought to be the precursor of the cells that resorb bone (see p. 3) (Volkman and Gowans 1965; Van Furth and Cohn 1968; Van Furth, Langevoort and Schaberg 1975; Gothlin and Ericsson 1976; Owen 1978). There is no evidence that cells of stromal and haemopoietic origin share a common stem cell (Friedenstein 1976; Owen 1978).

1. THE OSTEOBLAST

1.1. Evidence for stromal origin

It has already been said that the osteoblast is differentiated from a stromal cell derived from the primitive mesenchyme. The evidence for this is embryological, morphological, and experimental.

1.1.1. EMBRYOLOGICAL

This evidence has been described in Chapter 1. The earliest formation of bone in the perichondrial collar arises from cells that differentiate on the outer edge of the original mesenchymal condensation (see Fig. 1.2). These cells stain for alkaline phosphatase, the characteristic enzyme of the osteoblast.

1.1.2. MORPHOLOGICAL

Morphological studies have shown that osteogenic connective tissue cells of periosteal and endosteal surfaces and Haversian canals of bone are continuous with the stromal elements of the marrow—stromal cells merge into preosteoblasts and osteoblasts near bone surfaces (McLean and Urist 1968; Burkhardt 1970). Recently a study of the histology of marrow (Western and Bainton 1979) has shown that there are many stromal cells which show a strong reaction for alkaline phosphatase, an enzyme which is characteristic of bone forming cells.

1.1.3. EXPERIMENTAL

Several experimental systems provide evidence of the stromal origin of the osteoblast. Some of them have been briefly mentioned in the discussion of the Bone—bone marrow interaction in Chapter 1.

1.1.3.1. *Formation of bone from marrow fibroblasts*

First there are the extremely important studies of Friedenstein and his colleagues on the formation of bone from marrow fibroblasts (Friedenstein, Piatetsky-Shapiro, and Petrakova 1966; Friedenstein, Lalykina, and Tolmacheva 1967; Friedenstein, Petrakova, Kurolesova, and Frolova 1968; Friedenstein, Chailakhjian, and Lalykina 1970; Friedenstein 1973, 1976). They have shown that fibroblast colonies are formed from cell suspensions of a variety of tissues grown in monolayer cultures *in vitro* (Friedenstein *et al.* 1970; Friedenstein 1973; Friedenstein, Chailakhjian, Latzinik, Panasyuk, and Keiliss-Borok 1974; Friedenstein, Deriglasova, Kulagina, Panasyuk, Rudakowa, Luria, and Rudakow 1974). These cells can be passaged, harvested, and suspended in a suitable medium, placed in a diffusion chamber and implanted *in vivo*, for instance in the peritoneal cavity. If the fibroblasts were grown from marrow, bone formation occurred in the diffusion chambers, but no bone was formed from fibroblast cultures from other tissues (Friedenstein 1973; Friedenstein, Chailokhjian, Latzinik, Panasyuk, and Keiliss-Borok 1974; Friedenstein, Deviglasova, Kulagina, Panasuk, Rudakowa, Luria, and Rudakow 1974). Friedenstein called these cells present in bone marrow which are capable of spontaneous bone formation, Determined Osteogenic Precursor Cells, DOPC. These cells are considered to be components of the fibroblastic marrow stroma. Their morphology is not known. It is thought that they do not migrate via the blood stream and 'home' to particular sites like haemopoietic stem cells (Trentin 1976).

In addition to the DOPC there are other cells in the body that are capable of forming bone in certain circumstances. These again have been described by Friedenstein (1968, 1973) and called Inducable Osteogenic Cells, IOPC, since they are capable of forming bone in the presence of an inducing agent (see p. 54) and cease to form bone when the inducing agent is withdrawn (Friedenstein 1973). They are undifferentiated mesenchyme cells present in many different tissues. Inducable cells may be components of the fibroblastic stroma of the particular tissue in which ectopic bone formation occurs or may be brought there via the blood stream (Friedenstein 1976; Urist, Nogami, and Terashima 1975).

1.1.3.2. *Regeneration of primitive bone trabeculation*

In the discussion of bone — bone marrow interaction in Chapter 1 experiments were briefly mentioned where marrow was completely removed from the shaft of a long bone either by curettage or by perfusion. At first a blood clot fills the depleted cavity. Then active proliferation of connective tissue occurs, budding from the endosteal bone surfaces. As the blood clot contracts this connective tissue advances into the cavity and differentiates to form primitive bony trabeculae. The necessary bone-forming cells must have been derived from cells left on the endosteal surface of the bone following removal of the marrow (Patt and Maloney 1975; Patt 1976). Subsequently this primitive bone is resorbed and the space is filled by marrow tissue, the haemopoietic element being supplied by haemopoietic cells coming in with invading capillaries. Blood cells are distinguished from osteogenic cells by the fact of their mobility.

1.2. Morphology

In discussing the osteoblast it must always be remembered that the appearance of cells that form bone differs in the case of young bone from that in adult bone. Failure to recognize this difference has led to a great deal of confusion. Young bone is technically easy to cut in section: old bone, until modern techniques were developed, is extremely difficult. Figure 1.9 shows active osteoblasts and their precursors or osteoprogenitor cells on the surface of characteristic young bone where apposition is taking place; while Figs 1.10, 1.11, and 1.12 show characteristic 'resting osteoblasts' on the surface of adult bone where new bone is not being laid down, though even on adult bone active osteoblasts that take up tritiated thymidine may be found in small numbers (Kimmel and Jee 1977, 1978a). There is no evidence that the so-called resting osteoblast is not capable, after appropriate stimulation, of performing the same functions as the active osteoblast of young bone.

1.2.1. OSTEOBLASTS OF ACTIVELY GROWING BONE

The active osteoblast tends to be columnar in shape with the nucleus at the

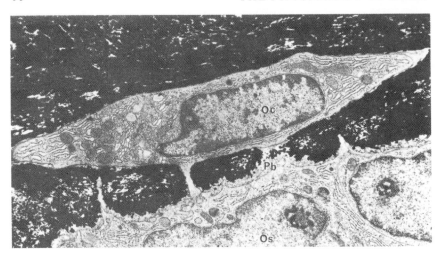

Fig. 2.1. Electron micrograph of a young and relatively flat osteocyte (Oc) in its lacuna in calcified bone. Below it are osteoblasts (Os). A process from the osteocyte connects with an osteoblast in the plane of section. Parts of processes of osteoblasts are also seen. Some osteoid tissue (prebone), labelled Pb, is present between the osteoblasts and the calcified bone but very little of it can be discerned between the osteocyte and the wall of its lacuna. (From Ham and Cormack (1979) by courtesy of authors and publishers; also courtesy M. Weinstock.)

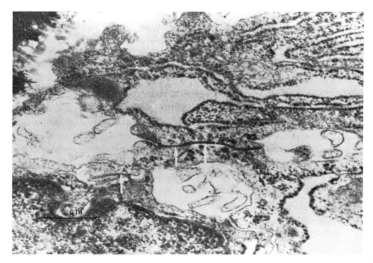

Fig. 2.2. Electron micrograph of gap junctions (arrows) between bone cell processes. (From Matthews *et al.* (1973) by courtesy of authors and publishers.)

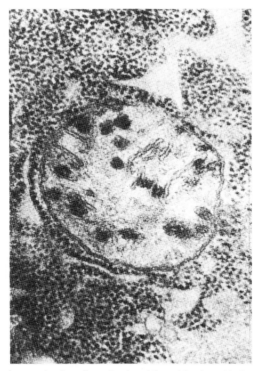

FIG. 2.3. Electron micrograph of swollen mitochondrion with mineral laden granules. Swelling of mitochondria accompanies mineral loading ($\times$ 56 250).

end furthest from the bone surface. The cell shows an irregular contour, particularly on the matrix surface where there are many fine protoplasmic processes which penetrate the adjacent osteoid and mineralized matrix via canaliculae. These processes finally rest on the plasma membrane of deeper osteocytes, or upon the osteocyte processes that meet them within the canaliculae (Cameron 1972; Matthews, Martin, Kennedy, and Collins 1973; Ham and Cormack 1979) (see Fig. 2.1). These cell to cell junctions within bone have been described by Holtrop and Weinger (1971) and resemble 'gap' junctions associated with facilitated ion transport between cardiac muscle cells or smooth muscle cells (Fig. 2.2.). Osteoblasts contain an abundance of rough-surfaced endoplasmic reticulum, a prominent Golgi complex next to the nucleus, and mitochondria. They are rich in glycogen and alkaline phosphatase. The deep basophilic staining seen in conventional histological preparations is accounted for by the RNA protein of the microsomes. Electron dense granules thought to be calcium are often associated with the mitochondria (Fig. 2.3).

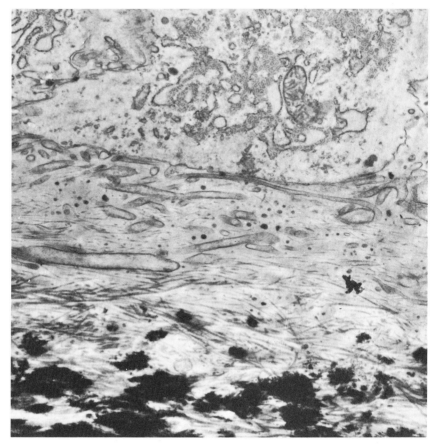

FIG. 2.4. Electron micrograph of osteoblast on left with processes reaching into the osteoid, which shows vesicles and collagen fibres and towards the right increasing area of calcification (× 16 740). (By courtesy of Dr E. Bonucci.)

Extensions from the osteoblasts within the osteoid have been described in some detail by many workers (Bernard and Pease 1969; Matthews and Martin 1971; Ham and Cormack 1979). Their significance and that of the vesicles noted by Anderson (1969, 1973, 1978) both in cartilage and bone matrix is discussed in more detail elsewhere (pp. 88, 106). Such osteoblast processes seen in section extending into the osteoid, together with matrix vesicles, are seen in Fig. 2.4.

Differentiation of osteoblasts from osteoprogenitor cells

The differentiation of the osteoblast from osteoprogenitor cells and the part the osteoblast plays in laying down bone matrix has been studied in a series of elegant experiments using autoradiographic techniques (Kember 1960, 1971; Young, 1962, 1963, 1964; Owen 1963, 1967, 1970, 1971, 1978; Owen and Macpherson 1963; Bingham, Brazell, and Owen 1969). Tritiated thymidine, which is taken up by the cell synthesizing DNA, was used to analyse cell differentiation and tritiated glycine, which labels matrix components, to estimate the rate of matrix formation.

Little (^{3}H) thymidine was taken up by the fibroblasts, which therefore play no significant role in increasing the cell population. The active proliferating cells which showed an initial high level of labelling proved to be the osteoprogenitor cells or preosteoblasts.

The majority, but not all, of these preosteoblasts subsequently divided to give rise to the osteoblasts, cells on the bone surface which contained only half the amount of label seen in preosteoblasts. About 3 days later a few of the cells embedded in the matrix adjacent to the mineral surface were labelled, and subsequently these labelled osteocytes increased in number as more labelled osteoblasts become incorporated into bone matrix. In the young rabbit an osteoblast may remain on the surface for approximately 3 days, during which time it will lay down 3 times its own volume of matrix.

1.2.2. OSTEOBLASTS OF MATURE BONE

Osteoblastic cells on the surfaces of adult bone differ morphologically from the osteoblasts on the surface of young periosteal bone where osteoid is being laid down on large areas of surface. They have been described by Pritchard (1972) as 'resting osteoblasts'. It is fashionable today to call them 'Lining cells' (Vander Wiel, Grubb, and Talmage 1978; Kimmell and Jee 1978a; Lloyd et al. 1977, 1978). They can be seen in Fig. 1.10 and 1.11, which are light microscope views of sections of human iliac crest, as a single layer of cells either adjacent to the mineral surface or to the separated marrow. They are seen at a much higher magnification in Fig. 2.8. They have long narrow dense nuclei lying in an even longer thin line of cytoplasm, and are very different from the plump upstanding cells seen in young bone. Woods and his colleagues (Woods 1973; Woods, Earnshaw, and Kanis 1977), however, consider that such cells should not necessarily be considered inactive. Looked at with an electron microscope both Matthews (Matthews and Martin 1971) and Talmage (Vander Wiel, Grubb, and Talmage 1978) describe the lining cells as having long thin processes extending back into the osteoid and mineralized bone. They have the appearance of fibroblasts with few intracellular organelles. Kimmell and Jee (1977 and 1978a,b), as already discussed, have made an extensive study at the light-microscope level of the character of the cells lining bone surfaces in young adult beagles and in young adult humans. They found the majority of the cells were of the lining cell type with long flattened nuclei. Some of these flat cells, on apparently quiescent surfaces were, however, found to be synthesizing DNA. DNA synthesizing flat cells were about three times as frequent as DNA synthesizing osteoprogenitor cells and ten times as frequent as DNA synthesizing osteoblasts—a surprising and at present unexplained finding (Kimmell and Jee 1977). In a later paper Kimmell and Jee present evidence that 1·5 hours after injection of tritiated thymidine, bone lining cells showed a labelling index in one young dog of 1·3 per cent, while that for osteoprogenitor cells was about 1·6 per cent (Kimmell and Jee 1978a). These results are difficult to understand. It is clear, at least, that these thin, flattened, cells can no longer be considered 'resting osteoblasts' as they have often been in the past. They are cells capable of proliferation since they synthesize DNA and are therefore at risk from carcinogens, particularly bone seeking radionuclides. Indeed, such cells irradiated by α particles have been reported to give rise to fibrosarcoma (Lloyd et al. 1977–8; 1978–9). There is no evidence that they cannot, with appropriate stimulation, perform the same functions as the osteoblast of young bone.

1.3. Function

It has long been recognized that the outstanding function of the osteoblast is to lay down osteoid (Owen 1963). Osteoblasts synthesize the collagen and some of the carbohydrate protein complexes which make up osteoid. They may concentrate certain plasma proteins which are found in matrix. The part they play in producing the peptides and lipids found in the non-collagenous organic matter of bone is not known. The peptides may be breakdown products and the lipids cellular in origin (see Chapter 3). More recently the osteoblast has been implicated in the deposition and exchange of calcium and other ions (Talmage and Grubb 1977; Anderson 1978; Matthews, Vander Wiel, and Talmage 1978).

1.3.1. SYNTHESIS OF COLLAGEN

Osteoblasts rapidly incorporate into matrix tritium-labelled amino acids injected intravenously. These labelled compounds are first found on the bone surface (Canneiro and Leblond 1959; Leblond and Weinstock 1971; Owen 1963) and later in a clearly defined line in the osteoid at varying depths, depending on the time after injection and the rate of growth. In Fig. 2.5 is seen part of the periosteal surface of a cross-section from the femur of a 2-week-old rabbit. The rabbit was given a single injection of tritiated glycine and killed 4 days later. The glycine (Gly) outlining the position of the periosteal surface and the neighbouring canals at the time of injection is in the region indicated by the arrow. In Fig. 2.6 is seen a higher magnification of region R in Fig. 2.5; it shows the glycine band in the matrix outlining the periosteal surface on neighbouring Haversian systems at the time of injection, while in

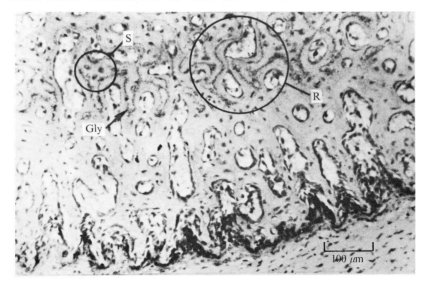

FIG. 2.5. Part of the periosteal surface of a cross-section from the femur of a 2-week-old rabbit. The rabbit was given a single injection of tritiated glycine and killed 4 days later. The glycine (Gly) outlining the position of the periosteal surface and the neighbouring canals at the time of injection is in the region indicated by the arrow. Detail of regions R and S are shown in Figs 2.6 and 2.7. (From Owen (1963) by courtesy of author and publisher.)

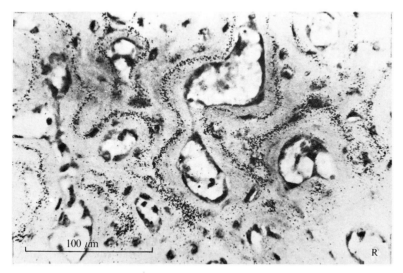

FIG. 2.6. A high magnification of region R (Fig. 2.5), shows the glycine band in the matrix outlining the periosteal surface and neighbouring Haversian systems at the time of injection. (From Owen (1963) by courtesy of author and publisher.)

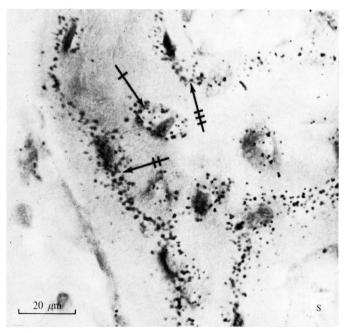

Fɪɢ. 2.7. A high magnification of region S (Fig. 2.5) illustrates glycine uptake in the cytoplasm of the osteocyte (arrow 1). Bands of glycine taken up on the neighbouring bone surfaces are shown (arrows 2 and 3). (From Owen (1963) by courtesy of author and publishers.)

Fig. 2.7 the glycine uptake in the cytoplasm of the osteocytes, in the lacunar walls and neighbouring bone surfaces can be seen.

In Table 2.1 are shown the tritiated amino acids that Young (1964) found incorporated into osteoblasts 30 minutes after injection and the relative proportion of each found in osteoblasts and osteoclasts. These proportions are in keeping with the amounts found in collagen.

The osteoblast is thought to synthesize procollagen within the cell. This is then extruded and cleavage to collagen and assembly into the fibril is achieved extracellularly (see p. 62) (Prockop, Kiuirikko, Tuderman, and Guzman 1979).

1.3.2. SYNTHESIS OF CARBOHYDRATE PROTEIN COMPLEXES

As discussed in Chapter 3 a variety of carbohydrate protein complexes are found in bone matrix. Some are synthesized by the osteoblasts, others reach the bone from the plasma via the bone fluid (see p. 75).

Protein–polysaccharide synthesis. ^{35}S is rapidly incorporated into growing bone and part, at least, of this is found in the chondroitin sulphate fraction (Lea and Vaughan 1957; Kent *et al.* 1956). At the level of the electron micros-

TABLE 2.1

Average number of silver grains for nucleus over osteoblasts and osteoclasts
30 minutes after injection of various tritiated amino acids†

Tritiated amino acid	Number of silver grains‡		Ratio
	Osteoblast	Osteoclast	
Glycine	52·9	3·4	15·6
Proline	55·3	7·4	7·5
Alanine	25·1	6·5	3·9
Arginine	22·9	10·1	2·2
Serine	49·0	31·8	1·5
Lysine	44·9	34·1	1·3
Leucine	38·6	24·7	1·6
Valine	22·8	15·7	1·5
Phenylalanine	10·5	7·4	1·4
Isoleucine	26·1	20·3	1·3
Methionine	44·4	28·6	1·6
Tyrosine	28·3	22·2	1·3
Histidine	25·0	16·7	1·5

† (From Young (1964) by courtesy of author and publishers.)
‡ Total number of grains divided by total number of nuclei appearing in the cells analysed.

cope ^{35}S is seen to be taken up by the Golgi apparatus of the osteoblast and the sulphated mucopolysaccharide is probably released into the extracellular matrix by way of Golgi derived vesicles (Leblond and Weinstock 1971).

Glycoprotein synthesis. Tritium labelled fucose and glucosamine have been used to study glycoprotein synthesis (Owen and Shetlar 1968; Leblond and Weinstock 1971). Both are components of bone sialoprotein, a matrix constituent. They can be demonstrated in the osteoblasts immediately after injection and subsequently in the osteoid. Triffitt and Owen (1973) have demonstrated the uptake of ^{14}C glucosamine by the more acidic components of the non-collagenous constituents of bone matrix, namely sialoprotein, and also by a number of at present uncharacterized glycoproteins not found in plasma and presumably, therefore, synthesized by the osteoblast. Plasma glycoproteins found in matrix presumably pass like other macromolecules between the osteoblasts (Matthews and Martin 1971) or are taken up from the blood as it passes from the marrow to the periosteal surface (see p. 75).

1.3.3. CALCIFICATION PROCESS

The osteoblast may play at least three roles in the mechanism of calcification. First as the origin of matrix vesicles (Anderson 1976, 1978) (see p. 88), secondly, by exerting some control on the movement of calcium ions in and out of bone fluid as proposed by Talmage and his colleagues (Talmage 1970; Talmage and Grubb 1977; Matthews, Vander Wiel, and Talmage 1978) and

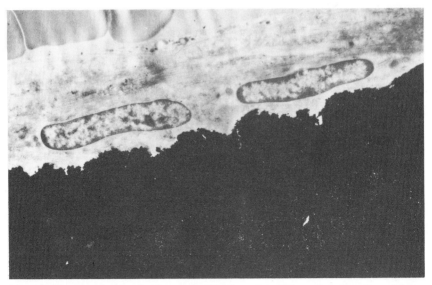

FIG. 2.8. Electron micrograph of an undecalcified section of the endosteal surface of femur obtained at amputation from a 65-year-old man at a site 15 cm proximal to the knee joint. The bone was considered to be normal with no evidence of bone disease. Three distinct regions can be seen here: (1) bone mineral which appears black—bottom half of the picture; (2) a layer of connective tissue shows collagen fibrils in which two cells with flattened nuclei but scant cytoplasm are clearly visible; and (3) fatty marrow at the top left. (From Lloyd and Henning (1978–9), courtesy of authors and publishers.)

thirdly, by its capacity to store calcium in its mitochondria and possibly pass it on into the matrix (Matthews and Martin 1971; Posner 1978b).

1.3.4. MAINTENANCE OF MINERAL HOMEOSTASIS

Many workers have shown (Matthews and Martin 1971; Bygrave 1978) that the osteoblast, particularly in its mitochondria serves as an available source of Ca^{2+}, as seen in Fig. 2.3, p. 31. The possible contribution of the osteoblast to the maintenance of mineral homeostasis is discussed on page 37.

1.4. Factors affecting osteoblast behaviour

Factors at present known to affect the behaviour of the osteoblast are discussed in detail elsewhere. They are the parathyroid hormone (p. 156), possibly vitamin D metabolites (p. 147) and thyroid hormone (p. 188). The dramatic effect of testosterone on the growth of antlers—presumably by its stimulating action on chondroblasts and osteoblasts is discussed on page 91.

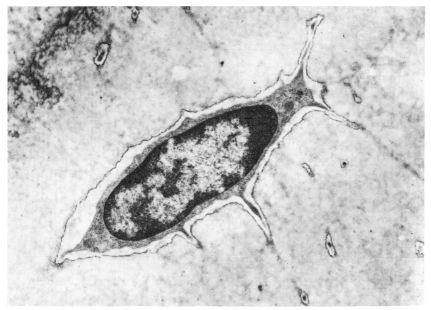

Fɪɢ. 2.9. Electron micrograph of part of a decalcified section of bone, showing an osteocyte in its lacuna with the proximal parts of four of its cytoplasmic processes extending into canaliculi. Two canaliculi with processes cut in cross section are indicated by arrows. (From Ham and Cormack (1979) by courtesy of the authors.)

2. THE OSTEOCYTE

2.1. Origin and subsequent fate

In a study of RNA synthesis in osteogenic cells in young rabbits using (^{3}H) uridine, Bingham, et al. (1969) showed a rapid uptake of label into both preosteoblasts and osteoblasts, reaching a maximum after 24 hours and then declining slowly, whereas the mature osteocyte already embedded in matrix took up no label. A few days after injection, labelled osteocytes were seen near the growing bone surface. These cells acquired their nuclear label before they became buried by freshly formed matrix. After burial they lost their label. The cell presumably dies within its lacunae or is in some way digested in the process of bone resorption since at no time has release of intact osteocytes been seen (Tonna 1966, 1972; Jande and Belanger 1973). There is no evidence to support the view, put forward by Rasmussen and Bordier (1974), 1966, that the osteocyte can revert to an osteoblast, or become an osteoclast by fusion.

2.2. Morphology

In young woven-bone osteocytes are present as closely but irregularly packed cells, rich in cytoplasm, almost indistinguishable from the osteoblasts from which they have been derived. Their processes are relatively few and short. In mature lamellar bone the osteocytes are flattened and ovoid, and possess numerous fine branching processes, Fig. 2.9. They tend to be evenly spaced and uniformly orientated with respect to the long and radial axes of the lamellar systems they occupy. It is probable that no osteocyte is further than $0.1–0.2$ mm from a matrix capillary (Ham and Cormack 1979). They are surrounded by a capsule of non-mineralized osteoid (Matthews and Martin 1971). The young osteocytes almost fill the lacunae in which they lie; older osteocytes are separated from the surrounding walls by a zone of amorphous material and loose collagen fibres. Wasserman and Yaeger (1965) described a capsule that contained both granular and fibrillary material. Immediately beyond this capsule they noted an osmiophilic lamina distinct from the rest of the matrix surrounding a lacuna. The cytoplasmic processes of the osteocyte extend through their canaliculae to communicate with neighbouring osteocyte processes and, if near the bone surface, with osteoblast processes (see Fig. 2.1) (Holtrop and Weinger 1971; Matthews et al. 1973; Weinger and Holtrop 1974). These processes are said by some observers to contain no organelles (Weinger and Holtrop 1974); others describe microtubules. Ham and Cormack (1979) considers the processes have actin-containing filaments, so they may well be capable of contraction. Tight junctions between processes have been found by many observers (Holtrop and Weinger 1971; Weinger and Holtrop 1974). Examination of electron microscope preparations show an extensive endoplasmic reticulum, a large juxta nuclear Golgi apparatus and numerous vesicles and vacuoles (Doty and Schofield 1971). Membrane-bound vesicles, probably lysosomes, may be seen (Jande and Bèlanger 1973; Ham and Cormack 1979). On the whole osteocytes have a smaller complement of the same organelles than the osteoblasts and do not appear to develop new ones. Those they have when first surrounded by bone gradually become less prominent with age (Jande and Bèlanger 1971; 1973). They contain small amounts of a very large number of enzymes, though, with the exception of 5-nucleotidase, less than either osteoblasts or osteoclasts.

2.3. Function

The function of the osteocyte is still extremely controversial. Some workers consider it is concerned only with the proper maintenance of bone matrix (Ham and Cormack 1979). Others that it plays an important part in mineral homeostasis, possibly under the influence of PTH (Baud and Boivin 1978; Talmage and Grubb 1977; Matthews et al. 1978). A third group who speak of osteolysis, regard the osteocyte as involved in both matrix and mineral metabolism, creating what Baud and Boivin have recently described as a mini remodelling cycle (Baud and Boivin 1978). Both Parfitt (1976a,b) and Chambers (1980) consider that the osteocyte shows two types of bone resorption: one the periodic removal and replacement of perilacunar bone, and second the resorption affecting bone beyond the perilacunar region. The latter is described as always occurring in close juxtaposition with osteoclastic resorption.

2.3.1. MAINTENANCE OF BONE MATRIX

It has long been recognized that osteocyte death is synonymous with bone death. As already described, no osteocyte is further than 0·1 to 0·2 mm from a capillary that could serve as a source of nutrients and, further, its processes running through the canaliculae bathed in bone fluid are another source of necessary nutrients (see Fig. 1.6). The lacuno-canalicular system bathed by bone fluid, forms, according to Baud (1968), an exchange area of 250 mm^2 per mm^3. This communicates directly with the submicroscopic interfibrillar spaces of the bone matrix representing an exchange area of 35 000 mm^2 per mm^3. Doty and Schofield (1972) have shown that horseradish peroxidase injected into the circulation can penetrate the lacunae and canaliculi of rat bones. Owen and her colleagues (1977) have given experimental proof that albumin is removed from blood plasma and concentrated in matrix as blood passes through bone from the endosteal to the periosteal surface. It would appear, therefore, that the osteocyte network is well equipped for the maintenance of bone matrix.

2.3.2. MATRIX FORMATION

It has already been said that autoradiographic studies have shown tritiated glycine label both in the youngest osteocytes and their lacunae walls in experiments involving young bone. The osteocyte at this point in its career is only an imprisoned active osteoblast and it is not surprising to find it still capable of forming and excreting collagen. No such label is seen in the older osteocytes. The only evidence that, apart from these very young cells, the osteocyte contributes to matrix formation, is the fact that tetracycline given to a rat produces fluorescence of all lacunar and canalicular surfaces within thirty minutes (Baylink and Wergedal 1971).

2.3.3. MINERAL HOMEOSTASIS

Recently, much stress has been laid on the part played by the osteocyte in association with the osteoblast in maintaining a constant minute to minute level of plasma calcium (Parfitt 1976a,b; Talmage and Grubb 1977; Matthews et al. 1978; Baud and Boivin 1978). Matthews and Martin stated in 1971 'In the normal animal it is probable that continuous exchange of calcium and inorganic phosphate between bone and tissue fluid is mediated by osteoblasts and osteocytes rather than osteoclasts'. This movement of ions is thought to be controlled by PTH which it is known can both stimulate calcium uptake and calcium loss dependent on circumstances.

2.3.4. ALKALINE EARTH LONG-TERM EXCHANGE

A rather different mechanism by which osteocytes might participate in long-term exchange rather than minute to minute release of calcium has been proposed by Marshall and Onkelinx (1968). They concluded, in a mathematical analysis of calcium exchange mechanisms, that a slow diffusion of alkaline earth ions into the practically solid matrix surrounding the canaliculi of bone, provides the probable mechanism for the diffuse uptake of calcium and other alkaline earth ions into bone and for long-term exchange as postulated in Marshall's mathematical models (see Chapter 8). He considers that the calcium ion must reach the volume of bone by passing through tiny canals; subsequent diffusion outwards from these canals will take place in cylindrical rather than plane geometry. Diffusion from lacunae cannot be expressed mathematically but diffusion from canaliculi can. He pictures radial diffusion from each canaliculus into its surrounding territory of calcified matrix as involving penetration of alkaline earth ions through the collagen, water, ground substance, amorphous component, and embedded bone crystals. The diagram in Fig. 2.10 is taken from his paper. This diffusion mechanism, Marshall considers, is sufficient to explain the rapid uptake of tracer in the diffuse component seen in autoradiographs as well as the long-term retention (p. 126). Most of the skeleton can be reached by short distances of diffusion into canalicular territory, so that a very large mass of calcium in the bone may exchange with an extremely small mass of calcium in the blood and in the rest of the initial calcium pool. In addition, retention is enhanced by the geometry of the cylinder, because once an ion has left the cylinder axis it is very improbable that it will return by a random-walk process. In Marshall's view, therefore, the intracellular and extracellular fluid in the canalicular system provided by the osteocyte is basic to the constant 'exchange' of calcium atoms between blood and bone.

2.3.5. OSTEOLYSIS

The word osteolysis was proposed by Bélanger and his colleagues in 1963 (Bélanger, Robichon, Migicovsky, Copp, and Vincent 1963) to define 'an active physiological phenomenon taking place within the intimacy of the bone under the influence of osteocytes, whereby bone matrix is modified and bone salt is lost'.

No satisfactory evidence has yet been given that osteocytes are capable of modifying bone matrix, nor is there anything in their lineage to suggest that

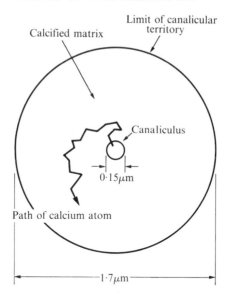

FIG. 2.10. Radial diffusion of an atom of calcium or other alkaline earth from a canaliculus into the surrounding territory of calcified matrix. The dimensions are from Baud's (1962) electron-microscope measurements of mouse bone. (From Marshall and Onkelinx (1968) by courtesy of authors and publishers.)

they are cells capable of modifying the constituents of matrix. The modest part they may play in minute to minute calcium homeostasis must still be left an open question.

2.4. Factors affecting osteocyte behaviour

There is no satisfactory experimental evidence that any of the hormones and other factors like Vitamin D metabolites affect the osteocytes though Talmage and his colleagues, as already discussed, have proposed that the osteocytes associated by their processes with the surface osteoblasts respond to changing levels of plasma calcium by releasing calcium from their lacunar walls to maintain mineral homeostasis (Talmage and Grubb 1977; Matthews *et al.* 1978). Both Talmage and Matthews suggest that the osteocyte will be affected by calcitonin and PTH. Changes in the ultrastructure of osteocytes have been described following administration of PTH (Krempin, Friedrich, and Ritz 1978).

3. THE OSTEOCLAST AND MONONUCLEAR CELLS THAT RESORB BONE

There is increasing evidence that the classical multinucleated osteoclast lying in Howship's luna on a bone surface is not the only cell involved in bone resorption. Other mononuclear cells found on bone surfaces also resorb bone. Further it is recognized that certain locally produced agents, osteoclast stimulating or activating factor (OAF or OSF), prostaglandins and possibly other lymphokinines, quite apart from hormones, are involved in the process. As discussed on page 52 when the problem of osteopetrosis is considered, it is further possible that a helper thymic cell may, at least under some circumstances be required.

3.1. The classical osteoclast

3.1.1. MORPHOLOGY

The classical osteoclast found lying in Howship's lacuna on the resorbing bone surface is multinuclear and has a 'ruffled' or 'brush' border. The largest cell may contain up to at least 100 nuclei, the smallest two, the majority have about 10 or 20. Recent electron microscope studies suggest that a distinction must be made between the 'ruffled border' and the 'brush border'. Ham and Cormack (1979) describes the ruffled border as a *cause* of resorption, i.e. it is composed of fine finger-like cytoplasmic processes fanning out from the cell to terminate upon the bone surface, while the brush border is an *effect* of resorption. It is composed of the straight collagenic fibrils of calcified bone or cartilage at sites where they are disposed more or less at right angles to a surface undergoing resorption, in which process the mineral between the fibrils is removed so that they are freed from it (Ham 1979). In Fig. 2.11 is shown an electron micrograph of the ruffled border of an osteoclast applied to the surface of the bone. On the left-hand corner is the bone and, applied to the surface at each end, is what Ham describes as the clear zone, enclosing as if with a girdle, the ruffled border. Behind is a region of membrane-bound vesicles: probably lysosomes and vacuoles. Not shown in this figure, are the nuclei, which lie further back in the cell behind the vesicles. The cytoplasm associated with the nuclei contains mitochondria, a fair number of ribosomes and polyribosomes, some endoplasmic reticulum and many prominent Golgi saccules, which suggest the osteoclast is a secreting cell. It has been suggested that the clear zone serves to anchor the osteoclast to the bone surface since this zone contains actin fibres (Ham and Cormack 1979), but it has been shown that marker molecules in tissue fluid can pass between the bone and the site of a clear zone.

One of the most remarkable features of the osteoclast is its high degree of mobility, while bone continues to 'melt away' after the osteoclast has moved from its original site of action (Gothlin and Ericsson 1976). This activity is illustrated in Figs 2.12 and 2.13, which show areas of active resorption following an injection of (^{3}H) glucosamine. At one hour following injection, the

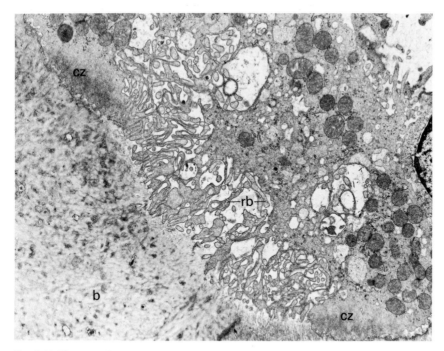

FIG. 2.11. Electron micrograph (× 3995) of ruffled border (rb) of an osteoclast, showing also its clear zone (cz). The bone (b) that it is eroding is seen as a light area at the lower left corner. The basal part of the cell, seen at upper right extending to lower right, contains numerous mitochondria. Note also the vesicular region between the ruffled border and the basal region. (From Holtrop and King (1977) by courtesy of author and publisher.)

label is concentrated at the junction of the cell and the bone surface, and there is very low label on the rest of the surface. Six hours after injection of (^{3}H) glucosamine some labelling is still present on the osteoclast surface, but a heavily labelled area is present adjacent to the osteoclast (Owen and Shetlar 1968). The possible significance of this label is discussed on page 77.

3.1.2. ORIGIN

It was thought for many years that the osteoblast and the osteoclast shared a common stem cell. As was stated in Chapter 1, all the evidence suggests that they differentiate from different stem cells. In 1962 Fischman and Hay raised the question as to whether the osteoclast might be derived from the mono-nuclear cell of the blood. They showed in regenerating newt limbs, that osteoclasts that at one stage actively engaged in resorption, appear to differen-tiate from a precursor cell with characteristics similar to those of a mono-nuclear blood cell, since osteoclast nuclei were labelled only at a time when

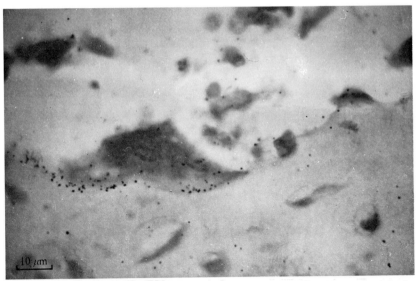

FIG. 2.12. Incorporation of ³H-glucosamine by an osteoclast. Labelling 1 hour after injection of ³H-glucosamine. Note concentration of label at junction of the cell and the bone surface and very low label on the rest of the surface. 10 days exposure. (From Owen and Shetlar (1968) by courtesy of authors and publishers.)

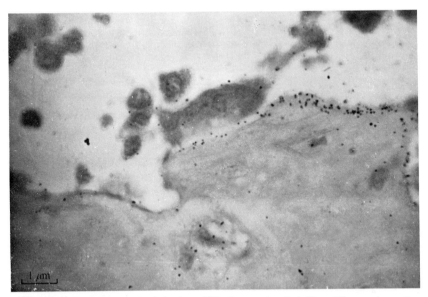

FIG. 2.13. Labelling 6 hours after injection of ³H-glucosamine. Labelling still present on osteo-clast surface; a heavily labelled area of the non-osteoclast surface is present adjacent to the osteoclast, while the rest of the non-osteoclast surface is barely labelled. 10 days' exposure. (From Owen and Shetlar (1968) by courtesy of authors and publishers.)

such mononuclear cells were labelled. In 1963 Jee and Nolan made the same suggestion following the injection of carbon molecules into rats. As would be expected, some carbon particles were taken up into macrophages, and about 15–35 days later, particles could be seen within undoubted osteoclasts. This might mean that carbon-laden macrophages fused to form osteoclasts, or that osteoclasts already on a bone surface had taken up some wandering carbon particles. The evidence that the osteoclast is indeed derived from the mononuclear cell of the blood and not from a bone-forming precursor can be summarized as follows:

(1) *Embryology*. In the first chapter, when a brief account was given of the embryological development of bone and bone marrow, it was shown that the cells that formed bone, the early osteoblasts, were derived from an undifferentiated mesenchyme cell, while the cells that formed the haemopoietic element of the marrow came originally from the yolk sac and, having colonized the liver, reached the developing bone within the penetrating capillaries. This haemopoietic element gives rise to the granulocytes, the megakaryocytes, the erythrocytes, the lymphocytes and monocytes of the peripheral blood.

(2) *Quail chick chimaeras*. Further evidence for the separate origin of the osteoclast has come from elegant experiments using quail-chick chimaeras. The nuclei of quail and chick cells are sufficiently different from one another to enable a morphological distinction to be made between them. This difference has been used to study the developmental relationship between osteoblasts and osteoclasts (Jotereau and Le Douarin 1978). Limb buds or femur rudiments from chick embryos were grafted into quail embryos and similar quail fragments into chick embryos. Endochondral ossification with the development of a marrow cavity proceeded normally. In grafts which were implanted before the development of myelogenesis, the osteocytes and osteoblasts all continued to show nuclei of the graft donor type, while the osteoclasts showed nuclei of host origin. If the graft was implanted later, when the femur contained myeloid tissue, the osteoclasts showed nuclei of both chick and quail type at first, but later, as donor marrow was replaced by host marrow, the osteoclasts contained entirely host nuclei. These experiments, with quail chick chimaeras, show that osteoclasts are derived from blood born precursors, and that osteocyte and osteoblast nuclei do not contribute to their formation (Kahn and Simmons 1975).

(3) *Parabiosis experiments*. Gothin and Ericsson joined a pair of inbred rats by skin flaps, so establishing a cross circulation. They irradiated one animal with a dose sufficient to destroy all haemopoietic tissue and shielded the other. The right femur of each rat was fractured, the cross circulation was arrested and tritiated thymidine injected into the shielded rat. The cross circulation was shortly reestablished. When

sections of the healing fractures were examined seven to twenty-eight days later, in the shielded animal both osteoblasts and osteoclasts were labelled, while in the irradiated animal only osteoclasts were labelled. These experiments indicated that osteoblasts are derived from a local precursor while osteoclasts are derived from circulating cells.

(4) *Osteopetrosis*. Osteopetrosis is discussed further on p. 52. It is a rare disease in man, but occurs in certain strains of mice and rats. It is characterized by a failure to resorb bone during growth. It can be cured in mice (mi/mi), by parabiosis with a normal mouse (Walker 1973), or by injection of normal marrow (Loutit and Sansom 1976). The osteopetrosis in these mice can also be cured by infusion of haematopoietic stem cells from 'beige mice' (bg/bg) (Ash, Loutit, and Townsend 1980b). The strain is characterized by having giant lysosomes. Giant lysosomes were found in the osteoclasts and granular cells in recipient animals, none were seen in osteoblasts or osteocytes, again demonstrating that osteoclasts are different in origin from osteoblasts and osteocytes.

The fact that the osteoclast is derived from a haemopoietic cell is now generally accepted. This cell is also thought to be the mononuclear cell from the haemopoietic marrow, which reaches the tissues via the blood stream to become a tissue macrophage; as was first described by Volkman and Gowans in 1965. Fusion of one or more such macrophages would result in the multinucleated osteoclast. The osteoclast rarely shows an uptake of tritiated thymidine into more than one nucleus (Tonna 1960, 1961). Labelled monocytes, however, appear in the blood of rats 10–18 hours after administration of thymidine, which would give time for the fusion of one or more macrophages to contribute to the labelling of osteoclasts (Whitelaw and Batho 1975).

Chambers (1978), who has made extensive studies of the macrophage, concludes that the available evidence supports the origin of the multinucleated osteoclast from mononuclear phagocyte precursors of haemopoietic origin (Van Furth 1975; Van Furth *et al.* 1975; Owen 1978). He suggests that poorly understood changes in the bone surface may lead to phagocytic recognition, since bone surfaces appear chemotactic for monocytes (Mundy, Varani, Orr, Gondek, and Ward 1978; Teitelbaum, Stewart, and Kahn 1979). The bone, in effect, becomes a 'foreign body' and leads to the formation of foreign body giant cells. The osteoclast, he finds, has certain differences from the tissue macrophage such as lack of some surface cell receptors (C_3 and Fe) and inability to take up opsonized, or complement coated red cells, but it also has certain common characteristics, like adherence to glass surfaces and uptake of latex particles (Chamber 1979).

3.1.3. FUNCTION

Exactly how the osteoclast exerts its resorptive effect on bone has resulted in an extensive literature, but no completely satisfactory account can be given, since there is no agreement between different workers. Today it is questioned by some workers as to whether the osteoclast does more than, by secretion of acids, dissolve the mineral and so release the collagen fibres to be digested by other mononuclear cells (Heersche 1978), as discussed on p. 50. Other workers consider that, in the process of resorption, the calcium is first removed and subsequently matrix constituents are ingested and digested by the many lysosomes present in the cytoplasm (Reymolds 1968; Hancox 1972). All reports describe both crystals and fragments of collagen lying free in the region of the 'ruffled' border, but some observers claim that collagen fibres are not seen within the lysosomes or vacuoles of the osteoclast and cannot therefore be digested by the osteoclast (Heersche 1978). The removal of apatite crystals has been attributed to the production of both citric and lactic acid, so freeing the collagen (Vaes 1968a,b) but the evidence, which has recently been reviewed, on the part played by both acid and enzymes in relation to organ and tissue culture experiments, is confused. Digestion of matrix constituents may, in part at least, be explained by the high content of acid hydrolases and other enzymes, many of them present in the lysosomes (Vaes 1968a,b, 1969, 1973; Doty and Schofield 1972) (see p. 209). Enzymes which have been found are acid phosphatase, aryl sulphatase, acid trimetaphosphatase, leucine aminopeptidase, β galactosidase and β glucosidase, and adenosine triphosphatase. Various neutral phosphatases have also been demonstrated, together with succinic dehydrogenase and cytochrome oxidase (Gothlin and Ericsson 1976). Collagenases have not been isolated from osteoclasts. This is perhaps odd, as macrophages are rich in collagenase, and how have they lost the enzyme in process of fusion? However, as discussed elsewhere (Chapter 12), collagenases are usually present in cells, together with an inhibitor, and are not necessarily stored in cells but are freshly synthesized on demand. Cathepsin B_1 (Burleigh, Barrett, and Lazarus 1974), a powerful collagenase, is known to have a lysosomal localization and to be present in bone. The part played by the osteoclast itself in digestion of collagen must at the present remain for further investigation. There is no question, however, but that it plays an essential part at some point in resorption, since so many of the factors like PTH, calcitonin, and the diphosphonates that affect resorption produce marked changes in both the appearance, the number and the behaviour of the osteoclast. Chambers (1980) suggests that the most plausible mechanism for osteoclast formation and function is that osteocytes alter bone locally in such a way as to lead to its phagocytic recognition by mononuclear phagocytes. These cells then accumulate on the altered bone surface, commence digestion and fuse in a similar way to that shown for other macrophage polykaryons.

3.1.4. FACTORS AFFECTING THE OSTEOCLAST BEHAVIOUR

The factors that affect the osteoclast are discussed in greater detail elsewhere (see p. 156). In summary, it can be said that the parathyroid hormone is the only factor that is at present recognized as increasing their number as well as their activity. Calcitonin decreases their number and effectiveness. 1,25-$(OH)_2D_3$ while not increasing their number, enlarges the size of the 'ruffled' border and their activity. The diphosphonates (see p. 111) have a dramatic effect on osteoclasts, reducing their numbers and their efficiency. How far these factors affect mononuclear cells that may also be concerned in resorption is not at present clear. Cortisol may well exert its effect on bone resorption by interfering with the synthesis of prostaglandins rather than by any direct effect on bone cells.

3.2. Mononuclear cells

Bone undergoing resorption has been shown to be chemotactic for monocytes. Electron microscope studies, as well as routine histology, show groups of mononuclear cells on bone surfaces, which because of their moth eaten character, are clearly undergoing resorption (Gothlin and Ericsson 1976; Mundy, Altman, Gondek, and Bandelin 1977; Earnshaw 1979). These mononuclear cells are thought to be tissue macrophages derived from monocyte precursors in the marrow (Volkman and Gowans 1965; Loutit and Nisbet 1979). Since the tissue macrophage itself is difficult to isolate and investigate, much work on its function has been done with the peritoneal macrophage or mononuclear cells concentrated from circulating blood (Kahn, Stewart, and Teitelbaum 1978; Teitelbaum *et al*. 1979; Yoneda and Mundy 1979). These mononuclear cells have the characteristics of tissue macrophages, as already discussed. They are surface adherent, ingest latex particles, and show non-specific esterase activity (Yoneda and Mundy 1979). They can be shown experimentally to resorb bone. (For reasons which are not at present clear mouse macrophages are more efficient than rat macrophages.) Bone resorption, as measured by net release of ^{45}Ca from matrix in tissue culture, is initiated as early as 3 hours after the addition of bone particles to a culture of peritoneal macrophages (Teitelbaum *et al*. 1979). This capacity to resorb bone is not surprising since macrophages are rich in collagenase. For resorption to occur it is essential that the cell is in contact with the bone surface (Kahn *et al*. 1978). Yoneda and Mundy (1979) conclude that the mononuclear cell or macrophage possesses multifaction capacities in bone resorption and may reveal each function separately or synergistically, depending on environmental conditions.

3.3. The fibroblast

It is suggested by Deporter (1979) that during chronic inflammatory disorders of bone, the fibroblast as well as the osteoclast and mononuclear cell may be involved in bone resorption (see p. 54).

4. AGENTS OTHER THAN CELLS AND HORMONES ASSOCIATED WITH BONE RESORPTION

At least two factors produced locally in areas of bone resorption are now recognized as playing a part in the process of resorption. There may be others. Those recognized are 'osteoclast stimulating factor' or 'osteoclast activating factor', and prostaglandins, more particularly prostaglandin-PGE_2. There are probably other less well characterized lymphokinines (Horton, Raisz, Simmons, Oppenheim, and Mergenhagen 1972).

4.1. Osteoclast stimulating or activating factor (OSF or OAF)

In 1972 Raisz and his colleagues (Horton *et al.* 1972) isolated from the supernatant fluid of leucocytes grown in tissue culture with phytohaemoglutin, a factor which stimulated resorption in foetal rat bone in organ culture. Chemically it is a protein-containing macromolecule which can be differentiated from other known stimulators of bone resorption such as PTH, metabolites of Vitamin D and prostaglandins (Raisz, Luben, Mundy, Dietrich, Horton, and Trummel 1975; Mundy, Chapiro, Bandelin, Canalis, and Raisz 1976). It appears to be more susceptible to inhibition by cortisol than PTH (Strumpf, Kowalski, and Mundy 1978). This inhibition of OAF may account for the effects of cortisol in preventing the hypercalcaemia associated with myeloma and other haematological bone neoplasms (Mundy *et al.* 1974). OAF appears to be produced by lymphocytes activated by prostaglandins of the E series which are synthesized and released by macrophages (Yoneda and Mundy 1979). The regulation of OAF production by prostaglandins is mediated by cyclic AMP (Toshiyoki and Mundy 1979).

4.2. Prostaglandins

All the classical prostaglandins and their metabolites so far studied are stimulators of bone resorption *in vitro* (Seyberth, Raisz, and Oates 1978), but those of the E series are the most potent. Tashjian and his associates in 1972 (Tashjian, Voelkel, Levine, and Goldhaber 1972) first showed that certain experimental tumours in the rabbit could produce bone resorption without invasion and that the tumours secreted a bone resorbing factor in culture, subsequently identified as a prostaglandin. It is now recognized that the hypercalcaemia associated with inflammation and more particularly with haemopoietic bone cancers and secondary deposits in bone is probably in some way dependent upon prostaglandins produced locally (Seyberth *et al.* 1978). The effects of prostaglandins on resorption are similar in some respects of those of PTH, both appear to act through cAMP, both are inhibited by calcitonin (Klein and Raisz 1970). On the other hand, the receptors for PTH and PGE in bone are different, and at low concentrations their action is not synergistic. PTH increases the number of osteoclasts as well as stimulating them, while prostaglandin stimulates the osteoclasts — as demonstrated by enlargement of 'their ruffled borders' — but does not affect their numbers (Holtrop and Raisz 1979). Cortisol only influences the effect of PTH in high doses (Raisz, Trummel, Wener, and Simmons 1972), but has a strong inhibiting action on prostaglandins at low doses. Since cortisol is known to interfere in the synthesis of prostaglandins, it is possible that its inhibiting effect on bone resorption is dependent on an effect on prostaglandin synthesis.

The site of prostaglandin production is not established, nor its exact relationship to OAF. It is suggested that the production of OAF by lymphocytes is dependent on prostaglandin synthesized by monocytes or macrophages (Toshiyoki and Mundy 1979). Raisz and his colleagues (Raisz, Dietrich, Simmons, Seyberth, Hubbard, and Oates 1977) consider that it is probably not PG_{E2} itself which is the effective factor but that bone enzymatically converts the prostaglandin to some active metabolite, since there is no relationship found between PG_{E2} circulating level and the degree of hypercalcaemia.

5. OSTEOPETROSIS AND RESORPTION

Recent studies of osteopetrosis have emphasized the complexity of the factors involved in bone resorption, and lend additional support to the view that the osteoclast, is derived from a haemopoietic stem cell.

Osteopetrosis is a genetically determined disease recognized in human beings, mice, rats, rabbits, and birds. It is characterized by a marked increase of medullary bone due to failure of resorption (Loutit and Sansom 1976; Milhaud and Labat 1978; Chambers and Loutit 1979; Coccia, Kriuit, Ceruenka, Clawson, Kersey, Kim, Nesbit, Ramsay, Waruentin, Teitelbaum, Kahn, and Brown 1980). It has been studied experimentally in mice and rats. Some clinical observations have been made in children with infantile malignant osteopetrosis (Albers–Schonberg syndrome or marble bone disease) (Ballet and Griscelli 1978; Milhaud and Labat 1979; Coccia *et al.* 1980). The defect in the resorption process, though constant in any one strain of mouse and rat, appears to depend on different defects in different strains investigated (Loutit and Nisbet 1979). As Milhaud has said (Milhaud and Labat 1979) 'osteopetrosis is genetically heterogenous'. He has described a strain of rat (*op op*) where the osteopetrosis is cured by grafting the thymus of a normal sibling, while in the *mi mi* mouse the thymus does not appear to be involved

(Loutit and Nisbet 1979). The osteopetrosis has been corrected in certain strains of mice and rats by an infusion of histocompatible haemopoietic marrow without immunosuppression due to radiation (Walker 1953, 1975a,b; Loutit and Sansom 1976; Loutit and Nisbet 1979) or by parabiosis of affected mice and rats to normal siblings (Marks and Walker 1976). A few cases in children have shown remarkable improvement following compatible bone marrow transplants after immunosuppression by radiation (Coccia et al. 1980). Immunosuppression appears essential for engraftment. These observations all indicate that the cells responsible for a return to normal resorption are of haematogenous origin. The osteoclast itself has been shown to be abnormal (Marks and Walker 1976), but defects in the macrophage, and its precursor the monocyte, have also been demonstrated (Reeves, August, Humbert, and Weston 1979; Coccia et al. 1980; Ash et al. 1980b). Loutit and Chambers suggest that, in at least certain strains of mice (mi mi), the defect is due to a failure of recognition by the macrophage of bone as presenting a surface to be resorbed (Chambers and Loutit 1979). Certainly, following successful marrow engraftment in children, monocyte–macrophage function, which had been depressed, returned to normal, as did the resorbing activity of the osteoclasts (Coccia et al. 1980). In one case where compatible marrow from a brother was given to a sister with osteopetrosis, it was possible by appropriate techniques to show after the sister's recovery that her osteoclasts were of (donor) male origin, and her osteoblasts of (recipient) female origin, indicating clearly the haemopoietic and independent origin of the osteoclast discussed in more detail on p. 45.

In one strain of rat (op op) the interaction of a thymic lymphocyte also seems critcal (Milhaud and Labat 1978, 1979), but the thymus is not necessarily involved in all forms of osteopetrosis. One child, at least, transfused with foetal thymus, showed no improvement (Ballet and Griscelli 1978), and mi/mi mice are not cured by a thymic graft (Loutit and Sansom 1976). However, since thymic lymphocytes are known to 'activate' macrophages in certain natural inflammatory defences (Allison 1978) and macrophages are known to be involved in resorption, it is not unlikely that a thymic cell, i.e. a thymocyte helping function, may be involved in some forms of osteopetrosis.

6. THE FIBROBLAST

For the present it is convenient to call an undifferentiated cell present in connective tissue which retains mesenchymal potentiality: a fibroblast. It is a fusiform spindle-shaped cell with long tapering processes, or a more flattened spindle shaped cell with several slender processes. The nucleus is centrally placed, showing endoplasmic reticulum and a Golgi apparatus. The cytoplasm has many secretory vesicles and usually two long protoplasmic processes at each end of the cell. These are particularly obvious in tissue culture preparations. Though at present it is thought all fibroblasts look alike, they clearly have different potentials for differentiation. Fibroblasts cultured from marrow, for instance, can form bone in diffusion chambers. In such cultures it is not possible to distinguish the DOPC, the determined osteo-progenitor cell, already discussed (p. 28), nor the IOPC, the inducable osteoprogenitor cell (p. 29). Cultures of fibroblasts from other connective tissues will only form bone in the presence of an inducer (Friedenstein 1973; Urist, Mikulski, Nakagawa, and Yen 1977) (see p. 54). Such inducable cells (IOPC) (see p. 29) may be components of the fibroblastic stroma of the particular organ in which the ectopic bone formation occurs or may be brought there via the blood stream from the marrow (Friedenstein 1976; Urist *et al.* 1977). It is suggested by Deporter (1979) that the fibroblast plays a part in bone resorption in some chronic inflammatory diseases, particularly rheumatoid arthritis and peridontal disease. He proposes, as a result of electron microscope studies, that collagenase produced by the fibroblast destroys the bone collagen, while osteoclasts remove the mineral. Fibroblasts isolated from the synovium of rabbits with experimental arthritis produce a collagenase identical to the collagenase produced by normal rabbit fibroblasts (Werb and Reynolds 1975). Radionuclides present in bone may induce classical fibrosarcoma that contain no alkaline phosphatase (Bland, Loutit, and Sansom 1974). Some of these may occasionally arise from periosteal tissues (Price, Moore, and Jones 1972) but others probably arise from un-differentiated fibroblasts present in marrow.

The fibroblast, according to Ham, is a secretory cell, secreting procollagen, glycosaminoglycans, and proelastin. He considers it is derived from a cell he calls a pericyte, in the wall of capillaries. By many workers the so-called pericyte is a contractile cell (Rouget 1873; Backwinkel and Diddams 1970), i.e. a committed cell. It would appear acceptable to regard uncommitted cells in the walls of capillaries as the stem cell of the tissue fibroblast. The latter, however, is again probably an uncommitted cell with capacity for wide differentiation.

7. BONE-INDUCING SUBSTANCES

A number of agents capable of inducing bone formation in tissues containing undifferentiated mesenchyme cells have been described. They include transitional epithelium of the bladder (Huggins 1930), decalcified bone matrix and bone morphogenic protein described by Urist and his colleagues (Urist 1973, 1976; Urist and Iwata 1973; Urist *et al.* 1977). Urist has for many years studied the chemistry of an inducing substance isolated from bone.

Extraction of bone with EDTA (ethylene diaminetetraacetic acid) leaves a residue of about 88 per cent collagen and 6 per cent non-collagenous protein.

After implantation in muscle or a subcutaneous pouch, this residual matrix serves as a substration for the differentiation of migratory mesenchymal cells into cartilage, bone, and bone marrow. The matrix is morphogenic and capable of producing a spherical ossicle (Urist 1973). Demineralization of rat and guinea-pig bone in solutions of EDTA (ethylene diaminetetraacetic acid) is associated with loss of the bone morphogenic property. The loss is much greater at neutrality than in acidic solutions. The degradation of bone morphogenic protein (BMP) in a neutral solution is attributed to a hypothetical endogenous enzyme BMPase. The morphogenic protein is firmly bound to collagen. It is absent in lathyrism. Urist has postulated that urinary bladder epithelium, another bone inducing substance, may secrete a precursor substance to BMP. More recently, he has isolated from dense cortical bone a non-collagenous protein, different from BMP that he considers may also be concerned in the calcification process (Urist et al. 1977).

3. Chemistry of Bone Matrix

1. GENERAL CHEMISTRY OF BONE AND CARTILAGE

CERTAIN aspects of the character of the matrix components of bone are discussed in more detail than others since they are relevant to a consideration of the mechanism of calcification. This is particularly true of some carbo-hydrate protein complexes and certain plasma proteins concentrated in bone. On the other hand, no attempt is made to give a comprehensive review of the vast and ever-growing literature on collagen.

There are considerable gross differences in the composition of bone and cartilage according to the age of the bone and the part of the bone examined. In Table 3.1 is shown an analysis giving values for total ash, collagen, chondroitin sulphate, keratan sulphate, sialic acid, and other protein in bovine cartilage and bone. In Table 3.2 is shown a more detailed analysis of the organic composition of washed epiphyseal cartilage and bone in which data on the lipid content is also given. Sialic acid may be present in many glycoproteins other than sialoprotein, but in adult ox bone about 60 per cent of the sialic acid is present in bone sialoprotein (Herring and Oldroyd 1968). In Table 3.3. the most recent analyses of bovine cortical bone are sum-marized. This table indicates that there are significant amounts of non-collagenous organic material present in mature cortical bone, namely, about 11 per cent (Herring 1972). This is made up of proteoglycans, glycoproteins, plasma proteins, peptides and lipids, and is discussed in more detail, p. 69.

Pugliarello and her colleagues (Pugliarello, Vittur, de Bernard, Bonucci, and Ascenzi 1973) have recently summarized the structural differences in chemical composition at a microscopic level shown in Table 3.4. These differences indicate that the structural variety of bone tissue is correlated with a significant variability in the organic composition of matrix. (The areas of bone described as Mittelinien are layers of primary bone appearing in young animals, in both cross- and longitudinal-sections, as narrow lines regularly scattered in the outer, middle, and inner zones of the compacta and showing high X-ray absorption.)

The authors indicate that the figures in this table suggest that whenever intense and rapid calcification occurs, increased amounts of non-collagenous protein are present. Similarly, it is known that in the ossifiable cartilage

TABLE 3.1

Composition of bovine cartilage and bone

Tissue	Ash percentage in total dry tissue	Coll†	CS†	KS†	SA†	OP†	Total organic
		Percentage of dry, mineral-free weight of tissue					
		Calf					
Articular	6·2	63·7	25·3	3·69	0·52	9·6	102·8
Epiphyseal	25·2	56·2	33·9	4·36	0·69	14·7	109·9
1 spongiosa	69·7	75·8	1·9	1·29	0·41	10·6	90·0
2 spongiosa	69·3	79·5	1·1	0·70	0·35	6·6	88·3
Diaphyseal	70·6	79·2	0·8	0·86	0·25	4·7	85·9
		Foetus					
Articular	9·6	46·1	35·6	4·57	0·87	22·0	109·2
Epiphyseal	11·3	38·2	36·9	3·12	0·86	26·9	106·0
1 spongiosa	72·3	71·2	2·6	2·69	0·65	11·8	89·0
2 spongiosa	71·3	72·6	1·6	1·75	0·48	12·8	89·3
Diaphyseal	73·6	96·3	1·7	1·51	0·54	7·1	107·1

From the results of Campo and Tourtellotte (1967).

† Key: Coll, collagen; CS, chondroitin sulphate; KS, keratan sulphate (calculated from glucosamine values); SA, sialic acid; OP, other protein, calculated from total nitrogen — (collagen + hexosamine nitrogen). From Herring (1972) by courtesy of author and publishers.

matrix, collagen is also decreasing and proteoglycans increasing (Vittur, Pugliarello, and Bernard 1971, 1972).

2. COLLAGEN

The collagen of bone is synthesized in the form of procollagen in the osteoblast; the procollagen is extruded and cleavage to collagen and assembly into fibrils is achieved extracellularly (see p. 62).

As far as possible, the papers discussed are concerned with the collagen of bone and cartilage. As shown in Table 3.3 a high proportion of mature cortical bone by weight is collagen.

Collagen is the major macromolecule of most connective tissues, though its structure in different tissues is variable (Miller 1976; Prockop, Kivirikko, Tuderman, and Guzman 1979). It has recently become evident that genetic polymorphism is dramatically expressed in this structural protein, which suggests that perhaps collagen molecules and the fibres derived from them have other functions beyond their well-recognized structural role.

TABLE 3.2

Organic composition of washed epiphyseal cartilage and bone

Zone	Nondialyzable organic matter‖	Percentage of organic matrix§					
		Collagen††	Chondromuco-protein‡‡	Sialo-protein§§	Lipid	Sulphur	Nitrogen
Resting cartilage	(3) 93·9±5·8	(12) 60·1±1·4	(10) 40·7±2·3	(8) 3·43±0·06	(3) 1·00±0·12	(10) 1·54±0·04	(8) 10·80±0·36
Proliferating cartilage	(3) 62·8±2·0	(10) 39·3±1·1	(8) 59·2±2·5	(8) 4·69±0·10	(3) 4·86±0·90	(7) 2·07±0·15	(10) 9·78±0·20
Hypertrophic cartilage	(5) 33·6±3·4	(12) 23·3±1·3	(10) 41·8±0·05	(8) 4·49±0·05	(5) 7·70±1·49	(8) 1·40±0·03	(6) 10·25±0·52
Calcified cartilage	(5) 18·6±1·3	(13) 22·1±0·9	(8) 19·3±0·6	(8) 4·80±0·12	(5) 8·50±0·81	(8) 0·83±0·03	(6) 8·89±0·29
Cancellous bone	(2) 24·6±1·2	(12) 72·4±1·6	(10) 4·1±0·5	(8) 2·39±0·05	(4) 0·61±0·06	(6) 0·37±0·07	(6) 11·79±0·31

† Values are means ±standard error of means, the number of samples being in parentheses.
‡ From Wuthier (1969).
§ Organic matrix is freeze-dried weight minus ash content of washed tissues.
‖ Percentage of freeze-dried weight of washed tissue not dialyzable after demineralization with 0·5 M EDTA, pH 8·0.
†† Percentage hydroxyproline/0·141 (Eastoe 1955).
‡‡ [Percentage hexosamine−(percentage sialic acid × 0·45)]/0·264 (Luscombe and Phelps 1967; Herring 1964).
§§ Percentage sialic acid/0·171 (Herring 1964).

From Herring (1972) by courtesy of author and publishers.

TABLE 3.3

Composition of bovine cortical bone

	Percentage by weight		
	Fresh bone	Dry bone	Organic bone
Mineral	68·8	75·7	—
Organic	22·1	24·3	100
Water	9·1	—	—
Collagen	19·5	21·5	88–89
Non-collagenous organic	2·5	2·8	11–12
Non-collagenous components			
Chondroitin 4-sulphate	0·18	0·20	0·82
Bone sialoprotein	0·17	0·19	0·78
Insoluble CRF	0·20	0·022	0·89
α_2HS (or G_2B) glycoprotein[a]	0·08	0·09	0·42
Albumin[a]	0·06	0·07	0·33
Osteocalcin[b] (or Gla protein)	0·07	0·08	0·37
Lipids[c]	1·03	0·14	4·69
Peptides[d]	0·12	0·13	0·53
Others	0·63	0·68	2·2–3·2

[a] Ashton *et al.* 1974.
[b] Price, Otsaka, Poser, Kristaponis, and Raman 1976.
[c] Shapiro 1970, 1971.
[d] Leaver and Shuttleworth 1968.

2.1. General structure of the molecule

The biological activity of a protein depends on the folding of the genetically defined sequence of amino acids in a polypeptide chain into a three-dimensional conformation. In the case of collagen, the structure at two levels of organization is determined by the amino acid sequence. At the first level three polypeptide chains are folded into a rod-like triple-helical molecule about 300 nm long and only 1·5 nm in diameter. Lateral and longitudinal association of the triple-helical molecules into fibrils is involved at the second level (Fig. 3.1). Each of the three polypeptide chains of the collagen molecule, known as α chains, is coiled in a left-handed helix with about 3 amino acids per turn. The three chains are then twisted round each other into a right-handed super helix, so forming a rigid rope-like structure. The α chains contain about 1000 amino-acid residues and, with the exception of short sequences at the end of the chains, every third amino acid in each chain is glycine. $(X\text{-}Y\text{-}Gly)_{333}$ where X and Y represent amino acids other than glycine, can therefore be given as the molecular formula of an α chain. The triple helical conformation also depends on the presence of proline and hydroxy proline in the α chains. They are rigid cyclic amino acids and therefore limit rotation of the polypeptide background, so contributing to the stability of the triple

TABLE 3.4

Synopsos of analytical data concerning different structures of bone tissue*

	Total nitrogen	Hexos-amines	Hydroxy-proline	Non-col-lagenous nitrogen	Total phosphorus	Calcium
Bone powder	4·19±0·08 (32)†	0·23±0·01 (20)	2·70±0·04 (33)	0·80	12·12±0·10 (29)	—
Bone sections	4·54±0·04 (85)	0·24±0·01 (26)	3·23±0·04 (92)	0·48	11·46±0·30 (87)	21·14±0·48 (8)
Bone sections (vessel-free)	4·45±0·14 (6)	0·17±0·01 (9)	2·85±0·09 (6)	0·87	11·36±0·16 (6)	—
Osteones at the highest degree of calcification	4·42±0·16	0·28±0·01	3·31±0·14	0·25	10·11±0·26	21·58±0·76
Osteones at the lowest degree of calcification	6·29±0·32	0·31±0·01	3·62±0·17	1·81	7·27±0·49	16·17±1·00
Osteoid tissue	7·71±0·20	0·61±0·04	4·48±0·28	2·06	2·05±0·16	—
Interstitial periosteal lamellar bone	4·97±0·13	0·14±0·01	3·11±0·08	1·07	9·97±0·18	21·69±0·41
Mittellinien	3·78±0·39	0·19±0·01	2·72±0·04	0·37	9·62±0·65	21·78±0·96

* Data are expressed in percentage of dry weight (means ± standard error).

† Number of experiments.

From Pugliarello *et al.* (1973) by courtesy of authors and publishers.

helix. About two thirds of the X and Y positions are occupied by a variety of different amino acids, which decrease the stability of the triple helix but are essential for organization of collagen at the second level, the assembly of the triple helical molecules into collagen fibrils. These other amino acids are clustered in groups of hydrophobic and charged residues and since their side chains point out from the centre of the triple helix they determine how the different collagen molecules associate with one another. The collagen molecules aggregate so that each molecule is longitudinally displaced about one quarter of its length relative to its nearest neighbour. This staggering of molecules largely explains the characteristic 'D spacing' seen in collagen fibrils when examined in the electron microscope (see Fig. 3.1).

This longitudinal staggering of the molecules involves rather less than one quarter of the length and leaves a 'hole' between the end of one triple helix and the beginning of the next. This hole, it has been suggested, may form a nucleation site for calcium apatite formation (see p. 104). There is still some controversy, however, about whether microfibrils make up a fibril or whether

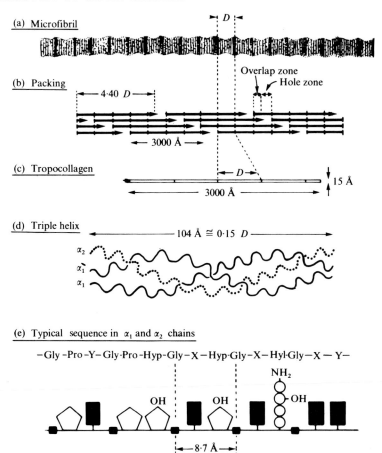

(a) Microfibril

D

Overlap zone
Hole zone

(b) Packing

4·40 D

3000 Å

(c) Tropocollagen

D

15 Å

3000 Å

(d) Triple helix

104 Å $\cong$ 0·15 D

α_2
α_1
α_1

(e) Typical sequence in α_1 and α_2 chains

−Gly −Pro −Y− Gly ·Pro -Hyp-Gly − X − Hyp·Gly − X − Hyl·Gly − X − Y−

NH$_2$

OH

OH

OH

8·7 Å

FIG. 3.1. Diagrammatic representation of collagen structure: (a) shows a stained microfibril of collagen exhibiting characteristic cross-striations with a regular repeat period (D) of approximately 680 Å; (b) is a two-dimensional representation of the packing arrangement of tropocollagen macromolecules in the microfibril. The drawing indicates the lateral displacement of tropocollagen molecules, but not the three-dimensional geometry of the microfibril. Veis and Bhatnagar (1970) discuss the limits imposed on the size of the microfibril by the three-dimensional geometry. In (c) each tropocollagen molecule has large numbers of darkly staining bands, and five of these, which are separated by a regular distance of 680 Å, account for the repeat period (D) in the microfibril. The NH$_2$-terminal and probably the COOH-terminal ends of the molecule are atypical and non-helical in structure; (d) indicates that each tropocollagen molecule consists of three polypeptides, two with identical amino-acid sequences (α_1 chains) and one with a slightly different amino-acid sequence (α_2 chain). Each α chain is coiled in a tight left-handed helix with a pitch of 9·5 Å, and the three chains are coiled around each other in a right-handed 'super-helix' with a pitch of about 104 Å; (e) shows that glycine occurs in every third position throughout most of the polypeptide chains, and there are large amounts of proline and hydroxyproline in the other two positions. X and Y represent any amino acid other than glycine, proline, hydroxyproline, lysine, or hydroxylysine. (From Grant and Prockop (1972), by courtesy of authors and publishers.)

TABLE 3.5
Structurally and genetically distinct collagens

Type	Tissue distribution	Molecular form	Chemical characteristics
I	*Bone*, tendon, skin, dentin ligament, fascia, arteries, and uterus	$[\alpha1(I)_2\alpha2]$	Hybrid composed of 2 kinds of chains. Low in hydroxylysine and glycosylated hydroxylysine.
II	*Hyaline cartilage*, cornea, vitreous body, and neural retinal tissues	$[\alpha1(II)]_3$	Relatively high in hydroxylysine and glycosylated hydroxylysine.
III	Skin, arteries, and uterus	$[\alpha1(III)]_3$	High in hydroxyproline and low in hydroxylysine; contains interchain disulphide bonds.
IV	Basement membranes	$[\alpha1(IV)]_3$	High in hydroxylysine and glycosylated hydroxylysine; may contain large globular regions.
V	Basement membranes and perhaps other tissues	αA and αB	Similar to type 4.

the cross sectional lattice of the fibril is dependent on random packing of individual molecules (Prockop *et al.* 1979).

2.2. Types of collagen in man

There are a variety of collagens found in man. They are all composed of polypeptides, with regions that are similar to the α chains just described, and have the general structure (X-Y-Gly) and large amounts of proline and hydroxyproline. Since they differ in the precise sequence of amino acids in the X and Y positions they are apparently the product of different genes. Recent studies have attempted to locate the collagen genes on different chromosomes using hybrids of human and mouse cells. The results are, however, conflicting. Genes for Type I collagen have been located on chromosome 17 and chromosome 7 by different workers (Sundar Raj, Church, Klobutcher, and Ruddle 1977; Sykes and Solomon 1978). In this connection, however, it must be remembered that under appropriate circumstances 'gene switching may occur' as discussed in relation to the collagens made by osteoblasts and chondroblasts (see p. 82). In Table 3.5 are shown a list of the different types of collagen at present recognized. Type 1 and Type 2 only will be discussed here, since they occur in bone and cartilage.

2.3. Synthesis of Type I and Type II collagen

The appropriate collagen is first synthesized in both osteoblasts and chondroblasts as a longer molecule, procollagen, that contains additional 'propeptides'. It is then secreted into the matrix for further processing and assembly of the fibrils into fibres.

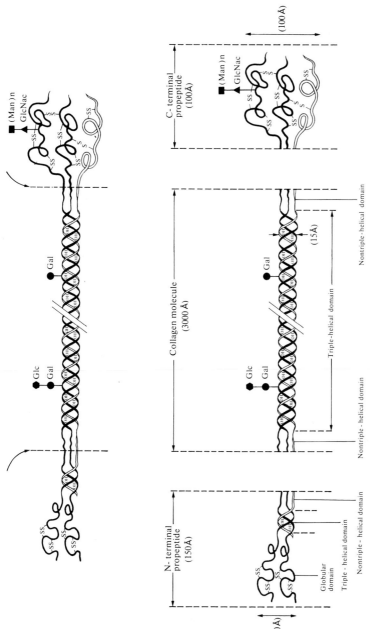

FIG. 3.2. Schematic representation of the structure of the procollagen molecule. Glc denotes glucose, Gal galactose, Man mannose, and GlcNac N-acetylglucosamine. (From Prockop et al. (1979) by courtesy of authors and publishers.)

(Man)n
GlcNac

Gal

Glc
Gal

N-terminal propeptide (150Å)

Globular domain

Triple - helical domain

Nontriple - helical domain

(20Å)

Collagen molecule (3000 Å)

Nontriple - helical domain

Triple-helical domain

(15Å)

Nontriple-helical domain

Gal

Glc
Gal

C-terminal propeptide (100Å)

(Man)n
GlcNac

(100 Å)

The known procollagens contain peptide extensions at both ends of their polypeptide chains (Fig. 3.2). These terminal propeptides are known as proα chains. In the case of Type 1 procollagen the two polypeptides are referred to as proα 1(1) and proα 2(1), or simply proα 2. The amino terminal propeptide of the proα 1(1) chain has a molecular weight of about 20 000 daltons and contains three different structural domains: a globular amino terminal domain, a central collagen-like domain, and another short globular domain. The carboxy terminal propeptides of both proα 1 and proα 2 chains have globular conformations without any collagen-like domains. The primary structure of the carboxy terminal propeptide of the proα 1 chain is different from that of the proα 2 chain. For further details of the chemistry of these terminal propeptides, and the different types of collagen, the paper of Prockop and his colleagues (1979) should be consulted.

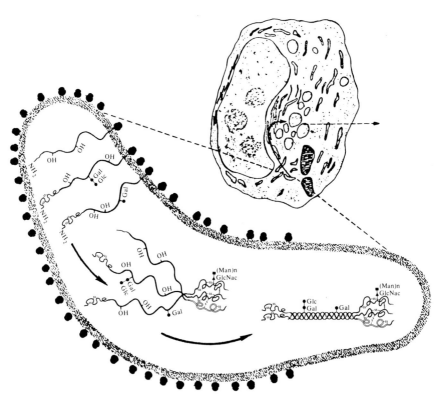

FIG. 3.3. Schematic representation of procollagen synthesis, post-translational processing and secretion by fibroblasts. Abbreviations are as in Fig. 3.2. As indicated, most of the processing occurs in the cisternae of the rough endoplasmic reticulum, but folding into the triple-helical conformation may occur at a later stage. The protein is secreted through the smooth vacuoles of the cell. The figure does not indicate synthesis and removal of 'pre' or 'signal' sequences. (From Prockop *et al.* (1979) by courtesy of authors and publishers.)

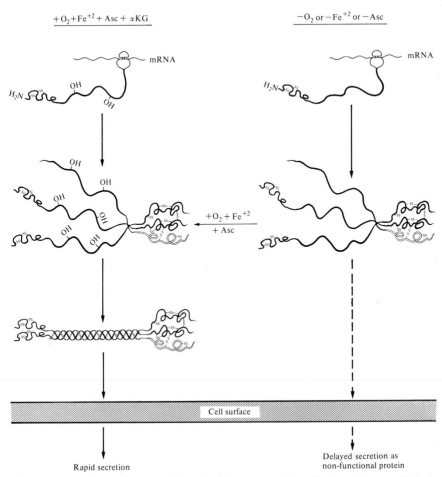

FIG. 3.4. Schematic representation of the role of the post-translational hydroxylations and helical conformation in the secretion of procollagen. In the presence of adequate oxygen (O_2), ferrous ions (Fe^{+2}), ascorbic acid (Asc) and α-ketoglutarate (αKG), proα chains of procollagen are hydroxylated, fold into the correct three-dimensional conformation and are rapidly secreted. If these cofactors for prolyl hydroxylase are not present in adequate concentrations, peptidyl prolyl residues are not hydroxylated to hydroxyprolyl residues. As a result the collagen domain cannot form a stable triple helix at 37 °C, and it is slowly secreted as a nonfunctional protein.
(From Prockop *et al.* (1979) by courtesy of authors and publisher.)

The propeptides account for about one-third of the procollagen molecule, but their function is still uncertain. It is suggested that they may (1) prevent premature fibril formation; (2) help to direct assembly of the protein into fibrils; (3) direct association of proα chains so that each molecule contains the correct three proα chains; (4) increase the rate and efficiency of folding the proα chains into a triple helical conformation; (5) or after they are cleaved from the molecule, they may function in a feedback mechanism to control the amount of procollagen synthesized by the cells. A schematic presentation of procollagen synthesis, post-translational processing and secretion by fibroblasts is shown in Fig. 3.3.

2.4. Intracellular processing of pro alpha chains

A great deal is now known about the intracellular processing of proα chains (Fig. 3.4). There is a separate m RNA for each proα chain. These chains are originally synthesized with additional 'pre' or 'signal' sequences at the amino terminal ends. These 'signal' sequences appear to direct movement of the polypeptides into the rough endoplasmic reticulum where the signal sequences are removed by a protease, or proteases. Three hydroxylases are also present, they require ferrous ions, molecular oxygen, and heto-glutarate and ascorbic acid as cofactors. They act on substrates according to unusual and specific requirements discussed in detail by Prockop and his colleagues (1979). The residue hydroxylated must be located in a peptide and must occupy the correct position in the amino acid sequence. The peptide must have a non-helical conformation. This requirement for a non-helical conformation is important. Addition of sugars to newly synthesized poly-peptides begins shortly after the N-terminal ends move into the cisternae of the rough endoplasmic reticulum and hydroxylysine is synthesized. The sugars in the propeptides of procollagen can be added when the proα chains are still non-helical. Another important step in the intracellular processing of the propeptides is the synthesis of both intrachain and interchain disul-phide bonds. The formation of interchain disulphide links in the propeptides is essential for folding into the triple helix. The helix does not form until after the proα chains are released from polysomes. Most helix formation occurs either in the rough endoplasmic reticulum or as the protein leaves the rough endoplasmic reticulum. It is possible that the helix does not form until the chains reach the Golgi complex. The rate of secretion of the procollagen depends on intracellular processing of the protein and specifically on folding of the collagen domain of proα chains into a triple helical conformation. Non-helical forms of procollagen are slowly secreted and tend to accumulate in the rough endoplasmic reticulum.

2.5. Extracellular processing

The conversion of procollagen to collagen, which takes place extracellularly, requires at least two enzymes, a procollagen aminoprotease that removes the amino propeptides, and a procollagen carboxyprotease that removes the carboxy propeptides. Collagen molecules produced by cleavage of procolla-gen spontaneously assemble into fibrils that are microscopically indistinguishable from the mature fibrils found in tissue. The immature fibrils, however, need to be cross linked by a series of covalent bonds, to acquire the necessary tensile strength. This is achieved by a variety of means. There is an intra-molecular crosslink that joins the α chains of the same molecule, formed by aldol condensation of two of the aldehydes, and there are a variety of cross links involving lysine (Prockop *et al.* 1979) and what has proved to be an extremely important lysyl hydroxylase, a copper-containing protein.

2.6. Collagen abnormalities

It is not surprising that errors in the complex biosynthesis of collagen should result both in genetic and other more transitory disorders.

2.6.1. GENETIC ABNORMALITIES

Only a brief mention is here made of some of the disorders of collagen biosynthesis that are recognized. It is probable that others will be found as increasing knowledge of the complex factors involved in the biosynthesis is applied to clinical problems.

2.6.1.1. *Ehlers–Danlos syndrome*

This is a generalized disorder of connective tissue. There is now a consider-able literature on the collagen defects in this condition (Prockop *et al.* 1979). In some patients there is a genetic defect in lysyl hydroxylase, the enzyme so important in the organization of cross-links. Others, with a different clinical picture, have a deficiency of Type III collagen dependent on a reduced rate of synthesis, and in yet others there is a genetic defect interfering with con-version of procollagen to collagen (Prockop *et al.* 1979).

2.6.1.2. *Osteogenesis imperfecta congenita*

This is a rare autosomal recessive skeletal disorder characterized by brittle bones. Other connective tissues are affected. It has been suggested by Müller and his colleagues (Müller, Raisch, and Matzen 1977) that Type III collagen as well as the usual Type I collagen is present in bone tissue. This has not been confirmed. All observers, however, find disturbances of cross-links. Trelstad, Rubin, and Gross (1977) describe a collagen unusually rich in hydroxylysine and glycosylated hydroxylysine and others a collagen with an increased ratio of immature, reducable cross-links to mature non-reducable cross-links (Fujii and Tanzer 1977).

2.6.1.3. *Marfan's syndrome*

This is a genetic disease affecting particularly the skeletal and cardiovascular systems. It has long been suspected that defective cross-linking of collagen is the basic lesion. This assumption is based largely on the observation that severe copper deficiency, or administration of nitriles such as β amino-propionitrile, to young growing animals produces deformities similar to Marfan's syndrome. Copper deficiency decreases lysyl oxidase activity *in vivo* because, as already described, the enzyme is a copper-requiring protein and the nitriles which produce 'lathyrism' in experimental animals also inhibit lysyl oxidase, both *in vivo* and *in vitro*, since they also chelate copper. Patients with the disease excrete an excess of hydroxyproline which might be due to defective cross-linkage and therefore excessive breakdown of collagen.

2.6.1.4. *Homocystinuria*

This is a metabolic disease inherited as an autosomal recessive. It is characterized clinically by widespread deformities and malfunction of connective tissue including severe osteoporosis. The basic defect is the deficient activity of an enzyme, cystathionine synthetase which results in the accumulation of homocysteine and other metabolites. High circulating levels of homocysteine are thought to interfere with the cross-linking of collagen (Kang and Trelstad 1973).

2.6.1.5. *Menkes' kinky-hair syndrome*

This syndrome is dependent on a genetic defect in copper absorption from the intestinal tract. Lack of copper necessary for the action of lysyl oxidase is thought also to be responsible for disturbances of collagen cross-links (Prockop *et al.* 1979).

2.6.2. TRANSITORY DISEASES

2.6.2.1. *Scurvy*

It was stated on p. 66 that ascorbate is required for the synthesis of hydroxy-proline by prolyl hydroxylase. Lack of the vitamin leads to the synthesis of proα chains that have a low hydroxyproline content and therefore cannot form a triple helix.

2.6.2.2. *Lathyrism*

This is a disease of the skeleton and connective tissues that occurs particularly in times of famine when people eat the seeds of a particular vetch. It is due to β APN (β-aminopropionitrile) which has been isolated from sweet-pea seeds. In addition its homologue aminoacetonitrile APN and a variety of unrelated chemicals may also give rise to lathyrism. They are thought to inhibit the enzymic formation of aldehyde cross-link precursors (Siegel, Pinnill, and Martin 1970).

2.6.2.3. *Heparin induced osteoporosis*

Patients on long-term treatment with heparin may develop osteoporosis (Griffiths *et al.* 1965). It has been suggested that this is due to the release of collagenase and therefore to destruction or disturbance of collagen (Sakamoto, Goldhaber, and Glimcher 1973). It should also be noted (see p. 75) that it has been suggested that maternal ingestion of anticoagulants during pregnancy may lead to foetal bone abnormalities (Hauschka and Reid 1978), due to interference with osteocalcin, a calcium-binding protein found in bone and related to the vitamin K-dependent blood coagulation factors (prothrombin, factors VII, IX, and X).

3. NON-COLLAGENOUS CONSTITUENTS OF MATRIX

The analysis of bone already discussed indicates that apart from mineral and collagen there is about 11 per cent of non-collagenous material present in mature cortical bone. This material though small in amount is extremely important, particularly in connection with the mechanism of calcification. Apart from lipids and peptides it is largely composed of carbohydrate protein complexes, many of them plasma proteins which become concentrated in bone matrix.

3.1. The carbohydrate protein complexes

The nomenclature of this group of substances is often confusing. They can be divided into two classes: (a) the protein–polysaccharides which are largely found in cartilage (Dorfman, Pei-Lee, Ho, Strom, Vertel, and Upholt 1977; Muir 1978) see p. 84, or proteoglycans; (b) the glycoproteins, which are largely found in bone matrix.

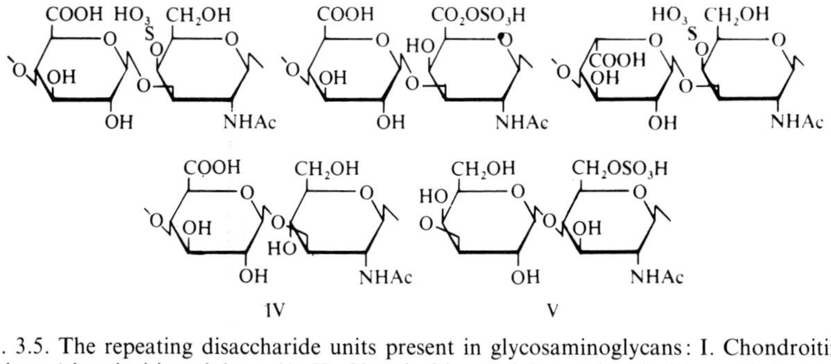

FIG. 3.5. The repeating disaccharide units present in glycosaminoglycans: I. Chondroitin 4-sulphate (chondroitin sulphate A). II. Chondroitin 6-sulphate (chondroitin sulphate C). III. Dermatan sulphate (chondroitin sulphate B). IV. Hyaluronic acid. V. Keratan sulphate. (From Herring (1968*b*), by courtesy of author and publishers.)

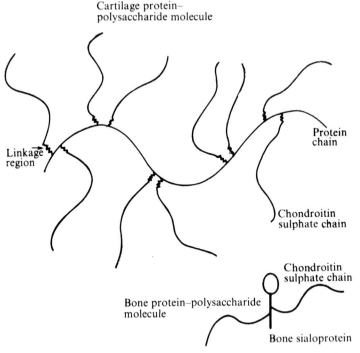

FIG. 3.6. Schematic representation of part of a protein–polysaccharide molecule and a possible structure for the bone protein-bound chondroitin sulphate fraction. (From Herring (1972) by courtesy of author and publishers.)

3.1.1. THE PROTEIN–POLYSACCHARIDES (OR PROTEOGLYCANS)

This group consists of a protein core or chain to which are attached a number of polysaccharide chains (the glycosaminoglycans). In Fig. 3.5 the repeating disaccharide units present in glycosaminoglycans are shown and in Fig. 3.6, a schematic representation of a protein–polysaccharide unit P, forming the core, to which are attached a number of polysaccharide chains.

3.1.2. GLYCOPROTEINS

Glycoproteins differ from protein–polysaccharides in the nature of the carbohydrate groups which (a) do not contain the regular repeating disaccharide group of the glycosaminoglycans; (b) usually contain a relatively small number of monosaccharide residues, and (c) have a wide variety of sugars including glucosamine, galactosamine, galactose, mannose, glucose, fucose, and sialic acid. These groups can be short, straight ones with only two or three residues in each or they can be larger, branching structures. The number of chains attached to the protein core can vary from one to as many as 800.

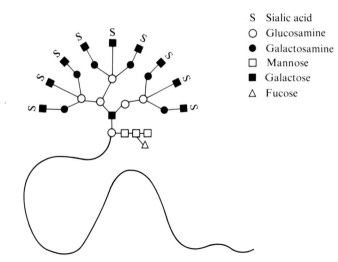

S   Sialic acid
O   Glucosamine
●   Galactosamine
□   Mannose
■   Galactose
△   Fucose

FIG. 3.7. Possible structure for the carbohydrate moiety of BSP. (From Herring (1972), by courtesy of author and publishers.)

In Fig. 3.7 is shown the possible structure for the carbohydrate moiety of bone sialoprotein (BSP), a glycoprotein to be discussed (see p. 71). To this sialoprotein it appears likely that, in bone, chondroitin sulphate may be attached giving a diagrammatic structure as shown in Fig. 3.6.

To illustrate the significance of this non-collagenous fraction of bone, some of the analytical data for bone at different stages of development are given in Table 3.5 (Herring 1972). A clear trend can be observed. Starting with osteoid or the most recently formed bone, there is a progressive decrease in the amount of non-collagenous constituents until mature and highly calcified bone is reached. There also appears to be a direct correlation between the amounts of non-collagenous material and sialic acid, which Herring (1972) suggested may be equated with the presence of glycoproteins.

A number of specific glycoproteins of bone matrix have now been isolated and further analysed. Of these, sialoprotein and osteocalcin appear to be synthesized by the osteoblasts, a large group of plasma proteins are concentrated in the matrix and there is a further, at present uncharacterized, group of glycoproteins. They clearly have many different functions in bone (Herring 1979). Some may have a role in collagen interactions, controlling fibril formation, as has been found in tendon (Anderson, Labedz, and Kewley 1977), and they are clearly associated with the complex processes involved in matrix calcification.

3.1.2.1. *Bone sialoprotein*

Bone sialoprotein, on the basis of present evidence, appears to be specific to bone (Herring 1968, 1976, 1979). Bone matrix contained more than 3 times as much sialic acid as tendon and the latter contained no bone sialoprotein (Herring 1976). Bone sialoprotein also differs in composition from serum orosomucoid. It does not resemble any of the plasma proteins. As yet no similar glycoprotein has been isolated from any tissue except dentine (Zamoscianyk and Veis 1966) from which a somewhat similar protein was recovered. It is perhaps significant that the dentine glycoprotein was also isolated from a highly mineralized tissue.

The molecular weight of bone sialoprotein is 23 000 (Andrews and Herring 1965). It has been calculated that the BSP content of bovine cortical bone matrix lies between 0·8 per cent and 1·15 per cent. There is considerable heterogeneity in the sialic acid content. This heterogenicity is greater in rabbit than in human or bovine bone (Herring 1969). It is at once obvious from the composition shown in Table 3.6 that the large number of carboxyl and sialic acid groups may account for its metal binding capacity. This metal binding capacity is illustrated in Table 3.7 where the binding of americium and plutonium, two surface seeking radionuclides, to certain matrix consti-

TABLE 3.6
The non-collagenous fractions of bone

Tissue	Percentage of total organic matrix				
	Coll†	MPS†	OP†‡	Rem†	SA†
Calf foetus:					
Primary spongiosa‡	71·2	2·6	11·8	14·4	0·65
Secondary spongiosa‡	72·6	1·6	12·8	13·0	0·48
Cancellous§	72·4	4	?	23·6	0·41
Diphyseal‡	96·3	1·7	7·1	−5·1	0·54
Calf:					
Primary spongiosa‡	75·8	1·9	10·6	11·7	0·41
Secondary spongiosa‡	79·5	1·1	6·6	12·8	0·35
Diaphyseal‡	79·2	0·8	4·7	15·3	0·25
Adult bovine diaphyseal‖	88	0·8	8	3·2	0·27
Calf diaphyseal osteones:					
Osteoid††	46·5	2·4	18·7	32·4	?
Partly calcified††	56·7	1·8	24·8	16·7	?
Highly calcified††	84·5	2·7	5·6	7·2	?
Bone in organ culture‡‡	28	2	50	20	?

† Key: Coll, collagen; MPS, mucopolysaccharide; OP, other protein (non-collagenous); Rem, remainder (material not accounted for; and SA, sialic acid.
‡ From Campo and Tourtellotte (1967).
§ From Wuthier (1969).
‖ Herring and Oldroyd (1968).
†† From Pugiarello *et al.* (1970).
‡‡ Fitton Jackson (1969).
    From Herring (1972) by courtesy of author and publishers.

TABLE 3.7

Composition of bone sialoprotein

Constituent	Bovine bone sialoprotein[†]		Rabbit bone sialoglycoprotein[‡] (% by weight)
	(% by weight)	(mole per mole of BSP)	
Sialic acid	20·5	15·3	5·8
Galactose	8·2	10·5	
Mannose	2·5	3·1	6·8
Fucose	0·7	1·0	1·0
Galactosamine	4·6	5·9	
Glucosamine	4·6	5·9	8·6
Phosphate	1·4	3·4	—
Protein	47·9	87·6	—

Amino acids	Bovine bone sialoprotein[†]		Rabbit bone sialoglycoprotein[‡] (% by weight of protein)
	(% by weight)	(mole per mole of BSP)	
Lysine	1·59	2·52	6·70
Histidine	0·74	1·07	5·93
Arginine	0·76	1·04	2·49
Aspartic acid	8·80	15·20	12·69
Threonine	5·02	9·70	4·57
Serine	3·20	7·00	4·15
Glutamic acid	12·80	20·09	22·95
Proline	2·15	4·27	6·94
Glycine	3·49	10·71	3·68
Alanine	1·36	3·51	6·46
Valine	1·38	2·71	6·29
Methionine			0·0
Isoleucine	1·25	2·19	2·91
Leucine	1·43	2·53	7·06
Tyrosine	1·54	1·95	2·75
Phenylalanine	0·72	1·00	3·56
Tryptophan	0·87	0·98	
Cysteic acid	0·81	1·10	0·83

† From Andrews *et al.* (1967).
‡ From Burckard *et al.* (1966).
From Herring (1972) by courtesy of author and publishers.

tuents is illustrated. Its capacity to bind yttrium and thorium was also shown by Williams and Peacocke (1967). In several ways BSP is an unusual glycoprotein, particularly in its high content of sialic acid, the presence of both glucosamine and galactosamine, and the large amounts of glutamic and aspartic acids. The possible structure of the carbohydrate moiety is shown in Fig. 3.7. The fact that this glycoprotein, peculiar to bone, is found as the protein core of 3 further acidic fractions, i.e. chondroitin sulphate, almost free of protein suggest that it may be playing some important role in the calcification process.

TABLE 3.8

Comparative binding of plutonium and americium to bone proteins and other macromolecules

	Molar protein : metal ratio	
	Plutonium 1:1	Americium 40:1
	(% of metal bound)‡	
Bovine γ-globulin	13·8 ± 5·1	0·7 ± 0·0
Human transferrin	18·9 ± 6·9	0·2 ± 0·0
Human albumin	1·2 ± 0·8	0·1 ± 0·1
Ovalbumin (chicken)	18·9 ± 2·7	0·5 ± 0·2
Bovine chymotrypsinogen A	1·7 ± 1·1	0·0
Sperm-whale myoglobin	1·6 ± 1·1	0·0
Bovine ribonuclease	0·5 ± 0·4	0·0
Cytochrome c (horse)	0·4 ± 0·2	0·0
Poly-L-Glu	68·7 ± 0·5	8·0 ± 3·0
Bone macromolecules§		
Sialoprotein	54·7 ± 9·3	10·4 ± 2·9
CP-S glycoprotein	36·6 ± 5·1	4·6 ± 2·9
Chondroitin sulphate protein	49·2 ± 3·0	14·9 ± 6·6
Protein-free chondroitin sulphate	13·2 ± 5·7	0·35 ± 0·3
Acidic glycoprotein fraction	30·0 ± 12·4	2·8 ± 0·9
Less acidic glycoprotein fraction	50·3 ± 9·1	5·1 ± 2·0
Soluble bone collagen	23·3 ± 4·3	0·6 ± 0·2

† Data from Chipperfield and Taylor (1968, 1970) and Chipperfield (unpublished results).
‡ Percentage recoveries of metal associated with protein following gel filtration. Means ± standard deviation or individual results.
§ A molecular weight of 25 000 is taken for all fractions.
  From Herring (1972) by courtesy of author and publishers (modified).

3.1.2.2. *Osteocalcin*

Osteocalcin is probably the fraction described by Ashton and his colleague as G2CF (Ashton, personal communication). It is also spoken of as bone Gla protein. It is a vitamin K dependent, calcium-binding protein, containing γ-carboxy glutamic acid. It is dependent on vitamin K for its synthesis. It has been isolated from chicken, bovine and sword fish bone. It differs from γ-CGLU containing plasma, and kidney calcium-binding proteins, by such criteria as molecular weight, amino acid composition, and primary sequence (Hauschka and Reid 1978). It has 4 γ-CGLU residues per 57 amino acid residues and binds 2 Ca^{2+} molecules per 6500 daltons. Barium and strontium do not compete significantly for the Ca^{2+} sites (Hauschka and Gallop 1977). Osteocalcin is about 20 per cent of total non-collagenous protein. It binds strongly to hydroxy apatite crystals, but less strongly to amorphous calcium phosphate (Price, Otsaka, and Posner 1977). It has been shown to be synthesized by embryonic chicken bones in culture and first appears exactly at the same time as histologically definable mineralization (Hauschka and Reid 1978). Lack of vitamin K reduces the amount of γ-CGLU by 30 per cent in three-week-old chicks. Its biosynthesis is warfarin-sensitive, and dicumarol decreases bone γ-CGLU by 80 per cent after 6 weeks (Hauschka, Lian, and Gallop 1975). It has been suggested that maternal ingestion of anticoagulants during pregnancy may lead to foetal bone abnormalities (Hauschka, Lian, and Gallop 1978). Osteocalcin is thought to be synthesized in bone — probably by the osteoblasts — rather than being synthesized elsewhere and transported to bone. A physiological role for this protein has yet to be established (Reddy and Suttie 1979) though it is suggested that it may serve as an inhibitor of calcium phosphate precipitation through its ability to interact with the hydroxy apatite crystal surface (Diamond and Neuman 1979). It has been described as strongly chemotactic for macrophages and may therefore play a part in bone resorption (see p. 50).

3.1.2.3. *Plasma proteins*

The spectrum of plasma proteins found in bone and dentine matrix is shown in Table 3.9 (Ashton, Höhling, and Triffitt 1976). They are present not only within the blood vessels and surrounding interstitium but also in bone fluid, and trapped within the calcified matrix (Lipp 1967; Owen and Triffitt 1972; Owen, Triffitt, and Melick 1973; Owen and Triffitt 1976; Ashton *et al.* 1976; Owen, Howlett, and Triffitt 1977). The two most important are albumin and α_2HS glycoprotein.

TABLE 3.9

Spectrum of plasma proteins present in human cortical bone and permanent dentine

	Amount of plasma protein present mg/100 g hard tissue	
	Bone	Dentin
Albumin	50 ± 8	33
α_1 antitrypsin	trace	2
α_1 antichymotrypsin	trace	trace
Transferrin	$5 \pm 1 \cdot 5$	3
α_2HS glycoprotein	25 ± 5	42
IgG	13 ± 4	5
Haptoglobin	trace	nd
Haemopoxin	trace	nd
Serum cholinesterase	trace	nd

From Ashton *et al.* (1976).
nd not detected.
Values represent mean $\pm$ SD of five samples of cortical bone and mean of two batches of dentin, each of which was prepared from teeth of 20 individuals.

3.1.2.3.1. *Albumin*. Albumin has been extracted separately from bone fluid and from calcified matrix and has in both cases been shown to be immunologically identical to serum albumin (Owen, *et al.* 1973). In calcified matrix it is probably permanently fixed, unlike that in soft tissues, and is not therefore available for exchange (Owen and Triffitt 1976). In young bone about 27 per cent of the albumin is in tissue fluid, about 57 per cent in calcified matrix, and about 16 per cent is intravascular. The total amount of extravascular albumin per unit mass of bone is similar to that in soft tissues (Owen and Triffitt 1976). The rate of clearance of the albumin from extravascular fluid in bone is approximately once every hour, while the amount incorporated into calcified matrix per day is calculated to be less than 0·5 per cent of the total albumin passing through the tissue fluid of bone every day (Owen and Triffitt 1976). It is of particular interest that in rabbits made vitamin D deficient, the retention of albumin was less than in healthy well-fed controls. When the passage of polyvinylpyrrolidone, a polymer of average molecular weight 35 000, though bone tissue fluid following injection was compared with that of albumin, it was found that none was retained (Owen *et al.* 1977). The retention and fixture of albumin in calcified matrix is attributed by Owen and her colleagues to the fact that albumin, like other highly charged proteins, adsorbs readily to hydroxy apatite (Triffitt and Owen 1977*b*), while PVP, a relatively neutral polymer, is not adsorbed nor incorporated into calcified matrix.

They consider the results from the vitamin-D-deficient rabbits support this view. The amount of albumin retained in calcified matrix in vitamin-D-deficient animals was much lower than in the controls, while extravascular albumin per gram of bone was approximately the same, so that entry of albumin into extravascular tissue does not appear to have been inhibited.

3.1.2.3.2. *$\alpha_2 HS$ glycoprotein*. α_2HS glycoprotein was first isolated from the major glycoprotein fraction prepared from an EDTA extract of bovine cortical bone in 1971 by Ashton and his colleagues (Ashton, Herring, Owen, and Triffitt 1971) and described as G2B glycoprotein. It was more fully characterized in 1974 (Ashton, Triffitt, and Herring 1974). It contained 78 per cent protein, 4 per cent sialic acid, 3 per cent hexosamine, and 14 per cent neutral sugars; it had an apparent molecular weight of approximately 50 000. It was found to be present also in bovine plasma, but to be highly concentrated in bone matrix. It was subsequently shown to be identical with a glycoprotein isolated from human and rabbit bone, the α_2HS glycoprotein (Ashton *et al.* 1976; Triffitt and Owen 1973). It is concentrated in human bone by factors varying from 30–100 times compared with plasma and this enrichment has been found in all species investigated. The enrichment of α_2HS glycoprotein in human bone and dentine is compared with other plasma proteins in Table 3.9. It is synthesized in the liver, but not by foetal rabbit calvaria in culture (Triffitt, Gebauer, Ashton, Owen, and Reynolds 1976). Levels of α_2HS glycoprotein and albumin in human foetal bone are at least an order of magnitude greater than those of adult cortical bone, even though plasma levels of the newborn are only 50 per cent and 10 per cent greater than in adults. Wilson and his colleagues have calculated, assuming the molecular weight of α_2HS glycoprotein is 49 000, that there would be one binding site for calcium per molecule (Wilson, Ashton, and Triffitt 1977).

α_2HS glycoprotein appears to be, in some way, at present not understood, associated with the process or mechanism of calcification in growing bone. The enrichment would appear to be a result of its preferential uptake from the bone tissue fluid by the developing mineral. α_2HS glycoprotein is concentrated, in comparison with serum albumin, in the mineral phase, following either the precipitation of apatite in serum samples or the addition of either apatite or amorphous calcium phosphate to serum (Wilson et al. 1977). Whereas the concentration of other non-collagenous material is lower in calcified, as compared with non-calcified material (Pugliarello, Vittur, and de Bernard 1970; Baylink, Wergedal, and Thompson 1972), the formation of calcium phosphate in vivo is accompanied by the accumulation of the specific plasma α_2HS glycoprotein from the tissue fluid (Triffitt, Owen, Ashton, and Wilson 1978). It is therefore suggested by Triffitt and his colleagues (Triffitt et al. 1978) that it may be associated with mineralization by forming calcium phosphate precipitates at sites of calcification by a process of adsorption. It has been suggested that it may in some way also be associated with resorption since it has been shown to be present by autoradiographic techniques on resorbing surfaces (Ashton, personal communication).

It is of interest that in Paget's disease, a condition in which both the formation and resorption of bone are elevated, the plasma α_2HS glycoprotein levels are decreased (Ashton et al. 1976). Other workers, using the fluorescein isothiocyanate-labelled-antibody to α_2HS protein, claim to have shown its localization in areas of mineralization in bone (Dickson, Poole, and Veis 1975). This observation awaits confirmation as does the observation of Van Oss, Gillman, Bronson, and Border (1974) that the glycoprotein has opsonic properties.

3.1.2.3.3. *Other uncharacterized glycoproteins found in bone.* There are other glycoproteins present in bone that are not yet characterized. Studies in which radioactively labelled glucosamine have been injected into the blood stream have shown that the radioactive material is found in two sites: first, in a position corresponding to the matrix synthesized immediately after injection (Triffitt and Owen 1973) and secondly on resorbing surfaces (Owen and Shetlar 1968).

It has been shown by appropriate techniques that there are several fractions in bone which can be labelled with radioactive glucosamine, one is in the more acidic fraction associated with sialoprotein and its fragments (Shetlar, Shurley, and Hern 1972), one is the α_2HS glycoprotein, a plasma protein already discussed (Triffitt and Owen 1973; Ashton, Höhling and Triffitt 1972), and there is a third, which is present in bone but not in plasma (Triffitt and Owen 1973). Owen and Triffitt (1972) have shown that this third fraction can be shown by autoradiographic techniques to be taken up in both osteoblasts and newly formed matrix and in osteoclasts and bone resorbing surfaces. In the latter the uptake of labelled material on the resorbing surface one hour after injection is concentrated at the junction of the bone surface and the osteoclast. In preparations where the osteoclast has been mechanically torn away from the surface the labelled material remains behind on the bone surface. The labelling of osteoclasts is always peripheral, no grains are seen over their interior. The cells and interstitial fluid of the extravascular soft-tissue layer, and the rest of the bone surface, which is not in contact with osteoclasts, is also labelled. This labelled material appears to be 'turned over' at this surface. By 2–3 days there is no label associated with the resorbing surface.

3.2. Peptides

The peptides in bone represent 0·55 per cent of the dried weight. They have been extensively analysed by Leaver and his colleagues (Leaver, Shuttleworth, and Triffitt 1965; Leaver and Shuttleworth 1966, 1968; Leaver, Triffitt, and Holbrook 1975). Some of them are probably collagen fragments attached to non-collagenous prolases, others may be what he describes as 'free and separate entities'. At least in human dentin he could find no evidence for a collagen-bound phosphoprotein (Leaver, Price and Smith 1975; Smith and Leaver 1978). Their function and importance in matrix is unknown.

3.3. Lipids

Lipids present in bone and calcifying cartilage are both intra- and extra-cellular. Though the amounts present are small, it is probable that they play

TABLE 3.10

Enrichment of $\alpha_2 HS$ glycoprotein in human bone and dentin

Tissue*	Concentration factor referred to different plasma proteins		
	Albumin	Transferrin	IgG
Bone	38	33	52
Dentin	97	98	220

From Ashton *et al.* (1976).

* Concentration factor $= \dfrac{[\alpha_2 HS] \text{ bone or dentin/[Reference protein] bone or dentin}}{[\alpha_2 HS \text{ serum}]/[\text{Reference protein}] \text{ serum}}$

Using values from Table 3.9 and taking serum concentrations of $\alpha_2 HS$-glycoprotein, albumin, transferrin, and IgG to be 60, 4400, 386, and 1500 mg/100 ml respectively.

TABLE 3.11

Distribution of lipid phosphorus among total phospholipids of calcifying tissues

	Cartilage				Bone	
	Resting	Proliferating	Hypertrophic	Calcified	Cancellous	Compact
	Percentage of total lipid P†					
(a) Neutral						
Sphingomyelin	6·3±0·4	5·0±0·6	5·9±0·7	6·0±1·2	10·8±0·8	9·1
Phosphatidyl choline	61·3±1·3	55·2±3·5	61·3±1·5	55·6±0·9	52·2±1·8	58·0
Lysophosphatidyl choline	2·5±1·1	1·3±1·0	0·8±0·5	2·0±0·3	3·4±0·4	1·3
Phosphatidyl ethanolamine	15·3±1·1	26·0±1·3	19·3±0·9	23·9±1·0	17·5±1·6	18·6
Lysophosphatidyl ethanolamine	4·0±1·0	2·6±1·8	1·5±0·8	0·6±0·3	1·1±0·6	1·3
Unidentified neutral phospholipids	0·0	0·0	0·0	0·0	0·2±0·0	0·0
Total neutral phospholipids	89·2±0·5	88·9±2·7	88·6±1·8	87·1±1·3	85·2±1·1	88·3
(b) Acidic						
Phosphatidyl serine	3·7±0·5	3·2±0·1	2·6±0·3	4·2±0·7	5·5±0·5	6·5
Lysophosphatidyl serine	0·0	0·0	0·4±0·3	0·3±0·1	1·0±0·2	0·3
Phosphatidyl inositol	4·1±0·4	4·0±0·5	2·6±0·4	3·2±1·0	3·0±0·8	1·1
Diphosphoinositide (tent.)	0·2±0·1	0·3±0·5	0·7±0·4	0·4±0·1	0·0	0·0
Phosphatidic acid	0·5±0·0	1·3±0·4	1·6±0·6	0·5±0·1	1·4±0·4	0·8
Diphosphatidyl glycerol	0·8±0·1	1·2±0·3	1·4±0·1	1·7±0·2	1·1±0·1	1·5
Phosphatidyl glycerol	0·4±0·3	0·4±0·2	0·3±0·2	0·7±0·1	0·7±0·2	0·4
'Chondrolipin'‡	0·1±0·0	0·4±0·2	1·2±0·3	1·0±0·1	0·5±0·2	0·0
Unidentified acidic phospholipids	0·9±0·3	0·8±0·5	0·6±0·2	1·0±0·7	1·6±0·6	1·2
Total acidic phospholipids	10·8±0·2	11·1±1·1	11·4±0·8	12·9±1·2	14·8±1·2	11·7
Number of samples	3	3	5	5	4	1

Each phospholipid includes both the diacyl and alkenyl-acyl forms. Percentage of the total lipid P was obtained by summation of P from each component on silica gel-loaded paper chromatograms, the recovery of total lipid P applied to chromatograms being 93·5–99·5 per cent. Values are means ± standard errors of means.

† Total lipid P is the summation of amounts from extracts 1, 2, and 3.
‡ This lipid may be a degraded form of phosphatidyl inositol.
From Herring (1972) by courtesy of author and publishers.

an important part in the mechanism of calcification (Irving 1965; Irving and Wuthier 1968; Posner 1978a), see p. 88.

Shapiro (1970, 1971) found that, of the total lipids released from bone, 65 per cent were removed prior to decalcification. Triglycerides comprised over 94 per cent of the pre-demineralized lipid extract: cholesterol esters were the predominant lipid of the post-demineralized extract. He postulates that a small proportion of the lipids, about 8 per cent, are probably bound to collagen by covalent forces.

The amount of lipid in dry cortical bone is small (1·14 per cent) (Herring 1977). Non-polar lipids, which are 2–5 times more abundant than polar lipids, consist mainly of triglycerides, free fatty acids, cholesterol, and cholesterol esters. The polar lipids include lecithin, sphingomyelin, phosphatidyl ethanolamine, serine ethanolamine, inositol ethanolamine, phosphatidic acid, and four unidentified lipids. The distribution of lipid phosphorus among total phospholipids of calcifying tissues is shown in Table 3.11 (Herring 1972).

The lipids concerned in calcification have been identified as calcium phospholipid phosphate complexes, the phospholipids being acidic phospholipids, principally phosphatidyl serine and phosphatidyl inositol (Posner 1978a). It is thought possible that they may be associated with a protein in the mineralizing region and loose the association in the extraction process. These complexes are richer in the more actively calcifying regions of bone and are absent from non-calcifying tissue in general. When extracted these complexes, which have a calcium to total phosphate molar ration of 1:1, can act as efficient nucleators of hydroxyapatite when dispersed in metastable calcium phosphate solutions. Their origin from matrix vesicles and the part they may play in calcification is discussed elsewhere, see p. 107.

4. Cartilage

IN the skeleton there is, throughout life, a close association between the two forms of connective tissue: bone and cartilage. However, cartilage is found in many sites where it is unassociated with bone and unlikely to calcify, as, for instance, in the trachea and larynx. Unfortunately, a prolific and easily obtainable source of cartilage is the nasal cartilage of large animals, and a great deal of work on the chemistry of cartilage is done on material that may not be of the same basic composition, nor behave in the same way, as that associated with bone. Certain general points about cartilage will first be discussed and then reference will be made in particular to epiphyseal cartilage and articular cartilage.

Cartilage tissue can grow both by apposition and by interstitial growth, while bone can grow only by apposition. Unlike bone, cartilage has no capillary blood supply and cartilage cells are nourished by dissolved substances diffusing through the wet jellied intercellular substance that surrounds them (Ham 1974). Most cartilage develops from mesodermal tissue but Hall (1978) describes Meckel's cartilage, part of the chondrocranium and visceral cartilage, as of neural crest origin. He classifies cartilage into four types.

1. TYPES OF CARTILAGE

1.1. Hyaline cartilage

Hyaline cartilage consists largely of proteoglycans held in a net of collagen fibres. It is characteristically found covering the articular surface of bones formed by endochondral ossification and epiphyseal growth. There are complex factors involved in the development of certain joint surfaces, particularly those of the mandible (Blackwood 1966) and the clavicle. These are discussed by Hall (1978).

1.2. Elastic cartilage

Elastic cartilage is characterized by the presence of elastic fibres in the extra-cellular matrix. This type is found for instance in the pinna, larynx, and epiglottis.

1.3. Fibrous cartilage

Fibrous cartilage has an increased collagenous fibre content in the matrix. It is found where ligaments and tendons are attached to bone, in intra-articular discs of joints and as articular cartilage at certain joint surfaces.

1.4. Intermediate tissue between bone and cartilage

Hall (1978) suggests that at certain sites, for instance in the development of the epiphyseal tubercle of the tibia by chondrogenic replacement of the pattelar ligament, a tissue intermediate between bone and cartilage is produced. He suggests that the growth of antlers is dependent on this type of tissue (see p. 91).

2. CARTILAGE CELLS

Three types of cartilage cell are often spoken of, the chondroblast, the chondrocyte and the chondroclast. Morphologically they are not well defined. The biology of cartilage cells has recently been discussed at length by Stockwell (1979).

2.1. Origin

In discussing endochondral ossification, the formation of a condensation of mesenchyme cells to form the early model of a long bone was described (p. 2). The cells in the centre became rounded and surrounded themselves with a matrix characteristic of mature cartilage, while the cells on the periphery developed the characteristics of osteoblasts and formed osteoid. It appears therefore that chondroblasts and osteoblasts share a common precursor. Dorfman and his colleagues (1977), and Von der Mark and Conrad (1979), have recently discussed in considerable detail the morphological, cytological, and particularly the biochemical events that occur during cartilage cell differentiation, with particular reference to collagen and proteoglycan synthesis. They indicate that at a very early stage in differentiation there are striking differences in both the collagen types and proteoglycans that are secreted by osteoblasts and chondroblasts, but that on the other hand in tissue culture the cartilage cell type is not necessarily stable. Collagen secreted by chondroblasts is Type II, that secreted by osteoblasts is Type I, and at a very early stage in embryonic development cartilage cells secrete Type II collagen. However, in tissue culture, a reversion to Type II collagen synthesis in sub-cultures of chondrocytes which had already changed to Type I synthesis under the influence of whole embryo extract, has been reported. If such 'gene switching' occurs as readily *in vivo* as it does *in vitro* it may be an important phenomenon in acquired diseases of connective tissue (Prockop *et al.* 1979). Hall (1978) suggests that the factor that determines whether the osteoprogenitor cell, which has both osteogenic and chondrogenic potential, develops as a chondroblast, is mechanical. For instance compression may result in changes in cyclic AMP. Ham and Cormack (1979) on the other hand, while recognizing a common progenitor cell, think that the microenvironment will determine whether differentiation leads to an osteoblast or a chondroblast. If there is a plentiful oxygen supply, owing to the presence of capillaries, the cell will become an osteoblast; if the microenvironment is avascular, cartilage forming cells will develop.

2.2. The chondrocyte

The chondrocyte, the characteristic cell of cartilage tissue, is easily recognized histologically. It occurs as scattered cells lying in lacunae with basophylic matrix. According to Stockwell (1978) the chondrocyte has many typical features, but nevertheless the cell type is difficult to define in structural terms. Identification, in practice, often depends on recognizing its synthetic and secretory products. Typical chondrocytes are ovoid cells ranging in maximum diameter from 10 μm in articular cartilage to about 30 μm in other hyaline cartilage. The cell has a scalloped surface and occasional cell processes that may reach beyond the lacunae are seen. The predominant cytoplasmic organelles are the granular endoplasmic reticulum and the Golgi apparatus. Mitochondria are common in young cells but rarer in old cells. Glycogen and lipid are common inclusions. The cell is embedded in a metachromatically staining extracellular matrix. It is unique in its ability to synthesize greater amounts of chondroitin sulfate proteoglycans and collagen than almost any other cell type, and also because these distinct gene products each have structures which make them unique from the collagens and proteoglycans made in small amounts by other tissues (von der Mark and Conrad 1979).

2.3. The chondroclast

Thyberg and his colleagues (Thyberg and Friberg 1972; Thyberg 1975; Thyberg, Nilsson, and Friberg 1975) in an analysis of cellular events in the uppermost part of the primary spongiosa of the metaphysis, differentiate between osteoclasts and chondroclasts on the basis of the location of the cells, i.e. whether associated with mineralized bone or mineralized cartilage. The so-called chondroclasts are distinguished by the abundance of lysosomes containing acid phosphatase and aryl sulphatase. In many cases they have a characteristic ruffled border. These cells are actively phagocytic of injected colloidal thorium dioxide, which suggests that, like the osteoclast, they may be of macrophage origin rather than derived from a cartilage-forming cell.

3. CARTILAGE MATRIX

Cartilage matrix, consists of proteoglycans and collagen but, while collagen represents about 89 per cent of diaphyseal bone matrix dry weight, it is only 56 per cent of the epiphyseal cartilage dry weight. The total non-collagenous material in bovine diaphyseal bone is 11·5 per cent and in cartilage it is 54 per cent, the great part being proteoglycan, rich in chondroitin sulphate (Rosenberg 1973). The chemistry of cartilage matrix in the epiphysis changes depending on the level at which the sample is taken. These changes are illustrated in Table 3.1 (p. 57). The amino-acid analysis of articular and epiphyseal cartilage is given by Campo and Tourtellotte (1967).

3.1. Collagen

The collagen of cartilage is known as Type II collagen $(\alpha2(II))_3$. It has three $\alpha1$ chains, which differ from $\alpha1$ chains found in collagens of other tissues, (Miller 1976). Among mesenchymal tissues, cartilage is the only one which contains and synthesizes Type II collagen *in vivo* and *in vitro*, though some epithelial tissues have been found to do so (Von der Mark and Conrad 1979). The fibrous components of cartilage are in general small (10–20 nm in diameter) and often fail to exhibit a well-defined cross-striation pattern characteristic of native collagen fibres in other tissues. Miller (1976) suggests that this collagen has evolved for the purpose of providing a fine network of small fibres, allowing maximum dispersion of the fibres throughout the proteoglycan components of the tissue. This arrangement would account for the remarkable mechanical properties of load-bearing cartilages.

3.2. Proteoglycans of cartilage

The proteoglycans of cartilage have recently been reviewed by Muir (1978). This review does not discriminate between epiphyseal and articular cartilage, but is based largely on work with articular or nasal cartilage. As Muir says 'Proteoglycans are found throughout connective tissue but those of cartilage have certain features that distinguish them from proteoglycans of other connective tissue. Proteoglycans exert a swelling pressure that is constantly restrained by the collagen in which they are entrapped.' In cartilage as many as 50–100 chondroitin sulphate chains are attached laterally to a protein backbone that comprises about 10–15 per cent of the weight of the molecule. In addition, fewer but variable numbers of keratin sulphate chains are attached to the same core protein. In any given cartilage, proteoglycans are heterogeneous and exhibit a range of chemical composition and molecular size. All sulphated glycosaminoglycans, with the exception of keratin sulphate, are attached to protein via a trisaccharide sequence of neutral sugars, in which xylose is glycosidically attached to the hydroxyl group of serine residues on the protein core. A unique feature of cartilage proteoglycans is their ability to form multimolecular aggregates of very high molecular weight, of the order of 50 millions. This aggregation depends on a highly specific interaction of proteoglycans with hyaluronic acid (Hardingham and Muir 1972). This interaction with hyaluronate appears to be unique to cartilage proteoglycans and is entirely specific to hyaluronate. The interaction with hyaluronate leads to a large increase in viscosity and hydrodynamic size. A single chain of hyaluronate can bind as much as 250 times its weight of proteoglycan. The effective binding site is of limited size, and of precise shape, enabling the maximum number of subsite interactions to take place in a small area of the molecule. Proteoglycans that interact with hyaluronate form a series in which the hyaluronate binding region is present in molecules of all sizes.

Muir (1978) states that the biological function of proteoglycan aggregation is unknown, but as it is apparently restricted to the proteoglycans of cartilage its role is presumably peculiar to the function of cartilage. She suggests, firstly, that the size of the aggregates immobilizes them very effectively in the collagen network: secondly that aggregates may be less compressible than monomers and may therefore make a greater contribution to the compressive stiffness of cartilage; thirdly since aggregates are more resistant to attack by proteinases than monomers, they may be catabolized more slowly; fourthly they may also indirectly play some part in regulating proteoglycan synthesis by chondrocytes, since free hyaluronic acid, but not that bound up in aggregates, inhibits proteoglycan synthesis (Wiebkin, Hardingham, and Muir 1975).

4. EPIPHYSEAL CARTILAGE AND ITS RELATION TO CALCIFICATION

The growth in length of the long bones is dependent upon the proliferation and subsequent calcification of the epiphyseal cartilage (Kember 1960; Sissons 1971).

The mechanisms involved in the calcification process are extremely complex, and, in spite of extensive investigation, still confused. Some of the observed facts will be described, but no entirely satisfactory account can yet be given. The problems are also discussed in Chapter 5. A photomicrograph of a longitudinal section of an epiphyseal plate is shown in Fig. 4.1. The reserve, or resting zone, consists of a narrow band of rounded chondrocytes widely separated by matrix. These cells take up little, if any, tritiated thymidine. In the next, or proliferating zone, the cells appear flattened and are arranged in longitudinal columns separated by both longitudinal matrix septa and narrower transverse septa. They take up much tritiated thymidine. In the next, or hypertrophic zone of maturing cartilage, the chondrocytes become progressively hydrated and together with their lacunae greatly

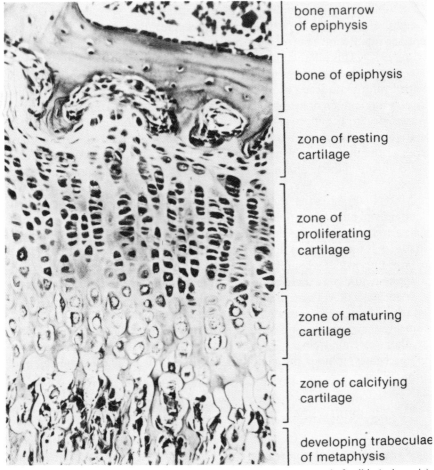

bone marrow
of epiphysis

bone of epiphysis

zone of resting
cartilage

zone of
proliferating
cartilage

zone of maturing
cartilage

zone of calcifying
cartilage

developing trabeculae
of metaphysis

FIG. 4.1. Photomicrograph of the epiphyseal plate (disc) at the upper end of a tibia (guinea pig) showing various zones of cartilage in the plate. (From Ham and Cormack (1979) by courtesy of authors and publishers.)

enlarged, and in the final zone the chondrocytes disintegrate while the longitudinal septa become calcified. Up into this zone press the invading vessels, stroma and cells of the encroaching diaphyseal marrow, forming what is known as the primary spongiosa. Some osteoid is laid down at first round calcified remnants of cartilage matrix by osteoblasts in the invading stroma and subsequently osteoid, free of cartilage, which is rapidly calcified, is formed. At the same time the osteoclasts present in the invading marrow are active. This combined activity of osteoblasts and osteoclasts leads to extensive remodelling and formation of the secondary spongiosa of the metaphysis

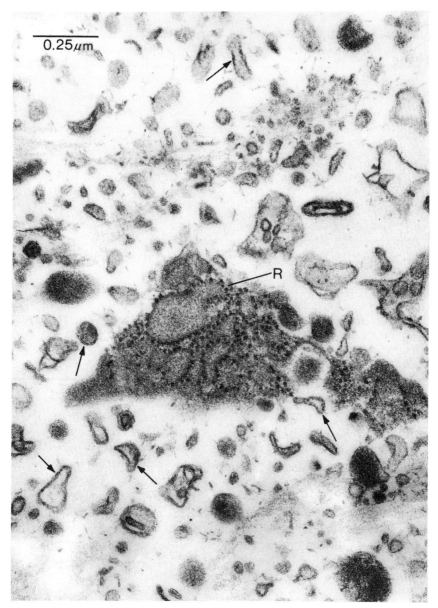

FIG. 4.2. Matrix vesicles upper hypertrophic zone. Ribosomes (R) are evident within a large cytoplasmic fragment. Several vesicles contain internal vacuole-like structures. Arrows indicate sectioned vesicles with typical three layers unit membranes. (From Anderson (1969) by courtesy of authors and publishers.)

(Sissons 1971). The cellular changes in the chondrocytes in the length of the plate are accompanied by complex chemical changes in the matrix, particularly in the hypertrophic zone associated with the process of calcification (Williamson and Vaughan 1967; Serafini-Fracassini and Smith 1974). These chemical changes, due to breakdown of the proteoglycans of the chondrocyte matrix, result in an appreciable increase in free anionic sites available to bind calcium in the region of the hypertrophic cartilage cells, where calcification begins in the longitudinal septa. In Chapter 6 where the mechanism of calcification is discussed in detail, the important part played by matrix vesicles in the calcification process is emphasized (see p. 107). Such vesicles, indeed, were first described in the epiphyseal plate (Anderson 1969; Bernard and Pease 1969; Bonucci 1971). An electron micrograph at high magnification of such vesicles in the cartilage plate is shown in Fig. 4.2. They are present in small numbers in the reserve zone, but become increasingly abundant in the proliferative and hypertrophic zones. In cartilage, as in the case of bone, they are thought to bud-off in some way from the membranes of the chondrocytes into the matrix. The vesicular membrane is enriched in phospholipids, probably the calcium phospholipid phosphate complex ($Ca-PL-PO_4$) described by Boskey and his colleagues (Boskey, Goldberg, and Posner 1978; Boskey 1978) which is capable of initiating hydroxyapatite formation. They also contain alkaline phosphatase, pyrophosphatases and ATPase (Anderson 1978; Bernard 1978). Any ionic calcium liberated from vesicles will readily be bound by the free anionic sites made available by the breakdown of the proteoglycans already described.

As long ago as 1964 Hjertquist (1964a,b) demonstrated the presence of free ionic calcium in the different regions of the epiphyseal plate. He found 1·5 per cent on a dry weight basis in the non-calcified areas, compared with 10 per cent in the zone of provisional calcification. Inhibitors of calcification are also present in the hypertrophic cell regions. Howell and his colleagues (Howell, Pita, Marquez, and Gatter 1969; Howell 1971; Howell and Pita 1976) by micropuncture techniques have obtained extracellular fluid from the distal hypertrophic cell zone of rat tibial cartilage. This fluid they say is distinctive for calcifying sites in several respects including the presence of an alkaline pH, an acid resistant nucleational factor for calcium phosphate mineral formation and an inhibitor of calcification. As Howell himself concludes 'No final comprehensive hypothesis of the chain of events involved in the inhibition of calcification can be constructed at the present time.'

5. ARTICULAR CARTILAGE

The type of tissue which forms the articular surface at a synovial joint appears to depend on the mode of development of the bone on which it lies. The surface tissue is hyaline cartilage in bones formed exclusively by endochondral ossification, whereas ossification in membrane, or in precartilage, results in an articular surface formed predominantly by dense white fibrous tissue or fibrous cartilage (Serafini-Fracassini and Smith 1974).

5.1. Hyaline articular cartilage

5.1.1. THE CELLS

In adult life, articular cartilage is dependent on appositional rather than interstitial cell proliferation. Mitotic rates in articular cartilage are only one-twentieth of those in the growth plate during development. No thymidine labelling can be detected in the normal adult. Cell proliferation is, however, resumed if tissue damage occurs or if cells freed from their matrix are grown in culture (Stockwell 1978, 1979).

Cellularity in human cartilage is reduced sevenfold during maturation from birth to adult life. This is largely due to the secretion and interposition of new matrix between cells. Cell distribution is not uniform within the adult tissue. At a microscopically local level cells lie either singly or in groups, while decreasing gradients of cell density are observed from the tissue periphery to its centre. The maximum cell density found in the superficial zone of articular cartilage must be attributed to proximity to synovial fluid and its contents. Overall cell density varies enormously between different species. Femoral condylar cartilage shows a 25-fold difference between small species (mice), which have a very cellular cartilage, and man. A similar range of cellularity is found between small and large joints of a single larger species. Hence a scale is involved: the overall cellularity of the tissue is inversely related to a common factor, cartilage thickness. It follows, therefore, that the total number of chondrocytes nourished by diffusion from a unit area of tissue boundary (for example the synovial fluid bathing the articular surface) is of the same order in all cartilages and that the degree of separation of cells, is probably due to other, mechanical, factors (Stockwell 1978).

5.1.2. THE MATRIX

Something has already been said (p. 84) of the chemistry of cartilage matrix. The water content of articular cartilage decreases with age from a value of 80–90 per cent in the foetus to about 70 per cent in an adult. Collagen on the other hand increases with age. In cattle, collagen forms 37 per cent of dry weight in the foetus, 58 per cent in the calf, and 67 per cent at 2 years of age (Campo and Tourtellotte 1967). In man there is no significant increase after the age of ten. The concentration of collagen is maximum close to the gliding surface where it forms a high percentage of the dry weight (Muir, Bullough, and Maroudas 1970). Earlier workers tended to regard the collagen fibrils of cartilage solely as tensile elements in a mechanical system designed to resist compressive forces which influenced their interpretation of fibril orientation (Serafini-Fracassini and Smith 1974). It is more likely that the collagen forms a sort of net to contain and anchor the proteoglycans (Muir 1978). Proteoglycans are closely bound to the collagen fibrils (Prockop *et al.* 1979). The glycosaminoglycans tend to be smaller in amount in articular than in other hyaline cartilage (Peters and Smillie 1971). They may be as low as 3 per cent of dry weight in the superficial layers while progressively increasing towards the bone-cartilage function. The proportions of the individual glycosamine glycans as a whole vary with age. The concentration of chondroitin 6-sulphate remains fairly constant, that of keratin sulphate increases, while that of chondroitin 4 sulphate falls (Serafini-Fracassini and Smith 1974). There are also regional differences.

5.1.3. NUTRITION

Articular cartilage acquires its nutritive material and discharges its metabolites by exchange with synovial fluid. Serafini-Francassini and Smith (1974) quote some evidence which suggests that blood vessels of adjacent bone marrow may play a part, but this is not generally accepted. Maroudas (1970) has shown that though small molecules diffuse readily through the tissue, with diffusion coefficients of about 40 per cent of those in aqueous solutions, large molecules are restricted, their diffusion coefficients being inversely related to their molecular size. This dependence on the molecular size of the solute is largely an expression of the excluded volume effect exercised by the glycosaminoglycans of the tissue. It has been claimed that it is possible to isolate from cartilage a low molecular weight cationic trypsin inhibitor which prevents the invasion of cartilage by endothelial cells, so accounting for its lack of capillaries (Sorgente, Kuettner, Soble, and Eisenstein 1975).

5.2. Fibrous articular cartilage

Fibrous articular cartilage has been studied particularly in the mandibular joint.

In this material the region adjacent to the bone is occupied by a layer of hyaline cartilage in which the cells are similar to the hypertrophic and degenerative cells of the radial zone of hyaline articular cartilage.

The regularly arranged collagen fibrils in the superficial part of a fibrous articular surface appear to be orientated in those planes which would be subject to maximal tensile stresses during compression of the surface, so differing from the random orientation of collagen fibrils in hyaline articular cartilage.

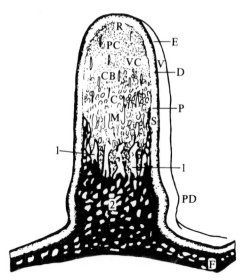

FIG. 4.3. An idealized drawing of a growing antler. The longitudinal relationships are closely approximated, while the lateral relationships are expanded for clarity. Although the relationship of a young, growing main beam is indicated, the distal (above the pedicle) longitudinal relationships apply to all growing tips. V velvet; E epidermis; D dermis; VC vascular channels; P periosteum; R reserve mesenchyme; PC prechondroblastic zone; CB chondroblastic zone; C chondrocytic zone; M mineralized cartilage; S sleeve bone; 1 primary spongiosa; 2 secondary spongiosa; PD pedicle; F frontal bone. (From Banks (1974) by courtesy of author and publishers.)

6. TISSUE INTERMEDIATE BETWEEN BONE AND CARTILAGE

The explosive and complex growth that results in the antlers of various ungulates under the influence of testosterone (see p. 178) was described in the white tailed deer by Banks in 1974. Mesenchymal tissue appears to differentiate as a cartilaginous supportive tissue that is finally replaced by osseous tissue. Chondroclasia and osteoclasia are responsible for remodelling and removal of mineralized cartilage and woven bone, which is replaced by lamellar, cancellous and compact bone. The elongation of the antler is achieved through a modified form of endochondral ossification, while the thickening is achieved through intramembranous mechanisms. This complicated process is illustrated in Fig. 4.3. Banks concludes that 'though there are differences between the architecture of the antler and typical somatic structures, the basic mechanism of endochondral and intramembranous ossification is similar' (see Fig. 4.3).

5. Chemistry of Bone Mineral

BONE is distinguished from other connective tissues by the fact that in its normal healthy state it is calcified. The basic matrix is impregnated by calcium apatite crystals or amorphous calcium phosphate.

1. CHEMICAL CHARACTER

The principal chemical constituents of bone mineral are calcium phosphate and carbonate, with lesser quantities of sodium, magnesium, and fluoride. They are present as a mixture of hydroxyapatite crystals and amorphous calcium phosphate (Eanes and Posner 1970).

1.1. Hydroxyapatite crystal

The whole hydroxyapatite crystal, regardless of size, can be generated, at least conceptually, by translationally periodic repetitions of a basic structural pattern of the constituent ions known as the unit cell. The unit cell for hydroxyapatite is a right rhombic prism which when stacked in the manner just described forms a simple hexagonal lattice. The atomic contents of the unit cell are given by the formula $Ca_{10}(PO_4)_6(OH)_2$. For further discussion of the chemistry and structure of hydroxyapatite as found in bone the reviews by Eanes and Posner (1967, 1970), and Posner (1978a) should be consulted.

Direct visual observations of bone apatite crystals with the use of the electron microscope have not been in complete agreement with the X-ray diffraction findings. The two prevalent viewpoints consider bone crystals to be either needle-like or, in contrast, plate-like. 'Bone crystals never grow in average largest diameter above 400–500 Å, while the two other dimensions are in the range of 200–300 Å and 25–50 Å respectively' (Posner 1978a). The size of the crystals appears to increase with age (Menczel, Posner, and Harper 1965). The initial growth of apatite crystals is rapid, occurring in a matter of minutes or less (Eanes and Posner 1965). The division of the bone mineral into submicroscopic particles results in a very large interfacial content between the mineral and the rest of the osseous tissue. A layer of water, termed the hydration shell, is thought to be bound to the surface of the crystals and through it ions are transferred to and from crystal surfaces (Neuman and Neuman 1958; McCarty, Hogan, Gatter, and Grossman 1966). There are

TABLE 5.1

Summary of present evidence concerning participation of ions in hydroxy-apatite solution interaction

Ion	Hydration shell		Crystal surface	Crystal interior	Ion displaced
	Water only	Bound-ion layer			
K^+	+	—	—	—	—
Na^+	+	—	+	—	
Mg^{2+}	+	+ ?	— ?		
UO_2^{2+}	+	+	— ?	—	Ca^{2+}
Sr^{2+}	+	+	+	+	
Ra^{2+}	+	+	+	+	
Ca^{2+}	+	+	+	+	
Cl^-	+	—	—	—	—
$Citrate^{3-}$	+	+ ?	— ?	—	
CO_3^{2-}	+	+	+	—	PO_4^3
PO_4^{3-}	+	+	+	+	
F^-	+	— ?	+	+	OH

From Neuman and Neuman (1958) by courtesy of author and publisher.

thus three zones in the crystals—crystal interior, crystal surface, and the hydration shell—all of which present surfaces available for the exchange of ions. Exchange in the interior of the crystal is probably slow, but that on the surface or in the hydration shell can be rapid. In Table 5.1 is a summary of what in 1958 Neuman and Neuman considered was the position of different ions in hydroxyapatite. They presume that any ion in solution can, and will, penetrate the hydration shell, but that only specific ions tend to congregate there. A greater and different specificity is required of ions penetrating the surface, and of these only a few are sufficiently similar to normal lattice ions to enter the crystal interior. The area of this surface may be as large as 180 m^2 g^{-1} (Eanes and Posner 1967) or 440 000–550 000 m^2 *in toto* (Howell 1971). Rowland (1966) concluded from autoradiography that only about 0·65 per cent of the bone calcium in humans is part of an exchangeable pool, whereas *in vitro* studies on bone mineral indicated that 27 per cent of the calcium is potentially exchangeable (Neuman and Neuman 1958). The question of the movement of calcium ions in or out of the skeleton is discussed in Chapter 8. Studies of surface bonding in apatite crystals suggests to Posner that a chemical linkage probably exists between the mineral in bone and certain free polar groups of collagen, thus contributing to the resistance of the skeleton to traumatic mechanical damage, but not associated with calcification mechanisms (Posner 1978a).

Traces of iron, copper, lead, manganese, tin, aluminium, strontium, and boron have been detected in bone (Eastoe 1961). There is considerable variability in the composition of the hydroxy-apatite itself. Woodard (1962) found that the Ca/P molar ratio ranged from 1.37 to 1.71. The ratio was age-dependent, with the lowest values being obtained for the bones of children and the elderly. It is known that sodium, strontium, and lead can be substituted in the calcium positions of apatite. Fluoride and chloride can chemically substitute for hydroxyl ion, though the replacements are not strictly isomorphous (Young and Elliott 1966). Ions such as potassium, which cannot be accommodated by the apatite lattice are probably adsorbed on its surface (Eanes and Posner 1970). The structural role of the carbonate has been a matter of controversy. It is the third-most-abundant ion in bone mineral and constitutes about 5 per cent of the total weight of ashed bone (Eastoe 1961). Eanes and Posner (1970) assume that most of the *in vivo* carbonate is adsorbed on the surface of the mineral. In fact many workers consider that the readily exchangeable surface carbonate in bone apatite may be needed to help maintain a constant serum pH, in conditions such as, acidosis. There are considerable difficulties in determining the underlying structural basis for the observed chemical stoichiometry of bone mineral involving the two major constituents, calcium and phosphorus. These are discussed in detail by Eanes and Posner (1970). Bone mineral apatite is not an equilibrium phase and is slowly perfecting itself chemically and in crystal size. It is this lack of perfection resulting from crystalline imperfections due to: (a) the presence of carbonate, sodium, and other ions, and (b) the deficiency in Ca and OH which combine to make bone mineral metabolically active (Posner 1978a). The most distinguishing features of bone apatite are a small crystal size, lack of chemical perfection and internal crystalline disorder. All these qualities satisfy the teleological need of a bone mineral which is insoluble enough for stability, yet is reactive enough to allow for normal resorption needs (Posner 1978a).

1.2. Amorphous calcium phosphate

As a result of electron microscope studies, Robinson and Watson (1955) reported the appearance of an amorphous 'haze' in areas immediately preceding the 'calcification front' and concluded that much of the inorganic component of infant bone may be non-crystalline. Hancox and Boothroyd (1966) later described granular material obscuring the fibrils of the preosseous matrix of embryonic fowl skull bone which they thought might represent bone mineral deposits. Subsequent X-ray defraction studies (Harper and Posner 1966; Termine and Posner 1967) indicated that this amorphous phase is a major component of bone mineral.

Posner and his colleagues find the amorphous phase distributed throughout the bone (Harper and Posner 1966). Approximately 40 per cent of the mineral in the femurs of adult human, cow, and rat is non-crystalline. The amorphous phase, however, does decline with age.

The spatial organization of the ions comprising the amorphous material is unknown. The amorphous calcium phosphates, like the synthetic apatites, do not have a rigidly defined chemical composition. The molar Ca/PO_4 ratios are found to vary from 1·44 to 1·55 depending on the conditions of preparation. Converted apatite, however, invariably had a higher molar Ca/PO_4 ratio than its amorphous precursor.

The rate of conversion of the amorphous into the crystalline form is controlled by the apatite product and not by the amorphous precursor. In synthetic systems this conversion rate has proved to be strictly proportional to the number of apatite crystals already formed and not to the amount of amorphous material remaining. The relation of amorphous calcium phosphate to the formation of calcium apatite crystals is discussed in detail by Eanes and his colleagues (Eanes and Posner 1970; Eanes, Termine, and Nylen 1973). They consider that, once formed, the amorphous salt becomes the controlling source of ions for the precipitation of apatite crystals.

A number of chemical species can stabilize ACP or prevent its conversion to hydroxy apatite, among them pyrophosphate, diphosphonates, adenosine triphosphate, ATP, and Mg. There is a synergistic effect on amorphous calcium phosphate when ATP and Mg are present together.

Most electron microscope studies suggest that in the process of mineralization the calcification front is probably characterized by the presence of amorphous calcium phosphate and that the apatite crystals arise later in bone as it becomes more mature (Posner 1978a). The presence of fully formed apatite crystals, which has been described by Anderson (1973) in the calcified vesicles of young bone, is probably due to an artefact induced by preparation of the material. The vesicles contain amorphous calcium phosphate but transformation into apatite is prevented by the presence of Mg and pyrophosphate (see p. 106).

1.3. Changes induced by chronic renal disease

It is of some interest that changes in the character of bone mineral have been described in chronic renal disease. X-ray diffraction analyses of bone from chronically uraemic non-acidotic rats with normal blood calcium levels and hyperphosphataemia showed smaller apatite crystals and in increase in amorphous calcium apatite compared to controls (Russell, Termine, and Avioli 1973).

2. INORGANIC CONSTITUENTS OTHER THAN HYDROXYAPATITE AND AMORPHOUS CALCIUM PHOSPHATE

A variety of elements other than the classical constituents of hydroxyapatite are found in bone. Some of the cations can substitute for calcium in the crystal lattice; others are only adsorbed on the surface of the crystal or in the hydration shell. It is not surprising that the alkaline earths, radium, strontium, and barium can replace calcium. It is not altogether clear why lead can do this. Sodium is also thought to be able to replace calcium, but potassium cannot.

2.1. Fluoride

Fluoride may be a normal constituent of the apatite crystal of bone, depending on the amount present either naturally or by artificial addition to the water supply (Posner, Eaves, Harper, and Zipkin 1963).

Fluoride is readily absorbed from the gastrointestinal tract. It may also reach the body by inhalation (Faccini 1969). Its distribution in the skeleton is similar to that of calcium since fluoride may replace OH^- in the calcium apatite lattice as a contaminant and is one of the most avid of the bone-seeking elements. It is thought to be incorporated by exchange with OH^- in the surface layers of existing crystals, and by incorporation in place of OH^- in the lattice of new crystals. F^- and OH^- are almost exactly the same size and have the same charge. When F^- intake is low the bone mineral is said to convert the apatite to fluorhydroxyapatite and so protects the body fluid and cells against the toxic effect of high concentration. The fluorhydroxyapatite crystals have been described as of larger size than calcium apatite crystals (Posner 1978a). It has been suggested that as the rate of reaction between a crystal solid and a solution is inversely proportional to the size of the crystal, the larger crystal size of the bone apatite, resulting from fluoride ingestion, produces a more stable mineral system. In addition, as the substitution of fluoride for hydroxyl ions produces a compound less soluble in water, it is suggested that fluoride has a stabilizing effect on bone and that it reduces the susceptibility of enamel and dentine to dental caries for the same reasons.

Excess of fluoride, dependent on natural high fluoride content of water supplies, or industrial contamination and hence of herbage, results in remarkable bone changes in both man and animals, often described as fluorine osteosclerosis (Faccini 1969). The compact bone is usually of normal width but lined on its periosteal surface with osteoid and a cell-rich periosteum; trabecular bone is also lined with osteoid, while osteoclastic resorption of the compacta may produce many resorption cavities containing fibrous tissue. Exostoses are frequently described. The histological appearance of the bones is in some cases not unlike that seen in hyperparathyroidism. Indeed, raised levels of circulating PTH have been described in both man (Teotia and Teotia 1973) and sheep (Faccini and Care 1965), though the plasma calcium may be normal. This is thought to be a compensatory phenomenon in order to keep the plasma calcium normal in spite of the abnormal calcium apatite.

Fluoride is damaging to the kidney, and it has been suggested that some of its effects on bone may be secondary to interference with vitamin D metabolism in the kidney. It is also known to have an inhibiting effect on many enzymes.

Fluoride has been used therapeutically in the prevention of dental caries and in osteoporosis. Jowsey and her colleagues think it is only effective in the latter condition if it is given in conjunction with vitamin D and calcium (Riggs, Jowsey, Kelly, Hoffman, and Arnaud 1973).

2.2. Sodium

The amount of sodium in bone is quite large, about $270 \, \text{mM} \, \text{kg}^{-1}$ varying a little from bone to bone. Davies, Kornberg, and Wilson (1952) record an average content of $239 \, \text{mM} \, \text{kg}^{-1}$ in rib and $300 \, \text{mM} \, \text{kg}^{-1}$ in the femur, while Edelman, James, Baden, and Moore (1954) noted $215 \, \text{mM}$ in the vertebrae and $237 \, \text{mM}$ in the skull. From 25 per cent to 60 per cent of bone sodium is rapidly exchangeable, and it is thought it may serve as a source of buffer in metabolic acidosis (Lehmann, Litzow, and Lennon 1966).

2.3. Potassium

Neuman (1969) suggested that bone potassium is largely in bone tissue fluid. More recently Morris and his colleagues (Morris *et al.* 1979) claim that it is largely in bone cells. It is not associated with the bone crystal (see p. 94).

2.4. Magnesium

Magnesium is discussed in Chapter 7 (p. 118). It is largely intercellular rather than associated directly with bone mineral.

2.5. Strontium

Strontium is the alkaline earth that follows calcium in the series of alkaline earths. It behaves in bone in many ways like calcium. Owing to the fact that both ^{89}Sr and ^{90}Sr are present in radioactive fallout resulting from atomic bomb explosions, the behaviour of strontium in the skeleton has received intensive study. The pattern of distribution of strontium in bone follows that of calcium. Its metabolic behaviour differs somewhat from that of calcium, as discussed in Chapter 8 (p. 128). Further, there is evidence from both animal and tissue culture experiments that bone, like the kidney and the intestine, discriminates against strontium in favour of calcium (Kshirsagar, Lloyd, and Vaughan 1966; Triffitt, Jones, and Patrick 1972). This discrimination is in part dependent upon the presence of living cells but also occurs at

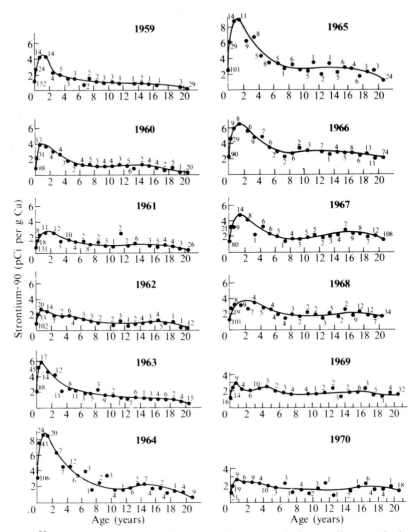

FIG. 5.1. ^{90}Strontium in human bone plotted according to year (the figures adjacent to the dots indicate the numbers of samples on which the means are based) United Kingdom Atomic Energy Authority results 1959–68. (Medical Research Council (1973).)

the level of crystal formation (Likins, McCann, Posner, and Scott 1960).

The diet of adults contains about 2 mg of stable strontium a day. The total amount in the adult skeleton is about 0·35 g. Fallout ^{89}Sr has a short half-life and is largely ignored in fallout studies. The amount of ^{90}Sr, which has a long half-life in the skeleton, has been monitored on an international basis (Bennett 1972; Medical Research Council 1973). It rose to a maximum figure

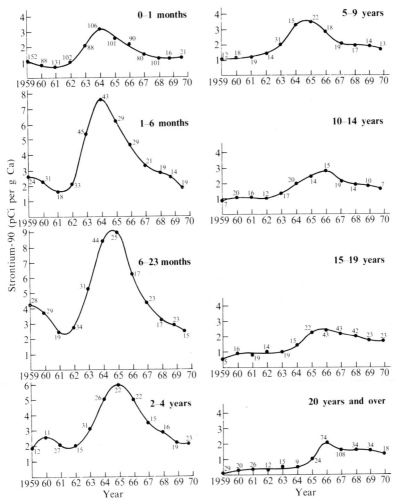

FIG. 5.2. ^{90}Sr in human bone plotted according to age (the figures adjacent to the dots indicate the numbers of samples on which the means are based) United Kingdom Atomic Energy Authority Results 1959–68. (Medical Research Council (1973).)

all over the world in 1964 and has since fallen (Fletcher, Loutit, and Papworth 1966; Bennett 1972) and, unless there are further large yield nuclear explosions in the atmosphere, it is expected to continue to fall significantly. The body burden varies somewhat in different parts of the world depending on fallout levels and dietary habits, but basically it follows the same pattern, affected by the age of the individuals studied (Bennett 1972). Values for the United Kingdom for the years 1959–70 are shown in Fig. 5.1, and the values according to age in Fig. 5.2. The levels at birth represent the level in the mother's plasma and tissue fluid. The rapid rise up to 6–12 months is dependent on the high milk intake and the considerable growth of the skeleton. Owing to differences in 'turnover' of alkaline earths in trabecular and cortical bone after growth has ceased, ^{90}Sr is concentrated 2–3 times more in vertebral than femoral samples. Bryant and Loutit (1963–4), from their analysis of both stable strontium and calcium and of ^{90}Sr in the skeleton of different age-groups over several years, calculate that in the first year of life skeletal turnover is 100 per cent and is still very high in the second year, while in older children it is about 10 per cent, decreasing to 1 per cent in the ivory bone of the femoral shaft in adults but to only 8 per cent in the vertebrae. The pattern of ^{90}Sr turnover in both adult bone and children is further discussed in Chapter 8 (p. 128) in relation to the movement of different ions in and out of the skeleton.

2.6. Radium and other α-emitters

All human bone is contaminated with trace amounts of radium and other α emitters (Turner, Radley, and Mayneord 1958) ingested with food and water. The levels appear to remain constant throughout life, and there is no evidence that the amounts found are sufficient to cause any pathological condition (Marinelli 1958).

2.7. Trace elements

Figures for trace elements in human bone were given by Tipton and her colleagues (Tipton and Cook 1963; Tipton and Shafer 1964; Tipton, Schroeder, Perry, and Cook 1965). Further figures have been obtained by Becker, Spadaro, and Berg (1968). These authors comment on the constant range of concentration of copper and zinc. Partridge (1968) has suggested that excesses and deficiencies of copper and possibly other trace metals exert their effect on the development of the connective tissue system, both collagen and elastin, by influencing the deaminative oxidation of lysine chains to aldehyde, and that these reactive aldehyde centres combine with further lysine side chains to form the cross-links of the stable fibre.

Many of the trace elements found in bone probably play an important part in the different enzyme systems involved in the functioning of the cells of bone and cartilage. Dixon and Webb (1964) give the following list of specific metal-ion enzyme activators: Na^+, K^+, Rb^+, Cs^+, Mg^{2+}, Ca^{2+}, Zn^{2+}, Cd^{2+}, Cr^{3+}, Cu^{2+}, Mn^{2+}, Fe^{2+}, Co^{2+}, Ni^{2+}, Al^{3+}. Molybdenum compounds also activate certain enzymes, but the ionic form of the activator is obscure. The activity of some enzymes is much influenced by the presence of anions, particularly the chloride ion, but with most enzymes the effects of anions are negligible at ordinary concentrations.

2.7.1. LEAD

Lead, which may reach the circulation either by inhalation or ingestion, is retained in the skeleton and, especially in children and industrial workers, may give rise to pathology (Goyer 1973).

2.7.2. ZINC

The importance of zinc in a variety of conditions is becoming increasingly recognized. Zinc deficiency besides leading to certain specific syndromes such as acrodermatitis/entropathica may lead to a general stunting in growth. Hurley and Swenerton (1971) reported that pregnant adult rats were unable to release sufficient quantities of bone zinc to meet the demand of the developing foetus during a 21-day period of dietary zinc deficiency and concluded that 'zinc in bone is not available to the rat even in the face of demonstrable need'. However, more recently Brown and her colleagues (Brown, Harrison, and Smith 1978) have shown that in male weanling rats zinc can be mobilized from the skeleton. This zinc mobilization appears to be independent of calcium and phosphorus. The femurs in the zinc deficient rats gained weight while the zinc decreased. The Ca:P ratio in the bones remained constant. Protection against zinc deficiency, has been shown to be possible, if excess zinc is fed before placing the experimental bird on a deficient diet (Harland, Spivey Fox, and Fry 1975). These observations are significant since they indicate that trace elements present in the skeleton, especially those which are required by particular enzymes, may prove to be extremely important as our understanding of metabolic processes increases.

2.8. Citrate

There is an unexpected amount of citrate in bones; 1 per cent of the fresh weight. The importance of bone citrate has been much discussed and is still not understood. The position of the citrate molecule in the bone crystal is undecided (Taylor 1960).

It was suggested by Armstrong and Singer (1956) that the citrate accumulates passively on the crystals of hydroxyapatite, perhaps by exchange with phosphate ions. On the other hand, the work of Dixon and Perkins (1952, 1956) suggested that the accumulation of citrate was the result of enzyme activity and that the presence of citric acid was essential for bone resorption. Citric acid is a powerful complexing agent for calcium, and this reaction, together with the liberation of H^+, has been suggested as responsible for the solubilization of the bone mineral and for the return of calcium to the bloodstream. Vaes (1968b) using embryo mouse calvaria studies the effect of resorption dependent on the action of PTH. Acid hydrolases were released and also citric and lactic acid. He concluded that while the hydrolases digested the matrix the acids released the calcium from the hydroxy apatite crystal. Jongebloed and his colleagues (Jongebloed, Vanden Berg, and Arends 1974) have indeed demonstrated the dissolution of single crystals of hydroxy apatite in both citric and lactic acid.

Citric acid, however, can probably accumulate without causing resorption; treatment of bone *in vitro* with fluoracetate or of the animal with oestradiol increases citric acid production by the bone without increasing solubility (Raisz, Au, and Tepperman 1961).

More recent experimental results are still somewhat unsatisfactory. Luben and Cohn (1976) working with organ culture of rat bone considered that PTH when added to bone in organ culture decreased up to 95 per cent the decarboxylation of ^{14}C citrate and increased up to 300 per cent the synthesis of hyaluronate while the addition of calcitonin or phosphate, either of which blocked the release of calcium, had no effect on citrate metabolism, suggesting that the actions of PTH on hyaluronate and citrate metabolism were not closely related. Franklin and his colleagues (Franklin, Costello, Stacey, and Stephens 1973) injected calcitonin into thyroparathyroidectomized rats and within thirty minutes noted a fall in plasma citrate and an increased excretion of citrate.

6. The Mechanism of Calcification

THE term calcification, as used in the present chapter, is concerned with the mechanisms involved in the deposition of both crystalline and amorphous hydroxyapatite within an organic matrix.

It would seem possible that the mechanisms of calcification in bone and cartilage may be somewhat different. There are substances present in the matrix of bone, such as the calcium binding proteins, which are not at present recognized in cartilage, while on the other hand they share common factors in matrix vesicles.

The early history of the many theories about the mechanism of calcification has been reviewed recently by Eanes and Posner (1970), Howell (1971), and Glimcher (1976).

The factors involved in calcification are divided by Posner into three broad groups which, however, overlap to some extent (Posner 1978a).

1. Raising the $(Ca^{2+}) \times (PO_4^{2-})$ solution ion product locally to levels at which spontaneous precipitation of mineral would occur.
2. Provision of substances that would create nucleating sites or remove barriers to these sites.
3. Presence of substances that prevent mineral formation that must be removed, or rendered inactive, to permit calcification.

1. RAISING THE $(Ca^{2+}) \times (PO_4^{2-})$ SOLUTION ION PRODUCT

1.1. Alkaline phosphatase and other enzymes

The $(Ca^{2+}) \times (PO_4^{2-})$ solution ion product in circulating blood is below the level needed for precipitation, which does not therefore occur. Robison (1923), as long ago as 1923, suggested that the enzyme alkaline phosphatase, which he found in excess in areas of calcification, hydrolyzed phosphate esters and produced an excess of free inorganic phosphate ions, thus elevating $(Ca^{2+}) \times (PO_4^{2-})$ ion product at specific calcification centres to a degree necessary to produce precipitations of apatite. The elevation of this enzyme in bone is still regarded as a marker of active tissue mineralization and its level in plasma is used as an indication of active bone metabolism. It is now known to play a vital part in the metabolism of matrix vesicles as one of the factors raising the $(Ca^{2+}) \times (PO_4^{2-})$ product (see p. 106).

1.2. Calcium binding and other glycoproteins

Posner (1978a) suggests that in bone matrix the calcium-binding proteins (see p. 71) may also be involved in raising the $(Ca^{2+}) \times (PO_4^{2-})$ product, raising the solution calcium phosphate supersaturation and so enabling apatite to be formed. He also includes the calcium-binding proteins as possibly being important as nucleation sites. Both the other glycoproteins and the calcium binding proteins are discussed under this heading on page 105. (Bernard, Furlan, Stagni, Vittur, and Zanetti 1976; Bernard, Stagni, Vittur, and Zanetti 1977.)

2. NUCLEATING SITES

The precipitation of the sparingly soluble salts involves the process of nucleation, i.e. the formation of the minimum grouping of ions capable of survival and growth. This nucleation is considered to be heterogeneous in the case of bone (Glimcher 1976; Posner, Betts, and Blumenthal 1976–7), i.e. the energy barrier to nucleation is lowered by the presence of a nucleating substrate.

2.1. Collagen

For many years Glimcher has emphasized the importance of collagen as the one and only important nucleation site in bone (Glimcher 1976). As he says 'the major mineralised structural components in bone tissue are the collagen fibrils, any hypothesis to explain the mechanism of calcification must account for this fact.' He considers there is a close relationship between collagen structure and the form and orientation of the apatite crystals which may find their place in the gap or 'hole' proposed in the structure of the collagen fibril (see p. 60). The view that crystals are found within the collagen fibril is not accepted by all electron microscopists (Cameron 1972) though many agree there is an alignment between collagen fibrils and apatite needles (Höhling, Kreilos, Neubauer, and Boyde 1971). In his recent extensive review of the mechanism of calcification, Glimcher (1976) is extremely critical of the view now held by many workers that cellular activity and the occurrence of matrix vesicles containing Ca and P is in any way associated with matrix calcification. He states 'The difficulty of explaining how the deposition of a solid phase of Ca–P in one tissue structure (mature vesicles, for example) facilitates or influences in any way the formation of new additional particles of a solid phase Ca–P in another spatially distant and distinct structure, collagen fibrils is not well appreciated.' Posner suggests that there is some evidence that galactose groups in collagen molecules may act as nucleating sites (Posner 1978a).

2.2. The glycoproteins of bone

The importance of the carbohydrate protein complexes of bone in the mechanism of calcification has become increasingly recognized, though the picture is still incomplete and indeed confused. They are included here, as possibly providing nucleating sites, without any great conviction that this is the right place for them. They may play probably a series of different roles. It is, however, abundantly clear that some of them, especially the known calcium-binding proteins like osteocalcin, must be concerned in some way with calcification. As already discussed (p. 71) some of these, for instance sialoprotein (Herring 1972; Zamoscianyk and Veiss 1966), and osteocalcin (Hauschka, Lian and Gallop 1978), appear to be peculiar to bone and dentin. Osteocalcin has a special affinity for Ca^{2+}. Other plasma proteins are selectively highly concentrated in bone but not in other soft tissues, like α_2HS glycoprotein (Triffitt et al. 1978) and others become incorporated in bone without concentration (Owen and Triffitt 1976; Triffitt and Owen 1977a). There are as yet uncharacterized glycoproteins found on both resorbing and active bone surfaces, which are not present in plasma (Owen and Triffitt 1972; Triffitt and Owen 1973).

It is not at present clear how the presence of these special glycoproteins can be given a role in calcification, together with the calcium accumulating vesicles, though it could perhaps be suggested that, in some way, when the vesicles burst liberating amorphous calcium apatite (Eanes and Posner 1970) certain of the matrix macromolecules, for instance sialoprotein as a polyanion–polycation complex, could act as an 'ion buffer' and release anions and cations under enzymic action. Such ions would then be available to make use of the nucleation site offered by the vesicle contents. There is evidence from the work of Vittur, Pugliarello, and Bernard (1971, 1972) and Baylink, Wergedal, and Thompson (1972) showing that considerable changes take place in the calcifying matrix that can be interpreted in part as a loss of non-collagenous protein, i.e. glycoprotein, as calcification increases. This finding adds support for the view that in different ways certain glycoproteins must be involved in the calcification mechanism, though not necessarily all in the same way since both α_2HS and albumin appear to be concentrated in areas of actual calcification, rather than in uncalcified osteoid. They appear to be associated with adsorption on crystal surfaces (Triffitt et al. 1978) and are thought by the workers who have studied them to be concerned in some way with calcification, since both α_2HS-glycoprotein and other plasma proteins which are adsorbed readily by calcium phosphates (Ashton et al. 1976) are likely to be associated with the mineral phase of bone matrix (Triffitt et al. 1978). Autoradiographs show incorporation of both albumin and α_2HS-glycoprotein at sites of bone formation. Posner (1978a) has suggested that the calcium binding proteins may play a double role in calcification, i.e. they may raise the $(Ca^{2+}) \times (PO_4^{2-})$ product and they may act as nucleation sites.

2.3. Matrix vesicles

Something has already been said about matrix vesicles. There is increasing evidence that both the osteoblast and the chondrocyte play a crucial role in the initiation of calcification of osteoid and cartilage matrix. They do this by being the source of matrix vesicles which may provide nucleating sites. An electron microscope picture of an osteoblast bordering recently secreted osteoid is shown in Fig. 2.4. In the clear osteoid are many electron dense bodies described as matrix vesicles, osteoblast pseudopodia cut in various directions, some uncalcified collagen fibres and further to the left calcified fibres adjacent to the more densely calcified mass of collagen. Such matrix vesicles were first described in growth plate cartilage (Anderson 1968, 1969) (see p. 88) but were soon recognized to occur also in bone osteoid tissue (Bernard and Pease 1969; Bonucci 1971), and in dentin (Slavkin, Bringes, Croissant, and Bavetta 1972; Slavkin, Croissant, and Bringes 1972). Their importance as nucleation sites is now recognized by the majority of workers though Thyberg and his colleagues (Thyberg and Friberg 1972; Thyberg 1972) maintain that these structures, described as vesicles, are only extruded lysosomes, fragments of cellular projections or disintegrating cells. This appears unlikely since they are smaller than cartilage cell lysosomes and lack the right enzymes (Rabinovitch and Anderson 1976).

The vesicles measure about 100 nμ in diameter and when reaching the matrix from the cell they are invested in a trilaminar membrane enriched in phospholipids, which are largely internal (see Fig. 4.2) (Majeska, Holwerda, and Wuthier 1979). Wuthier (1975) has described these vesicles as a Ca^{2+} trap, the calcium coming from the mitochondria. They are rich in phosphate, alkaline phosphatase, pyrophosphatase, ATP and magnesium. As Posner and his colleagues say (Posner *et al.* 1976–7), by regulating the Mg, the ATP and possibly ATPase levels, the cell can store or utilize amorphous calcium phosphate granules. Once extruded into the matrix the phospholipid membrane of the vesicle is broken, the magnesium, inhibiting apatite formation, is lost and the amorphous phosphate granules can either become apatite or meet other factors favouring apatite formation like the calcium binding proteins in the matrix (Posner 1978*a*).

The evidence for this is both morphological and biochemical. Electron microscope studies, particularly in the case of cartilage vesicles, have shown the vesicles budding from the plasma membrane (Bonucci 1971; Cecil and Anderson 1978) while biochemical studies of isolated vesicles show a high sphyngomyelin content, cholesterol to phospholipid ratio (Peress, Anderson, and Saydera 1974) and the presence of significant amounts of 5′ AMPase, all of which are thought to be good biochemical markers for plasma membrane. Calcium phospholipid complexes are found in all mineralized rabbit tissues and no such complexes can be isolated from non-mineralized tissue such as muscle or bone marrow. The proportion is always highest in tissues involved in active mineralization (Boskey and Posner 1976; Boskey et al. 1978; Boskey 1978). This description of the behaviour of matrix vesicles in the calcification process certainly applies to bone. Ca and P are thought to be present in the vesicle before it is budded from the osteoblast, probably in the form of a calcium–phosphorus–lipid complex. A rather different picture has been presented by some workers in the case of cartilage. Ali and his colleagues have made a careful study of matrix vesicle development in the longitudinal septa of the hypertrophic zone of the cartilage plate (Ali 1976; Ali, Sajdera, and Anderson 1970; Ali, Wisby, Evans, and Craig-Gray 1977; Ali, Wisby, and Gray 1978). They consider the vesicle, which there is now evidence is budded from the surface of chondrocytes (Cecil and Anderson 1978), initially contains no Ca^{2+} or PO_4^{3-} but subsequently incorporates small amounts of Ca^{2+} by active uptake, by passive diffusion and specific binding. PO_4^{3-} is present slightly later and through enzymic action there is an elevation of the $Ca \times P$ product and precipitation of apatite in and around the vesicle. Other workers, as already described, suggest that calcium and phosphate, derived probably from the store in the mitochondria, are present in the vesicle in the form of calcium–phosphorus–lipid complex, before it is actually budded off from the membrane. Pictures of apatite crystals in matrix vesicles, whether of bone or cartilage, are probably an artefact produced by processing procedures. The technical problems involved in studying the cellular details of calcification are immense (Anderson 1976, 1978), but whatever the mechanisms involved may prove to be, there seems little doubt, that in some way, matrix vesicles and their contents, serve as nucleation sites in both osteoid and cartilage matrix.

2.3.1. CALCIUM STORAGE

Osteoblasts and chondrocytes store Ca^{2+} and phosphate in their mitochondria (Martin and Matthews 1970; Borle 1973; Bygrave 1978; Lehninger, Reynafarje, Vercesi, and Tew 1978; and Posner 1978a). Some of the ions certainly pass from the mitochondria to the matrix vesicles. Whether they also pass through the cytosol directly into extracellular tissue is not known. Lehninger and his colleagues (1978) describe different types of binding sites in the mitochondrial membrane, one for influx and one for efflux of Ca^{2+}. Borle (1973) has described the mitochondria as the main regulator of cytoplasmic calcium activity and calcium transport. Clearly this available source of calcium adjacent to the osteoid must play a significant role in calcification even though the precise means by which this is achieved is still not clear.

3. SUBSTANCES PREVENTING CALCIFICATION

3.1. Magnesium in matrix vesicles

Magnesium is largely present in bone as an intracellular ion. It is suggested by Posner (1978a) that it exerts a powerful effect intracellularly and in matrix vesicles in preventing the formation of calcium apatite crystals from amorphous calcium phosphate.

3.2. The proteoglycans in cartilage

Posner (1978a) considers that the presence of very large proteoglycan molecules, particularly in the cartilage plate, can in some way delay or prevent apatite precipitation. Experiments on the growth plate suggest that the enormous proteoglycan aggregate molecules (molecular weight about 200 million daltons) are enzymatically cleaved to much smaller subunits as the calcification region is approached. The total proteoglycan concentration is markedly reduced in going from the proliferating to the calcifying zone (see also p. 88). This effect of proteoglycans has been further studied on *in vitro* hydroxyapatite formation (Blumenthal, Posner, Silverman, and Rosenberg 1979).

3.3. A specific inhibitor in cartilage

Howell and his colleagues (Howell *et al.* 1969; Howell and Pita 1976) using a micropuncture technique have obtained extracellular fluid from the distal hypertrophic cell zone of rat tibial cartilage, which they describe as containing 'an inhibitor of calcification'.

Posner has said in attempting to summarize our knowledge of the mechanism of calcification 'the following are in some way related to mineralization, alkaline and acid phosphatase and other enzymes, Ca binding proteins, collagen, lipids, the mitochondria of cells, extracellular matrix vesicles and the proteoglycans.' He adds: 'There is no reason why the mechanism cannot be independent and redundant rather than co-operative' (Posner 1978a).

3.4. Pyrophosphates

In the early 1960s Neuman and Fleisch became interested in substances that might inhibit the postulated nucleating activity of collagen (Fleisch and Neuman 1961). Human urine and plasma were found to contain inorganic pyrophosphate (PP_1) and this was shown to inhibit the precipitation of calcium phosphate from solution. Further work indicated that PP_1 might take part in the regulation of calcification of the soft and hard tissues. The inhibition of the precipitation of calcium phosphate occurred both in solutions of crystals and in the presence of preformed apatite crystals, while

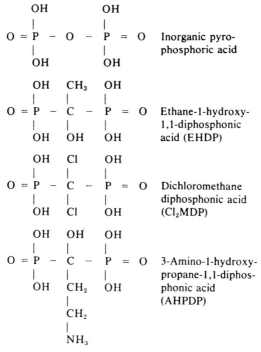

FIG. 6.1. The diphosphonates.

the conversion of amorphous into crystalline apatite was slowed. However, PP_1 had no effect on the formation of the amorphous phase. The marked effect of PP_1 on calcium phosphates *in vitro* at concentrations found in biological fluids suggested that PP_1 could protect soft tissues from mineralization, while in bone it might regulate the formation and dissolution of hard tissues (Russell and Fleisch 1976). The matrix vesicles, already discussed, have a high content of alkaline phosphatase (Ali *et al.* 1970) and alkaline phosphatases are known to possess pyrophosphatase activity. It is possible that the role of this enzyme is to hydrolyze PP_1 which would otherwise inhibit calcification (Russell and Fleisch 1976).

4. THE DIPHOSPHONATES

Attempts to use PP_1 and condensed phosphates for animal experiment proved unsatisfactory since these substances are not absorbed intact from the gut and are rapidly destroyed in the body when given by injection. However, the diphosphonates which possess P–C–P bonds, instead of a P–O–P bond of pyrophosphate (see Fig. 6.1), are much more stable to both chemical and enzymic degradation and are effective when given by mouth (Russell and Smith 1973). Early investigation showed that the diphosphonates inhibit the precipitation of calcium phosphate and also slow down the aggregation and dissolution of calcium phosphate crystals.

Most of the physicochemical effects of diphosphonates are probably related to the strong affinity they have for calcium ions and for calcium phosphates. They bind strongly onto the surface of crystals of hydroxy apatite — probably to more than one type of binding site — progressively displacing orthophosphate as they bind (Jung, Bisaz, and Fleisch 1973). The precise way in which diphosphonates exert their effects on calcium phosphates is not understood. It has been shown by Posner and his colleagues that diphosphonates have an important effect on the formation of calcium apatite by calcium phospholipid phosphate complexes found in matrix vesicles. The diphosphonates appear to act not only as an hydroxyapatite crystal poison but also as surfactants (substances that change the surface tension and/or surface change between two phases) (Boskey, Goldberg, and Posner 1979) so altering the ability of the vesicle membrane to induce hydroxyapatite formation and initiate calcification. Many diphosphonates have now been investigated but only three have hitherto been used in man, namely, ethane-1-hydroxy-1, 1-diphosphonic acid (EHDP); Dichloromethane diphosphonic acid Cl_2MDP; and 3-amino-1-hydroxy-propane-1, 1-diphosphonic (AHPDP); (Fig. 6.1) (Fleisch and Felix 1979).

Both animal experiments and clinical observations have shown that different phosphonates have different effects, and that the dose at which any phosphonate is given will influence its effect. Animal studies indicate that doses affecting bone resorption may be different from those affecting mineralization (Schenk, Merz, Fleisch, Muhlbauer, and Russell 1973; Miller, Jee, Kimmel, and Woodbury 1977; Lemkes, Reitsma, Frijlink, Verlinden-Ooms, and Bijvoet 1978).

Although Cl_2MDP has no effect on mineralization, AHPDP only affects it at much higher doses than those inhibiting resorption. AHPDP affects resorption more than other compounds (Reitsma, Bijvoet, Frijlink, Vismans, and van Breukelen *et al.* 1980). The use of both diphosphonates in the treatment of Paget's disease of bone have given important information on their possible mode of action (Hosking, van Aken, Bijvoet, and Will 1976; Frijlink, Bijvoet, Te-Velde, and Heynen 1979; Meunier, Alexandre, Edouard, Mathieu, Chapuy, Bressot, Vignon, and Trechsel 1979).

4.1. Clinical use

4.1.1. PAGET'S DISEASE OF BONE

Paget's disease of bone is a condition of unknown aetiology characterized by both excessive resorption and apposition. It responds well to treatment with both AHPDP (Reitsma, Bijvoet, Frijlink, Vismans, and van Breukelen 1980; Frijlink *et al.* 1979) and Cl_2MDP (Meunier, Alexandre, Edouard, Mathieu, Chapuy, Bressot, Vignon, and Trechsel 1979). Bone turnover is diminished, as indicated, by a decrease in both urinary hydroxyproline excretion and plasma alkaline phosphatase. Bone biopsy shows a decrease or even disappearance of abnormal osteoblasts and osteoclasts, while mineralization and plasma calcium return to normal. Bijvoet and his colleagues (Frijlink *et al.* 1979; Reitsma *et al.* 1980) suggest that the immediate effect on hydroxyproline excretion suggests an immediate blockage of osteoclast function and of new osteoclast formation, while the rise of osteoblastic formation is probably a result of the normal homeostatic mechanism (see p. 160) that maintains equilibrium between formation and resorption in many diseased states including Paget's. Kinetic studies showed increased calcium absorption from the gut but normal calcium excretion in the urine. Meunier and his colleagues (Meunier *et al.* 1979) have reported similar excellent results using Cl_2MDP. They found a transient increase in PTH in 13 out of 19 patients, which Bijvoet and his colleagues had suggested might occur as part of the normal homeostatic mechanism (see p. 160). It is clear that the two diphosphonates AHPDP and Cl_2MDP have an obvious anti-osteoclastic effect, without inhibiting bone mineralization. The decrease in alkaline phosphatase noted in clinical cases occurred about a month after a decrease in hydroxyproline excretion, showing that the antiosteoclastic effect precedes the reduction of osteoblast activity. The mechanism by which the diphosphonates selectively alter osteoclasts is still not clear. It is possible that because the diphosphonates are adsorbed on bone crystals, the osteoclasts are poisoned following phagocytosis of diphosphonated bone.

4.1.2. OSTEOLYTIC BONE DISEASE

In a small group of patients with osteolytic bone disease due to breast cancer or myeloma and associated hypercalcaemia, the serum Ca^{2+} dropped to normal levels accompanied by a decrease in urinary calcium and hydroxyproline, following treatment with AHPDP. It is suggested that this diphosphonate may inhibit tumour-induced osteolysis (see p. 11) Van Breukelin, Bijvoet, and van Oosterom 1979).

4.1.3. ECTOPIC CALCIFICATION

Diphosphonates have proved disappointing in the treatment of ectopic calcification such as occurs in myositis ossificans.

4.1.4. OSTEOPOROSIS

Bijvoet and his colleagues (Reitsma *et al.* 1980) have treated patients with osteoporosis (maintenance dose 3–6 μmol kg body weight^{-1} day^{-1}) with AHPDP. There was an initial improvement in calcium balance which appeared to be maintained.

4.1.5. BONE SCANNING

Apart from their therapeutic use, phosphonates are now used extensively, because of their strong affinity for calcified tissues, to effect localization of a γ-emitting isotope ^{99m}TC, by linking the tracer to the phosphorus compound. ^{99m}TC-diphosphonates, or ^{99m}TC-pyro/polyphosphonates, have now nearly completely replaced the previously used compounds for scintigraphy of bone (Fleisch and Felix 1979).

4.2. Fluoride

The part that fluorides may play in bone mineralization has been discussed in Chapter 5 (p. 96).

7. Calcium, Magnesium, and Phosphorus in Plasma and Urine

COMPLEX mechanisms are involved in maintaining a steady level of certain elements, particularly calcium, magnesium, and phosphorus, in plasma and the intracellular and extracellular fluids. These levels are discussed in this chapter, together with quantitative data about normal absorption from the food ingested and normal excretion. What is known of the mechanisms involved in maintaining these levels is discussed in later chapters.

1. CALCIUM

Many biological processes display specificities for calcium that must be attributable to highly selective calcium-binding sites. Structural evidence indicates that this specificity is largely due to the overall arrangements of suitable ligands at such sites. For those interested in calcium chemistry the symposium on calcium binding proteins and calcium function should be consulted (Wasserman, Corradino, Carafoli, Kretsinger, Maclennan, and Siegel 1977).

In attempting to study the physiology of bone the relationship of calcium to particular proteins constantly arises even if its significance is not always understood. The part played by calcium-binding proteins on the absorption from the gut is discussed on p. 144. A significant amount of the calcium circulating in the plasma is bound to albumin (see p. 76). The plasma glycoprotein $\alpha_2 HS$ is concentrated in bone and is considered in some way to be associated with the calcification process (see p. 76). Osteocalcin, a small Gla-protein which is found in bone (about 1 per cent of the total protein in chicken bone) and is vitamin K dependent, like prothrombin, is also a powerful binder of Ca^{2+} (see p. 74).

Hitherto, when the movement of calcium ions in and out of bone is discussed, the ionized calcium alone has been considered. The fact that albumin may also move into bone suggests that consideration may need to be given to the bound calcium as well (Owen *et al.* 1973) (p. 74).

Bone contains most of the body's calcium (Table 7.1). The other main constituent is phosphorus as inorganic phosphate (P_i). About 15 per cent of the body's phosphate lies outside the skeleton in body fluids and in tissues, mostly as organic phosphate compounds. In normal human adults the

TABLE 7.1

Distribution of calcium and phosphate in normal human adults

	Calcium†	Phosphorus (as P)†
Total body content for 70 kg human	1000–1500 g	700–1000 g
Skeleton	98%	85%
Skeletal muscle	0·3%	6%
Skin	0·08%	1%
Liver	0·02%	1%
CNS	0·01%	1%
Other tissues	0·6%	5%
Extracellular fluid	1%	1%

† Adapted from Widdowson and Dickerson (1964) by Russell (1976).

TABLE 7.2

The percentage of total calcium in the ionized form Ca^{2+}, the protein bound form CaPr, and the complexed form CaX, in body fluids

	CaPr	+	CaX	+	Ca^{2+}
Plasma	40%		10%		50%
UF	0		16%		84%
CSF	0		9%		91%
Urine	0		50%		50%

From Robertson (1976) by courtesy of author and publishers.

exchangeable pool of calcium, as measured by radioisotopes (^{45}Ca and ^{47}Ca), represents less than 1 per cent of total body calcium (in the region of 70 mg/kg) during the first few days after injection. About half of this is outside the skeleton, the rest within it. Calcium in body fluids is present in three forms: ionized, bound to protein, and complexed with organic acids such as citrate (Table 7.2) (Robertson 1976). The ionized calcium is diffusible, the citrate calcium, though not ionized, is also diffusible, the protein bound calcium is neither ionized nor diffusible.

1.1. Plasma (serum) levels

The normal level of calcium in the plasma is close to 10 mg per 100 ml. Measurements in a random sample of 85 women gave a range of 9·1–10·7 mg per 100 ml in 1960 (Smith, Davis, and Fourman 1960). Peacock and Nordin (1973) have more recently given a figure of 9·58 ± 0·06 mg per 100 ml as a mean figure in 25 normals. There are considerable diurnal variations in any one individual. The value goes up in the day when calcium is ingested in the diet and it falls during the night when there is no dietary intake. Knowledge of the true level of ionized calcium is essential to the clinician. Hitherto this has been difficult, for technical reasons, to estimate directly. Use has been made of the figures for total calcium and total albumin, employing a variety of corrections (Payne *et al.* 1979). Conceicao and his colleagues, having compared the direct method with four indirect methods in both normal and abnormal subjects conclude 'that calculation of the serum ionised calcium is not an adequate substitute for direct measurement' (Conceicao, Weightman, Smith, Luno, Ward, and Kerr 1978). The method of calculation may be reasonably satisfactory in normal subjects but of little value in patients with hypercalcaemia or hypocalcaemia. Both are seriously underdiagnosed when indirect methods are used. All four indirect methods were found to give closely similar results so it is unlikely that any refinement of the formulae used are likely to be helpful. Much of the error of the indirect methods is probably due to the variable binding of calcium to protein in different people. The figures given by Conceicao show that indirect estimation can lead to the serum ionized-calcium concentration being over estimated by up to 10 per cent.

The object of the complicated mechanisms involved in calcium homeostasis is to maintain the ratio of ionized calcium to phosphate in the plasma constant at a level just below that needed for precipitation. The relation between ionized calcium and phosphate in the blood is affected by the pH and the carbon dioxide of the blood which must also be kept constant.

1.2. Cell calcium and cyclic AMP

The weight of present evidence suggests that cyclic nucleotides directly or indirectly regulate cellular calcium metabolism (Rasmussen and Goodman 1977). Calcium is distributed asymmetrically within the various subcellular compartments, much of it is present in the mitochondria (Borle 1973; Wuthier and Gore 1977; Posner 1978*b*) or in microsomes as a non-ionic, rapidly exchangeable phosphate salt. Cytosol calcium concentrations are thought to be 100–1000 times lower than extracellular—i.e., in the range 10^{-5}–10^{-3} mol/l. The activation of cells by hormones or pharmacological agents is now thought to be associated with increases in intracellular calcium concentration derived from outside the cell or by release from mitochondria (Rasmussen and Goodman 1977). Hormonal activation is often associated with stimulation of adenylate cyclases specific to the target tissue (Russell 1976).

1.3. Absorption from the gut

The problems of absorption of calcium from the diet have been extensively studied. With the usual dietary intake of about 1 g/day of calcium the net amount absorbed is about 200 mg. Absorption takes place throughout the small intestine. It is quantitatively greater in the ilium than the duodenum even though active transport is more evident in the duodenum. The fraction of the dietary intake absorbed varies with the dietary content so that net absorption remains relatively constant. It takes place partly by simple passive ionic diffusion, partly by facilitated diffusion, and partly by active transport (Russell 1976).

The amount normally absorbed is thought to diminish with age in both sexes, starting at the age of 55–60 years in women and 65–70 years in men (Bullamore, Gallagher, Wilkinson, Nordin, and Marshall 1970). This decrease has been attributed to cholecalciferol deficiency. It may be associated with changes in sex hormone secretion (see p. 196). It is probable that the intestine has a peak capacity for calcium absorption, but that this is normally set well above the calcium intake from normal dietary loads (Wills 1973). The factors that control absorption are extremely complex and are discussed elsewhere in connection with vitamin D and PTH (pp. 144 and 160). The amounts absorbed are also influenced by a number of other substances that may be present in the diet, particularly phosphate, phytic acid, oxalic acid, and fatty acids (Wills 1973).

Bile and bile salts probably play a direct part in intestinal calcium absorption by increasing the solubility of calcium salts (Webling and Holdsworth 1966). Certain alginates given by mouth may reduce absorption (Sutton, Harrison, Carr, and Barltrop 1971), though their effect on strontium is greater than on calcium.

The epithelial cells of the gut discriminate against strontium in favour of calcium. Stable calcium decreases the net absorption of ^{90}Sr. On a low calcium intake the net absorption of ^{90}Sr averages 15·7 per cent and on a high calcium intake 4·9 per cent. However, the difference in the net absorption of ^{90}Sr on the two calcium intakes used is of low significance ($p < 0\cdot1$) (Spencer, Kramer, Samachson, Hardy, and Rivera 1973; Spencer, Warren, Kramer, and Samachson 1973).

1.4. Excretion of calcium

1.4.1. THE INTESTINE

Calcium is excreted into the gut in the gastric juice and the bile. There is some evidence that calcium secreted in bile is preferentially reabsorbed by the intestinal mucosa and that it does not mix significantly with the dietary calcium in the gut. Dolphin and Eve (1963) give a mean figure of 0·15 g calcium per day reaching the gut from the plasma.

Studies performed on the passage of calcium and strontium in the opposite direction, i.e. from the vascular space into the intestine, by administering tracer doses of ^{85}Sr and ^{47}Ca intravenously have shown that the plasma levels of ^{85}Sr and ^{47}Ca were similar in the first 24 hours. The 12-day cumulative faecal excretion of [85]Sr was only slightly greater than that of [47]Ca, indicating little discrimination against the passage of strontium from the vascular space into the intestine. The average [85]Sr/[47]Ca discrimination ratio of the intestinal excretions was only 1·22 (Spencer *et al.* 1973).

The measurements of faecal excretion of calcium usually include the endogenous calcium. The relatively small changes in the daily excretion of calcium are probably due to changes in the dietary intake which was not controlled (Carr, Harrison, and Nolan 1973). For discussion of the factors controlling calcium absorption see pp. 144, 160.

1.4.2. THE URINE

Excretion of calcium in the urine is more important than intestinal excretion as a regulator of plasma calcium (see p. 154). Factors controlling the renal excretion of calcium are discussed in the following chapters. It is probably regulated by PTH, though vitamin D metabolites may have a modulating effect (Parsons 1978). The excretion is usually less than 400 mg per day in men, less than 340 mg per day in women, and less than 6 mg per kg body weight in children (Bulusu, Hodgkinson, Nordin, and Peacock 1970; Davis, Morgan, and Rivlin 1970). The normal range of calcium excretion is wide. The figures quoted for adults by Davis and his colleagues were based on a study over 1 week of 75 men and 98 women, aged 20–69 years, who were all apparently healthy and taking their chosen free diet (see Fig. 7.1). The authors conclude that most of the variations in urinary calcium were due to variables

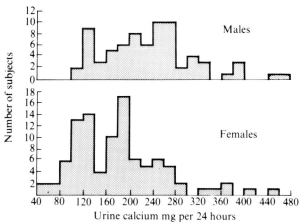

FIG. 7.1. The distribution of the values for the urinary excretion of calcium (mg per day) in 75 men and 98 women when the value for each person was calculated from the total number of collections from that person. (From Davis *et al.* (1970) by courtesy of authors and publishers.)

other than the dietary intake of calcium, the most important being variation in the efficiency of calcium reabsorption. Only in men over 50 was there any suggestion of a relationship between dietary calcium and urinary calcium. The urinary excretion diminished in men over 60 and in women over 50. In all subjects there was considerable day-to-day variation. This variability is confirmed by others (Nordin, Peacock, and Wilkinson 1972; Carr *et al.* 1973).

About 60 per cent of calcium in plasma is ultrafilterable at the glomerulus. This is reduced to 47 per cent by hypercalcaemia. Approximately 70 per cent of the filtered load is reabsorbed. Reabsorption occurs in both proximal and distal tubules (Dennis, Stead, and Myers 1979). Dennis states that it is not altogether clear that these effects are mediated through cyclic AMP, though some workers consider that control of calcium excretion by PTH is always affected through changes in cyclic AMP. The handling of calcium by the distal nephron is dissociated from sodium transport (Dennis *et al.* 1979) (see also p. 123).

1.4.3. SWEAT

Calcium loss in the sweat is appreciable and variable for different individuals. The mean ratio of the skin loss to the urinary output of calcium in one man was $(0\cdot072\pm0\cdot010)$ and in another $(0\cdot034\pm0\cdot001)$ (Carr *et al.* 1973).

2. MAGNESIUM

Magnesium is essential for life. It is present as an intercellular ion in all living tissue. It is an activator for a large number of enzymes, some of which are especially important in the skeleton, such as alkaline phosphatase and the pyrophosphatases (Rasmussen 1972). All enzymes that are known to be catalyzed by ATP show an absolute requirement for magnesium (Aikawa 1978). It may also affect other intracellular enzymic reactions, for instance it may prevent the formation of calcium apatite within matrix vesicles (see p. 88) (Posner *et al.* 1976–7; Wuthier and Gore 1977). The effects of magnesium on the skeleton are probably dependent upon its action on intracellular enzymes. Magnesium is the fourth most abundant cation in the skeleton. About 60 per cent of the body magnesium is in the skeleton (Aikawa 1978). An adult man of 70 kg body weight has a total body content of about 2400 meq compared to 60 000 meq of calcium. Only approximately 1 per cent of total body magnesium is extracellular. Under normal physiological circumstances in bone one third is absorbed on the surface of apatite crystals and is exchangeable, the rest replacing calcium in the apatite crystal (Alfrey, Miller, and Trow 1974; Brautbar, Lee, Coburn, and Kleeman 1979). Alfrey and his colleagues have calculated that in fresh human bone 30 per cent is surface-limited and freely exchangeable, though Foster (1968) said that only 2 per cent of bone magnesium was exchangeable. In Paget's disease exchangeable bone magnesium can be increased threefold. The magnesium requirement of adult man has been estimated by balance techniques to lie between 200 mg and 300 mg a day.

2.1. Plasma level

The plasma level is kept constant within narrow limits, remaining on the average $1.7 \, \text{meq} \, l^{-1}$ and varying less than 15 per cent from this mean value (Wacker and Paresi 1968). It is unaffected by sex or age. Approximately one third of extracellular magnesium is bound non-specifically to plasma protein. The remaining 65 per cent which is diffusible or ionized appears to be the biologically active component (Aikawa 1978).

2.2. Absorption from the gut

The average American ingests between 20–40 meq of magnesium a day and about one-third of this is absorbed. Faecal magnesium appears to be primarily magnesium from material that is not absorbed by the body rather than magnesium secreted by the intestine. Absorption takes place through the small intestine. Factors controlling absorption are not well understood though many have been suggested.

2.3. Excretion

Excretion of magnesium occurs through the kidney and the sweat.

2.3.1. KIDNEY

The kidney plays an important role in magnesium homeostasis. Massry (1977) states that approximately 1800 mg of magnesium is lost from plasma daily into the glomerulus, but only 3–5 per cent of filtered magnesium is excreted in the urine. It is not known whether active reabsorption occurs throughout the nephron. In studies carried out in the dog the major portion of filtered magnesium is reabsorbed by the proximal tubules and the reabsorption is isotonic or nearly so. In the rat reabsorption is less efficient. Massry considers that micropuncture studies and stop-flow experiments suggest that a very active transport mechanism for magnesium exists in the distal nephron and that, at least in the dog, it is dissociated from that of calcium and sodium. He lists the following factors which decrease tubular reabsorption, extracellular fluid volume expansion, renal vasodilation, osmotic diuresis, diuretic agents, cardiac glycosides, hypercalcaemia, alcohol ingestion, high sodium intake, growth hormone, thyroid hormone, calcitonin, and chronic mineralocorticoid effects.

The effect of PTH is at present confused. Massry (1977) considers it enhances tubular reabsorption. Dirks and Quamme (1978) think experimental results suggest that the administration of PTH significantly decreased the fractional excretion of magnesium in thyroparathyroidectomized rats. However, the acute administration of cyclic AMP, the proposed mediator of PTH action, failed to lower magnesium excretion. Chronic administration of mineralocorticoids causes increased urinary excretion of magnesium (Hanna and MacIntyre 1960).

2.3.2. SWEAT

Excretion in sweat is estimated to be about 15 mg per day. When men are exposed to high temperatures for several days, from 10 to 15 per cent of the total output of magnesium is recovered in sweat. Acclimatization does not occur as in the case of sodium and potassium. Under extreme conditions sweat can account for 25 per cent of the magnesium lost daily (Aikawa 1978).

2.4. Magnesium deficiency

It is difficult to achieve a significant magnesium depletion in normal individuals by simple dietary restriction because of the efficient renal and gastrointestinal mechanisms. Hypocalcaemia has been reported in man as a result of magnesium deficiency and also in a number of species (Massry 1977). The mechanisms underlying this hypocalaemia are not well understood. Massry considers they are multiple and suggests, relative or complete failure of the function of parathyroid glands, impaired skeletal response to PTH and abnormalities in the equilibrium between bone and extracellular fluid. There is some evidence of raised levels of PTH and hyperplasia of the glands during magnesium deficiency. Using foetal rat bone in tissue culture Raisz and Niemann (1969) found that decreasing magnesium concentration in the culture medium decreased resorption particularly in PTH treated bones without altering the loss from dead bone. They suggest that this shows that changes in ion concentration can alter bone resorption and its regulation by hormones.

Several histological studies have been made of the effect of magnesium deficiency in the bones of rats. Hunt and Bélanger (1972) fed both young and old rats a diet containing 0·8–2 mg per 100 g. No figures of plasma calcium are given. Within 18–21 days there was generalized medullary bone growth (osteomyelosclerosis) and also periosteal tumours of the desmoid type at the femoral linia aspera. The authors attribute these results to enzymic malfunction since this cation is such an important enzyme activator.

Smith and Nisbet (1968) describe osteoporosis and cessation of growth in rats with complete absence of magnesium from the diet. Retarded growth only, though associated with osteoporosis, occurred in rats whose magnesium intake was restricted. More recently Lai and his colleagues (Lai, Singer, and Armstrong 1975) have also described retarded growth in rats on a magnesium deficient diet. They also noted a decrease in acid and alkali phosphatase in the metaphyses of the deficient animals, which is not surprising in view of the fact that all enzyme reactions catalysed by ATP show an absolute requirement for magnesium. The addition of magnesium to the incubation media led to a greater increase in bone alkaline phosphatase in the deficient than in the control rats. Magnesium and phosphorus content of the deficient bone was abnormally low. A more detailed study of the effects of magnesium deficiency on bone cells has been reported by Schwartz and Reddi (1979). Demineralized bone matrix was implanted subcutaneously in young rats fed on a magnesium-deficient diet. When removed the implants showed retardation in cartilage and bone differentiation and matrix calcification with virtual absence of bone marrow. These data show that bone cell differentiation can occur in a severely magnesium depleted environment, though the onset of mineralization, bone remodelling, and marrow differentiation is impaired. Wuthier and Gore (1977) studying the part played by matrix vesicles in cartilage calcification consider that the binding of calcium to anionic phospholipid occurs within the vesicle but that the presence of abundant intracellular magnesium prevents the formation of calcium apatite until the vesicle membrane is broken (see p. 106) (Posner, Betts, and Blumenthal 1976–7).

3. PHOSPHATE

The importance of a proper understanding of phosphate metabolism has been increasingly recognized. Phosphate plays an important role in bone mineralization. Russell (1976) states 'The ability to produce mineralization is more than a simple function of the (Ca) $\times$ (P) product, although low products do tend to be associated with defective skeletal mineralization and high products with the ectopic deposition of calcium phosphate.' Defective skeletal mineralization can occur in some, though not all, situations where a low plasma phosphate exists, e.g. in phosphate deprivation syndromes or in inherited or acquired renal tubular disorders in which renal phosphate reabsorption is defective. Administration of phosphate alone may improve skeletal calcification. Dietary deprivation of phosphate is associated with increased absorption of calcium which is not seen in other hypophosphatemic states, perhaps because hypophosphatemia is able to stimulate the renal production of $1,25\text{-}(OH)_2D_3$. There is also evidence that phosphate can reduce the rate of bone resorption. How this is effected is not at present clear but it probably accounts for the useful therapeutic effect of phosphate in several hypercalcaemic states (Mundy 1979).

In rats, rickets does not develop with a lack of vitamin D alone unless phosphate deprivation is also present. This may be due to the fact that the high plasma phosphate found in rats may maintain skeletal mineralization even in the absence of vitamin D (Russell 1976).

Phosphate homeostasis depends primarily on mechanism governing the

TABLE 7.3
State of phosphate in normal human plasma

	mg per 100 ml	Percentage total
Free HPO_4^{2-}	1·55	43
Free $H_2PO_4^-$	0·34	10
Protein bound	0·43	12
$NaHPO_4^-$	1·02	29
$CaHPO_4$	0·12	3
$MgHPO_4$	0·10	3
Total	3·56	100

From Walser (1961) by courtesy of author and publishers.

renal excretion of phosphate (Bijvoet and Sluys Veer 1968; Dennis *et al.* 1979). The metabolism of phosphate is closely controlled or modulated by vitamin D metabolites and the parathyroid hormone (see p. 145). It also appears to be associated in some way which is not clearly understood with sodium (Dennis *et al.* 1979) (see p. 123).

3.1. Intake

Phosphate intake (expressed in terms of phosphorus) in adult man is usually in the range 0·5–2·0 g per day. The major part (about 80 per cent) is absorbed from the intestine, and in a healthy adult this amount appears in the urine each day.

3.2. Plasma levels

In contrast with calcium, most of the phosphate in plasma is in diffusible form. The state of phosphate in normal human plasma is shown in Table 7.3. The normal plasma level varies from 2·4 mg per 100 ml to 4·4 mg per 100 ml in healthy adults. It is higher in children and adolescents and has a circadian rhythm which is at least in part dependent on phosphate intake. Tissues are not nearly as sensitive to changes in phosphate as to changes in calcium levels in the plasma. Phosphate movements in and out of bone are approximately one half those of calcium in molar terms (Russell 1976).

3.3. Absorption from the gut

The factors controlling and affecting absorption of calcium from the gut have become increasingly understood in the last few years. The problems of phosphate absorption are at present less clear. The role of calciferol and its active metabolite 1,25-$(OH)_2D_3$ is firmly established in the case of calcium. The situation in the case of phosphate is still not completely clarified. Wasserman and Taylor (Wasserman and Taylor 1973; Taylor 1974) observed that phosphorus was rapidly translocated across all segments of the small intestine and that cholecalciferol stimulated the process in each segment. They were unable to detect the existence of a phosphate-binding protein comparable to the calcium-binding protein. In 1974 Chen and others (Chen, Castillo, Korycka-Dahl, and Deluca 1974) reported that cholecalciferol 25-(OH)D$_3$ and 1,25-(OH)$_2$D$_3$ — but not 24,25-(OH)$_2$D$_3$ — stimulated phosphate transport independently of calcium in the rat. Phosphate transport was highest where there was also some stimulation from the presence of calcium, but in the jejunum phosphate transport was completely independent of the presence of calcium. Such independent transport of phosphate by 1,25-(OH)$_2$D$_3$ has also been described by Norman (1978). The effect on phosphate transport occurs later than that on calcium transport. Norman concludes that the dramatic differences in time of the effect of 1,25-(OH)$_2$D$_3$ on calcium and phosphate transport indicate that they are dissociated from one another, though both may be influenced by vitamin D metabolites.

3.4. Excretion by the kidney

About 87 per cent of plasma phosphate is filterable at the glomerulus. Under conditions of normal diet and a normal PTH activity the mammalian kidney reabsorbs more than 80 per cent of the filtered load (Dennis et al. 1979). If plasma phosphate falls the efficiency of resorption can increase to nearly 100 per cent (Russell 1976). If radioactive phosphate is injected into the late part of the proximal loop 86 per cent is recovered in the urine when the parathyroid gland is intact, but only 50 per cent when it is absent. There has been intensive study of the site in the proximal tubules where phosphate reabsorption occurs. It is clear that the amount reabsorbed varies in the length of the tubules (Dennis et al. 1979). Although differences in reabsorption rates are demonstrable both in the presence and absence of the parathyroid gland, the earlier component appears to be less responsive to PTH than transport occurring in the later part of the tubule (Dennis et al. 1979). Though PTH increases excretion of phosphate by inhibiting phosphate reabsorption, the mechanism of inhibition is not known. There may be a small component reabsorbed in the distal convoluted tubules which is also influenced by the parathyroid. Dennis suggests that vitamin D in the form of 25-(OH)$_2$D$_3$ or 1,25-(OH)$_2$D$_3$ may influence phosphate excretion. How far this is a direct effect or whether it is mediated via effects on serum calcium and circulating PTH is uncertain. Reabsorption also appears to be highly dependent on the presence of sodium. This interaction between sodium and phosphate is not at present clear. It has been suggested that the link between phosphate and sodium may be that phosphate follows sodium as the counter ion. When the proximally rejected sodium phosphate reaches the distal tubule most of the sodium is reabsorbed but the distal tubular cell is relatively impermeable to phosphate which (accompanied by potassium and hydrogen) passes out into the urine (Staub, Hamburger, and Goldberg 1972).

3.5. Factors affecting renal reabsorption in kidney

Phosphate reabsorption is increased by growth hormone and in hypoparathyroidism, and in phosphate deprivation. It is diminished in hyperparathyroidism and in several inherited or acquired renal tubular disorders.

8. The Movement of Ions in and out of the Skeleton

STUDIES of the movement of ions in and out of the skeleton may be divided for convenience of discussion into two groups.

(i) In the first group are studies concerned with the overall pattern of uptake and retention of ions into the skeleton, the pattern of their distribution within the skeleton and the pattern of their loss from the skeleton. Quite apart from their value in clinical and physiological studies of calcium metabolism such studies are important to an understanding of the possible hazards dependent on the uptake of the bone-seeking radionuclides, which may reach the blood stream and finally deposit in bone.

(ii) In the second group are studies concerned with the maintenance of mineral homeostasis and the part that the osteogenic cells, under the influence of hormones, may play.

The maintenance of mineral homeostasis in the blood, particularly of Ca^{2+} and phosphate, is essential for the proper functioning of many cellular activities. It is achieved by the interaction of absorption from the gut, excretion by the kidney, and loss or increased uptake of Ca^{2+} from, or into, the skeleton. This interaction is under the control particularly of the parathyroid hormone, of vitamin D and its metabolites, and possibly calcitonin (see p. 138). PTH and calcitonin are considered to be the fast-acting components of the regulatory system (minute to hours), while vitamin D is responsible for adaptation over longer times (hours to days) (Russell 1976). Other hormones, however, play a part, largely indirectly through their effect on vitamin D metabolites (see p. 138).

1. THE OVERALL PATTERN OF MOVEMENT OF IONS

The earliest studies of the movement of calcium ions into and out of the skeleton were based on balance studies in which the difference between dietary intake and excretion of calcium was derived over a prescribed period. Such studies were inevitably beset with considerable experimental errors and will not be discussed further.

More recently, extensive use has been made of radioactive tracers and associated data analysis. Radioactive isotopes of the alkaline earths, notably

[85]Sr (Reeve and Hesp 1976; Reeve, Hesp, and Wootton 1976) have been used experimentally as a tracer for calcium and much information about the behaviour of the alkaline earths in animals and man has resulted from such studies. Another important source of information has been the study of the metabolism and bone deposition of [226]Ra after ingestion by radium dial painters and radium chemists and patients treated with radium (Vaughan 1973).

1.1. Use of radioactive tracers

In their original studies of calcium kinetics using radiocalcium, Bauer, Carlsson, and Linquist (1955, 1961) proposed that the rate of new bone formation, i.e. the accretion rate, A, could be measured after an intravenous injection of radiocalcium by its disappearance from the plasma and recovery in the excreta. They assumed that plasma calcium equilibrated with the exchangeable pool in bone and soft tissue and that accretion removed calcium from this pool at a steady rate. In the steady state, accretion was assumed to be balanced by resorption, implying that the subject was in exact calcium balance. Further work indicated, however, that this simple model could not be accepted. It provided considerable overestimates of the rate of bone turnover in man when compared with histomorphometric and radiotoxicity data (Marshall et al. 1972), and owing to the limited time span of most of these studies, slow exchange processes, which could be observed autoradiographically, were included in 'accretion' (Marshall 1969).

Since the original studies of Bauer et al. (1955, 1961) a variety of models have been used to analyse calcium kinetic data. Some workers exploited the fact that the radioactive calcium remaining in the subject at known times after an intravenous injection could be fitted by multi exponentials and proposed a variety of corresponding compartmental models (Heaney and Whedon 1958; Aubert and Milhaud 1960; Heaney 1963, 1976a; Cohn, Bozzo, Jesseph, Constantinides, Huene, and Gusmand 1965; Neer, Berman, Fisher, and Rosenberg 1967; Harris and Heaney 1969; Gonick and Brown 1970; Massin, Vallee, and Savoie 1974).

Other workers have criticized this approach on the grounds that simpler and computationally more tractable models can be used employing other mathematical functions such as power functions or integral equations (Anderson, Emery, McAllister, and Osborn 1956; Marshall 1964; Burkinshaw, Marshall, Oxby, Spiers, Nordin, and Young 1969; Marshall 1969; Reeve, Wootton, and Hesp 1976).

The potential and limitation of these techniques have been discussed recently by Reeve and his colleagues (Jung, Bartholdi, Mermillod, Reeve, and Neer 1978; Reeve, Veall, and Wootton 1978). Indeed Jung and his colleagues (Jung et al. 1978) have compared various compartmental and non-compartmental models using six sets of data from normal subjects. They conclude that one of the most striking results of this comparison was the great difference in the rate of new bone formation, A, i.e. the accretion rate, and the size of the exchangeable calcium pool, using different models. In some cases the coefficient of variation for A exceeded 100 per cent. However, Heaney (1976a) has stressed the clinical value of kinetic techniques and concludes that it is resorption, not mineralization which is in general, the prime measurement in all kinetic models.

Some of the difficulties that arise in interpreting the results of experiments using radioactive tracers are probably dependent, in part at least, on differences in the behaviour of the alkaline earths which are used in such kinetic studies.

1.2. Behaviour of the alkaline earths

In the study of the movement of ions in and out of the skeleton most attention has been paid to calcium for obvious reasons. The total mass of bone in a 70 kg standard man is 5000 g and the total body calcium is 1000 g. In soft tissue the calcium content is only 0·4 per cent and in blood only 0·03 per cent

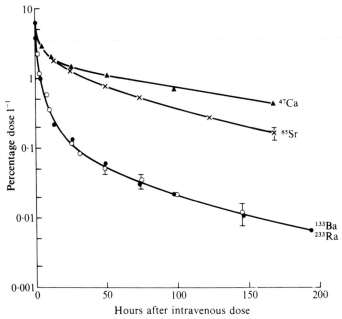

FIG. 8.1. Plasma concentrations for the four alkaline earths at various times after their respective intravenous dose. (From Harrison *et al.* (1966) by courtesy of authors and publishers.)

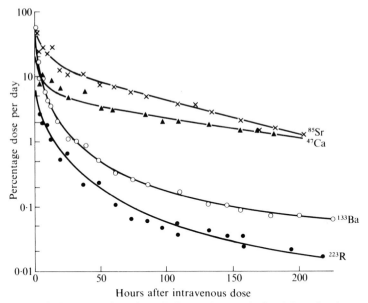

F<small>IG</small>. 8.2. Rate of urinary excretion of the alkaline earths over the first 8 days after the respective dose. (From Harrison *et al.* (1966) by courtesy of authors and publishers.)

of body calcium (International Commission on Radiological Protection 1972). The amount of calcium, therefore, that could be involved in the movement of ions in and out of the skeleton is large.

Broadly speaking, the four alkaline earths, calcium, strontium, barium, and radium follow a similar pattern of distribution in the skeleton. They are known as volume seekers since they are found throughout the bone mineral, but whereas the calcium content of the skeleton of standard man is 1000 g, the strontium content is about 300 mg, barium about 20 mg and radium occurs only as a trace element (Barnes *et al.* 1961; Harrison *et al.* 1967).

Though the patterns of absorption, excretion, and skeletal deposition of the alkaline earths in man have much in common, there are important differences between the way they are retained and further differences in their retention in different individuals. It is important to recognize this, especially, if experimentally radioactive strontium is used as a tracer for calcium.

The results of pooled short-term observations on several individuals indicate that strontium and calcium are largely excreted in the urine and barium and radium in the faeces (Harrison, Carr, Sutton, and Rundo 1966). In Fig. 8.1 the plasma concentration of the four alkaline earths at various short time intervals after an intravenous injection is shown. Figure 8.2 shows the rate of urinary excretion and Fig. 8.3 the percentage of the injected dose excreted over the first ten days. The difference between two individuals in

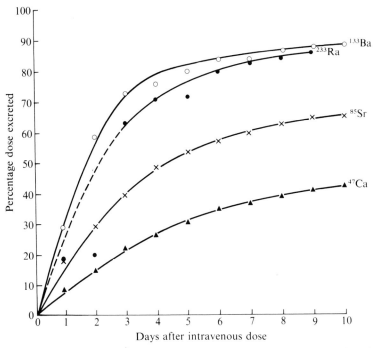

FIG. 8.3. Percentage of the respective dose excreted over the first 10 days. Ratio of total faecal to total urinary excretion after 8 days.

^{47}Ca	^{85}Sr	^{133}Ba	^{223}Ra
0·48	0·25	9·0	36

(From Harrison et al. (1966) by courtesy of authors and publishers.)

total retention of ^{45}Ca is shown in Fig. 8.4. Though the urinary excretion of calcium was very similar the faecal excretion differed by a factor of about two, thus giving a different retention pattern for the two individuals (Carr et al. 1973). Recently, a further analysis of the retention of the four radionuclides has indicated that turnover rates in bone for the four radionuclides are similar, and that differences in their late retention arise predominantly from differences in their early clearance from labile body pools (Newton, Rundo, and Harrison 1977). The data on which this conclusion is based is shown in Table 8.1 (Newton et al. 1977). The graph in Fig. 8.5 shows retention curves for calcium, strontium, barium, and radium between 6 days and 388 days expressed as three-component exponential functions with the parameters given in Table 8.1. Component 1, in the table, in the range 2·8–5·0 days is most probably related to the clearance of the activity from body fluids and soft tissues. Component 2, range 24–36 days, is tentatively attributed to the removal of labile activity from bone surfaces by an ion exchange process. Component 3 of half life 1100 days is assumed to be associated predominantly

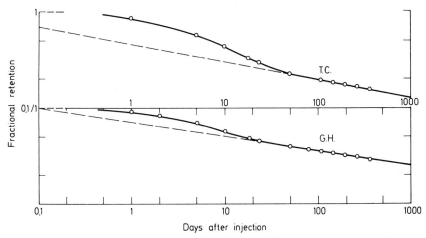

FIG. 8.4. Logarithmic plots of the fractional retention of ^{45}Ca against time (in days) for two subjects. (From Carr *et al.* (1973) by courtesy of authors and publishers.)

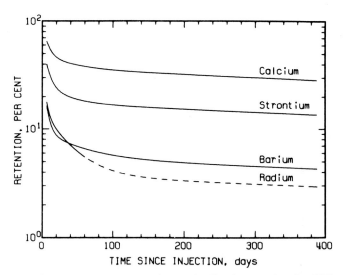

FIG. 8.5. Retention of calcium, strontium, barium, and radium between days 6 and 388 expressed as three-component exponential functions with the parameters given in Table 8.1. The dashed portion of the curve for radium indicates an extrapolation beyond the range of experimental observations. (From Newton *et al.* (1977) by courtesy of authors and publishers.)

TABLE 8.1

Parameters of three component exponential functions fitted to retention of calcium, strontium, barium, and radium in subject GEH, and excretory plasma clearance rates

Nuclide	Reference (original data)	Period after injection (days)	Component 1		Component 2		Component 3		EPC§ (1/day)
			%	Biological half-life (days)	%	Biological half-life (days)	%	Biological half-life (days)	
^{45}Ca*	Ca 73	6–388	41·9±1·4	4·9±1·4	13·1±1·5	29·5±4·0	35·9±0·4	1118±72	5·8
^{85}Sr†	Ru66	6–388	35·1±3·8	5·0±1·0	8·7±2·7	24·4±10·0	17·2±0·9	1118±450	10·9
^{133}Ba†	This study	6–388	22·5±1·9	3·6±0·3	4·2±0·2	35·9±4·4	5·4±0·2	1124±148	117
^{223}Ra*	Ha67	6–60	22·0±3·2	2·8±0·4	10·8±0·3	24·2±4·2	3·7±0·6	(1120†)	136

* Retention derived from measurements of excretion.
† Retention derived from body radioactivity measurements.
‡ Assumed value (mean of values for Ca, Sr, and Ba).
§ Total excretory plasma clearance at day 6, calculated from the time derivative of the three-component exponential function with the parameters shown, and measured concentrations in plasma (Ha67).

From Newton et al. (1977) by courtesy of authors and publishers.

with the turnover of activity bound in trabecular bone. Further analysis of the data for barium suggests there may be a fourth component possibly associated with removal from cortical bone.

The relatively long physical half-life of ^{133}Ba ($T_{1/2} = 10$ y) allowed whole body measurement to be continued for 15 years after the injection. Analysis of the retention curve over this period indicates a fourth component of biological half life about 8000 days which might well be associated with the removal of ^{133}Ba from cortical bone.

Thus experimental evidence has shown marked differences in the whole body retention of the four alkaline earths; while calcium and strontium are largely excreted in the urine following intravenous administration and the renal clearance of strontium is some three times that of calcium, barium, and radium are largely excreted in the faeces (Fig. 8.3). It is therefore evident that in *short term* studies strontium cannot be regarded as a good marker or as an alternative for calcium. Indeed there may also be a discriminating factor against strontium, relative to calcium, in the uptake from blood to bone in man, as there is in the rabbit (Kshirsagar *et al.* 1966; Lloyd 1968) (see p. 97). However, the results of *long term* investigations of body retention of the four alkaline earths suggest that these marked differences in whole-body retention, i.e. the retention in bone, are largely due to differences in the rates of clearance from plasma and soft tissue. When calcium, strontium or barium are incorporated into bone, however, they all appear to behave in a similar way. This is well illustrated by the close agreement in the value derived for the biological half-life of component 3 (in Table 8.1). These results suggest that strontium or barium, and may be even radium, is a suitable tracer for calcium when incorporated into bone, i.e. their turnover rates are then indistinguishable. Indeed Reeve and his colleagues (Reeve and Hesp 1976; Reeve, Hesp, and Wootton 1976) claim that ^{85}Sr is an adequate tracer for calcium for the study of skeletal kinetics provided that appropriate measures are taken to allow for the differences in their clearances from tissues other than bone.

The recent findings of Hauschka and his colleagues (Hauschka, Lian, and Gallop 1978) that one of the calcium-binding glycoproteins of bone appears to discriminate between calcium, strontium, and barium is perhaps of interest in view of this conclusion. Osteocalcin has a strong affinity for calcium apatite but not for barium or strontium. There is no information about radium, (p. 74).

In 1972 Marshall and his colleagues published models for the behaviour of the alkaline earth in adult man based on the kinetic and autoradiographic evidence then available. Papworth and Vennart have derived a simplified model applicable also to children and adults (Papworth and Vennart 1973). The predictions of the Marshall model for calcium are shown in Fig. 8.6. Similar results are given by the authors for radium, strontium, and barium. These models have proved useful, but in view of the recent actual observa-

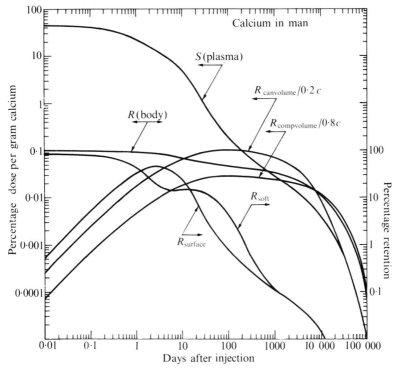

FIG. 8.6. Summary graph for calcium as of 30 December 1970. Arrows show which functions
are to be read on right-hand scale, and which on left. The whole body curve can be read on
both scales (with whole body calcium $c = 1000$ g). (From Marshall *et al.* (1972) by courtesy of
the publishers.)

tions on the long-term retention of barium already discussed (Newton *et al.*
1977), are perhaps in need of some revision, particularly in relation to barium,
as discussed by Harrison (1980).

1.3. Variability in different bones

Though most kinetic studies are concerned with the whole skeleton, it is
essential to remember that the behaviour of different parts of the skeleton as
far as the movement of ions is concerned, appears to be very different. In
considering the retention of alkaline earths in different bones, the Marshall
model (Marshall *et al.* 1972), for simplicity, divides bones into cancellous
and compact. But the 'turnover' rates in the movement of calcium and other
ions in and out of the body have been shown to be very different in different
bones. For example, in certain parts both of the long bones and of the skull,
these differences may have important pathological significance (Owen and

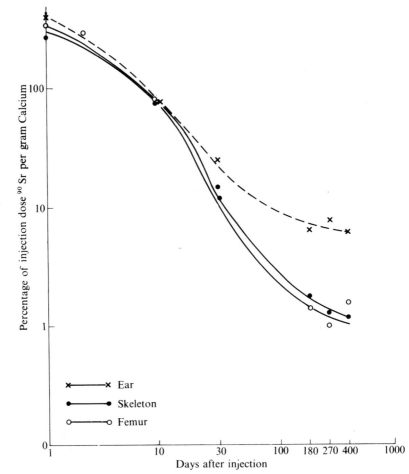

FIG. 8.7. Percentage injection dose ^{90}Sr per gram Ca in the skeleton, femur, and 'ear bone' of rabbits killed at different time-intervals after an intraperitoneal injection ($500\,\mu\text{Ci}\,\text{kg}^{-1}$) at 2 days old. (From Vaughan and Williamson (1969) by courtesy of authors and publishers.)

Vaughan 1959a,b; Kshirsagar, Vaughan, and Williamson 1965; Vaughan and Williamson 1967, 1969; Harris and Schlenker 1977–8).

The most recent figures for the relative incidence of osteosarcoma and carcinoma in humans carrying a significant radium burden, indicate that carcinomas of the sinuses of the skull are common and are likely to increase since the latent period for the epithelial tumours tends to be considerably longer than that for bone tumours (Littman, Kirsch, and Keane 1977–8). Experimental work with rabbits given ^{90}Sr suggests that this high incidence is in part dependent on the slow 'turnover rate' of alkaline earths in the bones of the skull, resulting in a high retention of the radionuclides (Kshirsagar *et al.* 1965; Vaughan and Williamson 1967, 1969). In the case of human patients exposed to radium, retention of radon in the enclosed space of the sinuses is also a contributory factor. Evans and his colleagues (Evans, Keane, Kolenkow, Neal, and Shanahan) reported in 1969 that the inner surface of the frontal bone of one patient who developed a carcinoma of his frontal sinus had a significantly higher ^{226}Ra concentration than the skeletal average elsewhere in the body. In the case of the rabbits given ^{90}Sr ($500 \, \mu\text{Ci kg}^{-1}$) when 2-days-old, measurement of the ^{90}Sr retained in the femur, the rest of the skeleton and the ear bone, as illustrated in Fig. 8.7, shows a significant retention in the ear bone. Measurement of the accumulated radiation dose in rads by an autoradiographic technique in another group of rabbits who developed osteosarcoma both in their ear bones and in mid-diaphysis of the femur, again shows a high radiation dose in those areas of bone where tumours were present.

1.4. Strontium

The behaviour of strontium in bone has already been discussed (pp. 128, 129).

1.5. Radium

All human bone is contaminated with trace amounts of radium and other α-emitters (Turner, Radley, and Mayneord 1958) ingested with food and water. The levels appear to remain constant throughout life, and there is no evidence that the amounts found are sufficient to cause any pathological condition even in areas where the water content is somewhat higher than the usual level (Marinelli 1958).

Particular attention has been given to the kinetic studies of radium in the skeleton, since there is a large population contaminated with radium available for study, and a large population still at risk in the uranium mining industry. The retention of ^{226}Ra in the skeleton is prolonged, as is shown in Fig. 8.8: an autoradiograph of a complete tibia cross-section from a patient with radium poisoning, given ^{226}Ra therapeutically for 1 year at the age of 46 years, who died 36 years later with an estimated body burden of $10 \, \mu\text{Ci}$. The different curves arrived at for whole body retention in man are shown in Fig. 8.9, in which the Marshall model is shown by the heavy curve. For further discussion of these curves and their variation from one another, the report of Marshall and his colleagues should be consulted (Marshall, Lloyd, Rundo, Liniecki, Marotti, Mays, Sissons, and Snyder 1972).

There is a relatively high retention of radium in soft tissues immediately after injection, 11·8 per cent at 3 days, which may explain some of the discrepancies noted in the early part of the curves of whole body retention. This

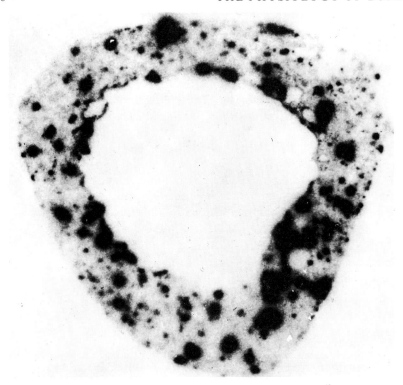

FIG. 8.8. A no-screen autoradiograph of a complete tibia cross-section from a case of radium poisoning (Case 118) given radium therapeutically for 1 year at age 46 years, estimated body burden 10 μg at death 36 years later. Note hot spots and diffuse reaction. (From Rowland and Marshall (1959) by courtesy of author and publishers.)

emphasizes the importance of the conclusions reached by Newton and his colleagues (1977) about the differences in early clearance from labile body pools of the alkaline earths.

1.6. Barium

The behaviour of barium has already been discussed on p. 132. It is of interest to note Ellsasser, Farnham, and Marshall (1969) have reported that the retention of barium on bone surfaces was much longer (certainly up to 6 days) than the retention of calcium, particularly round Haversian canals (Ellsasser *et al.* 1969).

2. THE PART PLAYED BY OSTEOGENIC CELLS IN THE MOVEMENT OF IONS

The part played by the osteogenic cells in the movement of ions in and out

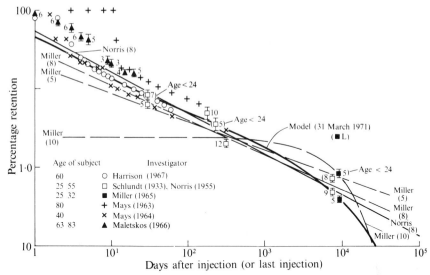

Fig. 8.9. Radium retention in whole body. Summary of virtually all data available for adult man. The heavy curve represents the Marshall model. Most of the points lie above the model curve for the first 1–2 days because no correction for faecal decay has been made. (From Marshall *et al.* (1972) by courtesy of the publishers.)

of the skeleton is extremely complicated. It has already received some consideration in Chapter 2, where the possible importance of both the osteoblast and the osteocyte in the movement of Ca^{2+} was discussed.

Many workers have studied the movement of ions in bone chips or bone powder and have ignored the important fact that both matrix and bone cells may be involved. For instance, Harrison and his colleagues (Harrison, Howells, and Pollard 1967) studied the uptake and elution of ^{45}Ca, ^{85}Sr, ^{133}Ba, and ^{223}Ra in rat bone powder. They found an increased retention of barium and radium compared to strontium and calcium; the exact reverse of that which occurs in *in vivo* experiments and could offer no explanation. The more recent work of Neuman and his colleagues suggests that this unexpected result may have been due to the fact that the cells and their membranes had been disturbed. They (Scarpace and Neuman 1976*a,b*) have emphasized how, in studying the movement of ions in relation to bone in culture, it is essential to use tissue where cells and their membranes are intact rather than cut bones or bone pieces. Embryonic bone in organ culture has in their hands proved valuable (see p. 14).

The factors that are recognized as controlling the activities of the osteogenic cells as far as mineral homeostasis is concerned are parathyroid hormone, possibly calcitonin and vitamin D metabolites, the action of which are altered in response to changes in plasma ionized calcium concentration (and phosphate in the case of vitamin D). Other hormones, e.g. thyroid hormones, growth hormone, adrenal and gonadal steroids have an effect on calcium metabolism but their secretion is determined primarily by factors other than changes in plasma calcium and phosphate. The importance of these factors is discussed in detail in Chapters 9 and 10.

2.1. Acute response to changes in plasma Ca^{2+}

It has become increasingly clear that the minute to minute or acute movement of ions in and out of the skeleton required to maintain a steady level of Ca^{2+} in the plasma and extracellular fluid, is probably achieved by the action of the osteoblast osteocyte system. How far this is entirely mediated through the parathyroid hormone as postulated by Talmage and his colleagues (Talmage and Grubb 1977), and how far it is dependent on the passive non-energetic influx and largely passive efflux, suggested by Neuman (Neuman, Neuman, and Myers 1979a,b) remains to be determined.

The study of Rowland (1966) on exchangeable bone calcium indicates that there is a constant exchange of Ca^+ ions on bone surfaces while a steady level of ionized calcium in plasma is maintained. Any minute-to-minute regulation by parathyroid hormone through the bone cells and kidney excretion he considers is superimposed on this exchange. Within seconds of a fall in plasma Ca^{2+} there is an increase in plasma PTH which decreases as Ca^{2+} rises (Russell 1976). Russell suggests this Ca rise is partly a passive process but that there is also a contribution from changes in PTH mediated osteolysis (see p. 156). There may also be an effect on the osteoblast since this cell is known to serve as a store for calcium and is also known to have surface receptors for PTH and to be influenced by the hormone (see p. 156).

In man, calcitonin is probably without effect on this minute-to-minute regulation under normal conditions, though it may play a bigger part in animals (Russell 1976).

2.2. Chronic response to disturbance of plasma Ca^{2+}

The response to prolonged changes in calcium metabolism inducing changes in plasma Ca^{2+} is mediated, not only by the bone cells, but also by changes in vitamin D metabolism and consequently in intestinal absorption of Ca^{2+}. A sustained fall in plasma calcium will result in increased parathyroid activity stimulating osteoclastic resorption and an increase $1,25\text{-}(OH)_2D_3$ synthesis, which in turn will both increase the intestinal absorption of calcium and the release of calcium from the skeleton (see p. 144). The action of the vitamin D metabolites on bone cells is at present confused though $1,25\text{-}(OH)_2D_3$ appears to have a clear effect on bone resorption (see p. 147).

9. Biological Factors in Mineral Homeostasis

The control of mineral homeostasis in both cells and body fluid is extremely complex, and many different factors are involved. Bone plays its part as the result of action by the metabolites of vitamin D, the parathyroid hormone (PTH) and calcitonin. The secretion of these hormones is altered in response to changes in plasma ionized-calcium and phosphate concentration. Other hormones, the thyroid, growth hormone, and the adrenal and gonadal steroids influence skeletal growth and development, and have effects on calcium metabolism, but their secretion is determined primarily by factors other than changes in plasma calcium and phosphate. The major sites of action of vitamin D, parathyroid hormone, and calcitonin are shown in Fig. 9.1.

1. VITAMIN D

1.1. Chemistry

Though still spoken of as vitamin D, it is now recognized that as an effective physiological agent vitamin D and its metabolites act as a steroid hormone.

In 1919 Mellanby showed that rickets can be produced by dietary manipulation and that this disease can be prevented by the administration of cod liver oil. Antirachitic substances were detected in several natural oils in 1925, and were designated vitamin D.

Cholecalciferol, or vitamin D_3, reaches the body in diets containing oily fish, eggs, animal livers, and dairy products. It is also formed in the skin by the action of sunlight on 7-dehydrocholesterol.

Holick et al. (1979) have recently described the skin as a unique endocrine organ responsible for the photobiosynthesis of vitamin D_3. When the epidermis is exposed to ultraviolet light skin stores of 7-dehydrocholesterol (provitamin D) are photolyzed, principally to previtamin D_3. Vitamin D_3 has greater than 1000 times higher affinity than previtamin D_3 for vitamin-D-binding protein, suggesting that the vitamin-D-binding protein preferentially transports vitamin D_3 from the skin into the circulation as cholecalciferol, leaving previtamin D_3 behind to continue its thermal equilibration to vitamin D_3 (Holick, McNeill, Clark, Holick, and Potts 1979). If it reaches the

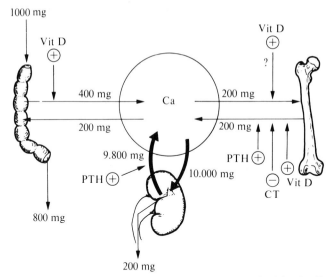

FIG. 9.1. Major sites of action of vitamin D, parathyroid hormone and calcitonin. (From Russell (1976) by courtesy of author and publishers.)

blood stream from the diet, cholecalciferol is absorbed in the intestine, either primarily in the upper intestinal tract (Schachter, Finkelstein, and Kowarsi 1964) or in the distal small intestine (Norman and DeLuca (1963)) depending on the form in which it is administered. Absorption in the small intestine probably requires the presence of bile salts (Avioli 1969). Before it can become biologically active, cholecalciferol has to be metabolized (DeLuca 1972; Avioli and Haddad 1973; Omdahl and DeLuca 1973). It is first converted in the liver to a 25-hydroxylated derivative (25-(OH)D$_3$). Whether this step is controlled by feedback inhibition is uncertain. It is then further hydroxylated in the kidney to 1,25-(OH)$_2$D$_3$ or 24,25-(OH)$_2$D$_3$, or even further to 1,24,25-(OH)$_3$D$_3$ (see Figs 9.2 and 9.3).

For a detailed discussion of the chemistry of vitamin D and its metabolites the reviews by Bell (1978), Holick and DeLuca (1978), and DeLuca (1977, 1978) should be consulted. The major site of storage of cholecalciferol itself appears to be adipose tissue. Little if any is stored in the intestine. Muscle and bone account for approximately 60 per cent or more of the accumulation of a single dose of calciferol and its metabolites. Little is excreted in the urine. The primary route of excretion is through the bile and hence the faeces (Holick and DeLuca 1978).

Under all normal physiological circumstances 25-(OH)D$_3$ is generally accepted as the most abundant circulating compound. It has a half-life of 2–3 weeks, once formed, which is much longer than that of ingested chole-

Vitamin D

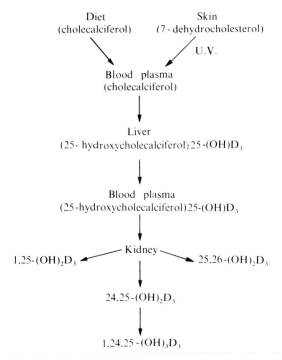

Diet
(cholecalciferol)

Skin
(7 - dehydrocholesterol)

U.V.

Blood plasma
(cholecalciferol)

Liver
(25- hydroxycholecalciferol) 25 -(OH)D$_3$

Blood plasma
(25 -hydroxycholecalciferol) 25-(OH)D$_3$

Kidney

1,25-(OH)$_2$D$_3$ 25,26-(OH)$_2$D$_3$

24,25 -(OH)$_2$D$_3$

1,24,25 - (OH)$_3$D$_3$

Fig. 9.2. Diagram of vitamin D metabolism.

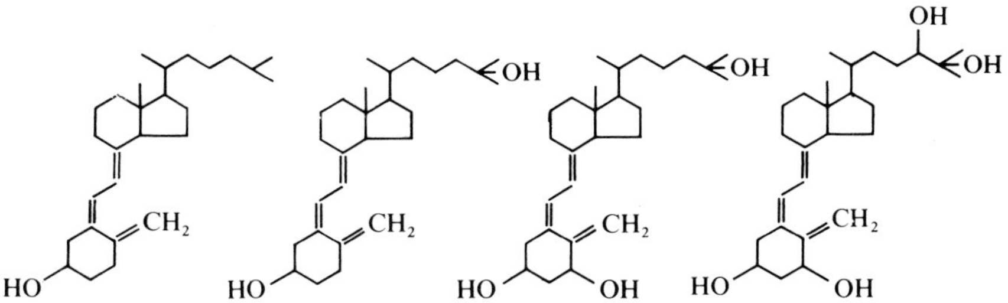

CH$_2$ CH$_2$ CH$_2$ CH$_2$

OH

HO   HO   HO   OH   HO   OH

Cholecalciferol
25 - hydroxycholecalciferol

1,25 -dihydroxycholecalciferol
1,24,25 - trihydroxycholecalciferol

Fig. 9.3. Structure of calciferol and some of its metabolites.

TABLE 9.1

Body weight and plasma concentration of calcium and inorganic phosphate of chicks treated with vitamin D derivatives

Treatment	Body weight (g)	Plasma Ca (mg per 100 ml)	Plasma Pi (mg per 100 ml)
Vitamin D_3	$264{\cdot}2 \pm 5{\cdot}3$	$10{\cdot}9 \pm 0{\cdot}40$	$6{\cdot}8 \pm 1{\cdot}22$
24,25-Dihydroxyvitamin D_3	$266{\cdot}7 \pm 9{\cdot}2$	$9{\cdot}4 \pm 0{\cdot}45$	$6{\cdot}3 \pm 0{\cdot}17$
24,25-Dihydroxyvitamin-D_3			
+ 1 hydroxyvitamin D_3	$289{\cdot}2 \pm 7{\cdot}9$	$10{\cdot}4 \pm 0{\cdot}22$	$6{\cdot}9 \pm 0{\cdot}31$
None	$211{\cdot}7 \pm 9{\cdot}0$	$6{\cdot}3 \pm 0{\cdot}12$	$5{\cdot}8 \pm 0{\cdot}17$

From Ornoy *et al.* (1978) by courtesy of authors and publishers.

calciferol (Parsons 1978). Individual plasma levels vary widely depending on diet and exposure to sunshine. Levels up to 80 ng/ml have been recorded, but the concentration must fall below 4 ng/ml before calcium metabolism is disturbed (Parsons 1978). The normal circulating level of $1,25{\text{-}}(OH)_2D_3$ is extremely low, reported figures between 32 ± 1 to 29 ± 2 pg/ml are given (Parsons 1978). It has a circulating half life in man of 14 hours (Mawer, Backhouse, Davies, Hill, and Taylor 1976). There are conflicting views as to the circulating level of $24,25{\text{-}}(OH_2)D_3$. Ornoy and his colleagues (Ornoy, Goodwin, Noff, and Edelstein 1978) think it the effective hydroxylated metabolite in normocalcaemic animals, as shown in Table 9.1, while rather lower levels have been reported by other workers (Haddad, Min, Walgate, and Hahn 1976; Taylor, de Silva, and Hughes 1977; Graham, Preece, and O'Riordan 1977). The three metabolites that appear at present to be of major regulatory significance are $25{\text{-}}(OH)_2D_3$; $1,25{\text{-}}(OH)_2D_3$ and possibly $24{\text{--}}25{\text{-}}(OH)_2D_3$.

In addition to the naturally occurring D_3 metabolites it has recently been shown that at least one synthetic vitamin D analogue, namely 1-α-hydroxy-cholecalciferol, can increase calcium absorption two- to threefold, raise serum calcium, and reduce serum alkaline phosphatase in patients with chronic renal failure in doses as low as 10 μg daily, as well as in the rachitic chick (Chalmers, Davie, Hunter, Szaz, Pelc, Kodicek 1973). This analogue is easy and simpler to make than $1,25{\text{-}}(OH)_2D_3$ and therefore has an important therapeutic future.

1.2. Regulation of vitamin D metabolism

Conversion of $25{\text{-}}(OH)D_3$ to $1,25{\text{-}}(OH)_2D_3$ is effected in the kidney by 1-α-hydroxylase, present only in renal mitochondria. Conversion to $24,25{\text{-}}(OH)_2D_3$ is controlled by a second hydroxylase, the 24-hydroxylase (DeLuca 1977). This latter enzyme has been demonstrated in human tissues other than the kidney (Haddad, Min, Mendelsohn, Slatopolsky, and Hahn 1977). The control of the production of $1,25\text{-}(OH)_2D_3$ is exerted by the integrated action of PTH, plasma phosphate levels, and $1,25\text{-}(OH)_2D_3$ itself.

1.2.1 THE EFFECTS OF PTH ON VITAMIN D_3 METABOLISM

The production of $1,25\text{-}(OH)_2D_3$ is stimulated by a low calcium diet resulting in hypocalcaemia and suppressed by administration of a high calcium diet as long as the parathyroid is intact. If the parathyroid glands are removed, hypocalcaemia results in excess production of $24,25\text{-}(OH)_2D_3$. Administration of PTH, however, restores the capacity to produce $1,25\text{-}(OH_2)D_3$ and correction of the hypocalcaemia.

In conditions of normal dietary intake the fraction of dietary calcium absorbed by the intestine is principally controlled by the circulating level of PTH through its modulating action on hydroxylation of calciferol in the kidney. Plasma levels of $1,25\text{-}(OH)_2D_3$ are almost doubled in primary hyperparathyroidism and halved in hypoparathyroidism (Haussler, Hughes, Baylink, Littledike, Cork, and Pitt 1977).

1.2.2. THE EFFECTS OF PHOSPHATE ON VITAMIN D_3 METABOLISM

Phosphate plays an important role in the regulation of $1,25\text{-}(OH)_2D_3$ biosynthesis (Haussler, Hughes, Baylink, Littledike, Cork, and Pitt 1977). Rats on a low phosphorus diet resulting in hypophosphataemia have a marked increase in serum and tissue $1,25\text{-}(OH)_2D_3$ even in the absence of the parathyroid glands. In response to hyperphosphatemia there is a significant reduction in plasma $1,25\text{-}(OH)_2D_3$.

Tanaka and DeLuca (1973) suggest that the renal tubular cell inorganic phosphorus level underlies the regulation of synthesis of $1,25\text{-}(OH)_2D_3$ in the kidney and that the parathyroid hormone and calcitonin regulate $1,25\text{-}(OH)_2D_3$ synthesis through their effects on renal cell inorganic phosphorus levels. The common denominator of the regulation of vitamin D metabolism in the kidney is, they suggest, cellular inorganic phosphorus levels. PTH, by inhibiting tubular phosphate reabsorption, may therefore reduce to low levels the tubular cell inorganic phosphorus levels and in this way bring about production of $1,25\text{-}(OH)_2D_3$.

1.2.3. AUTOREGULATION OF $1,25\text{-}(OH)_2D_3$

It has been suggested that $1,25\text{-}(OH)_2D_3$ in some way controls its own synthesis. There is a marked increase in renal $1\text{-}\alpha\text{-hydroxylase}$ activity in vitamin D deficiency states (Fraser and Kodicek 1970; Drezner and Harrelson 1979) and a disappearance of this enzyme activity after administration of physiological amounts of $1,25\text{-}(OH)_2D_3$ or $1\text{-}\alpha\text{-}(OH)_2D_3$.

1.2.4. OTHER HORMONES

Attempts have been made to implicate other hormones in the regulation of $1,25\text{-}(OH)_2D_3$ production. It is probable that at least in some cases their apparent action is secondary to permutations of calcium, phosphates, and PTH.

1.2.5. SEX HORMONES

It has recently become apparent that both oestrogens and androgens have an important effect on the metabolism of $25\text{-}(OH)D_3$ (see p. 194), more particularly oestrogen. The egg-laying hen has a high level of 1-hydroxylase in the kidney. A similar high level can be induced in the male bird by giving oestradiol, but not if the bird is castrated. Oestradiol stimulates the production of 1-hydroxylase, but suppresses the production of 24-hydroxylase. It is not at present clear how far a fall in oestrogen secretion at the menopause and lower levels with increasing age are possibly responsible for osteoporotic bone changes (Castillo, Tanaka, DeLuca, and Sunde 1977; Tanaka, Castillo, and DeLuca 1976).

1.3. Biological effects

The active metabolites of vitamin D_3 have three target organs: (1) the intestine; (2) the bone; and (3) muscle. The last is not for discussion here.

In several instances, notably in renal calcium reabsorption in the distal convoluted tubule of the kidney (Sutton, Harris, Wong, and Dirks 1977) and the transfer of calcium from the bone fluid compartment to the extra cellular fluid compartment (Holick, Garabedian, and DeLuca 1972), the active form of vitamin D, $1,25\text{-}(OH)_2D_3$, appears to work hand in hand with PTH, the two being interdependent on each other (Garabedian, Tanaka, Hollick, and DeLuca 1974; DeLuca 1978).

1.3.1. INTESTINAL ABSORPTION

1.3.1.1. *Calcium*

The early literature covering the investigation of the mechanism and control of calcium absorption in the intestine is too extensive to be discussed here. Orr and his colleagues noted in 1923 an excessive loss of calcium in the faeces of animals deprived of vitamin D and concluded the vitamin stimulates the absorption of calcium. This was confirmed by Nicolayson in the 1930s. Reviews of more recent experimental work and the part played by vitamin D metabolites are those of Norman (1978), Lawson (1978), Holick and DeLuca (1978). There is evidence that both $25\text{-}(OH)D_3$ and $24,25\text{-}(OH)_2D_3$ can stimulate absorption of calcium in the intestine (Kanis, Heynen, Russell,

Smith, Walton, and Warner 1977; Parsons 1978) but the important and most effective metabolite is $1,25\text{-}(OH)_2D_3$.

Norman concludes that the role of $1,25\text{-}(OH)_2D_3$ is firmly established in terms of its ability to stimulate or mediate an increased intestinal absorption, certainly of calcium and probably of phosphate, and that many of the 'black box' complications, illustrated in Fig. 9.4, for the multi-step process of transfer of these substances, have at least been identified as existing. There is, however, still confusion as to the exact processes underlying calcium absorption by the mucosal cells. Calcium is probably transferred by simple passive ionic diffusion, by active transport and by facilitated diffusion. The intestinal columnar epithelial cells have a unique morphology. The apical surface exposed towards the lumen is composed of a multitude of villi, thus increasing the surface area of the mucosa 600-fold, and is referred to as the brush border. A variety of carbohydrate hydrolases and an alkaline phosphatase are associated with this brush border (Norman 1978). Beneath the columnar epithelial and the goblet or mucus secretory cells, lie the vascular and lymphatic systems which also project into each villus, thus providing an efficient mechanism for the translocation of any substrate once it leaves the cell. The outermost surface of the columnar epithelial cell is covered with a filamentous polysaccharide coat, which may play a part in transferring ionic calcium (Norman 1978). It is known that $1,25\text{-}(OH)_2D_3$ is bound first in the cytosol and is rapidly transferred into the nucleus of the intestinal mucosal cell, where it binds to a specific binding site on chromatin, leading to the production of messenger RNAs that code for calcium transport proteins (see Fig. 9.4). These are then translated in the polysomes to the specific binding proteins described by Lawson and others (Drescher and DeLuca 1971; Wilson and Lawson 1977). These proteins are not the same as that originally described by Wasserman and Taylor in 1966. The protein described by Wasserman and his colleagues (Wasserman, Fullmer, and Taylor 1978) is extremely well characterized, but its importance in calcium transport in the intestine is still uncertain, since it is also present in many other tissues where its function is unknown, and it appears later at the brush border than the increased absorption of calcium-induced by $1,25\text{-}(OH)_2D_3$. Calcium finally leaves the mucosal cell from the inner surface at the same time as sodium enters as illustrated in Fig. 9.4.

1.3.1.2. *Phosphate*

$1,25\text{-}(OH)_2D_3$ also stimulates the transfer of phosphate across the ilium and jejunum, a process that is probably independent of the effects on calcium transport (Wasserman and Taylor 1973; Chen *et al.* 1974; Norman 1978). At least some of the phosphate transport dependent on $1,25\text{-}(OH)_2D_3$ is active (against an electrochemical gradient), but it is not at present clear whether facilitated diffusion, and a carrier mediated process are not also involved.

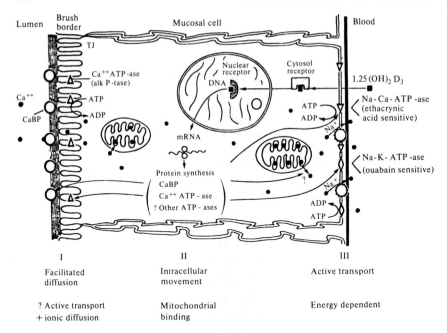

FIG. 9.4. Hypothetical intestinal mucosal cell to show some of the factors thought to be involved in calcium transport and in the stimulatory effect of 1,25-(OH)$_2$ vitamin D$_3$. CaBP=calcium binding protein; Ca^{2+} ATPase=calcium stimulated adenosine triphosphate. (From Coburn, Hartenbower, and Massvy (1973) by courtesy of authors and publishers.)

1.3.2. THE KIDNEY

1.3.2.1. *Hydroxylation of 25-(OH)D$_3$*

The kidney plays a key role in the metabolism of calciferol since it is the site of the hydroxylations which produce the active metabolites already described. Some at least of these metabolites, produced by the different hydrolases, exert an effect on the kidney. The possible autoregulation of 1,25-(OH)$_2$D$_3$ production has already been mentioned on p. 143.

1.3.2.2. *Excretion of calcium and phosphate*

Reabsorption of calcium, phosphate, and sodium in the renal tubules is probably influenced by calciferol metabolites. It has long been known that both the calcium-retaining and phosphaturic responses of the renal tubules to parathyroid hormone are diminished, though not abolished, in severe vitamin D deficiency (Sutton, Harris, Wong, and Dirks 1977).

Recent experiments indicate that if 1,25-(OH)$_2$D$_3$ is given to thyroparathyroidectomized rats renal reabsorption of calcium is increased (Steele, Engle, Tanaka, Lovenc, Dudgeon, and DeLuca 1975). Puschett and his colleagues (Puschett, Fernandez, Boyle, Gray, Amdahs, and DeLuca 1972) claim to have isolated a calcium-binding protein, in the kidney, which is decreased in vitamin D deficiency and increased after administration of the vitamin. How far these observations are significant, since 99 per cent of the filtered calcium is anyhow reabsorbed, is questionable. DeLuca (1978) concludes that $1,25\text{-}(OH)_2D_3$ and PTH 'working hand in hand, being inter-dependent on one another, stimulate calcium absorption in the distal con-voluted tubules.'

Parsons (1978) questions whether vitamin D plays a controlling role in the excretion of calcium and phosphate in the urine and considers it may only exert, what he calls, a modulating effect, the controlling influence being PTH.

1.3.3. SKELETON

Since the classical experiments of Mellanby (1919), it has been known that mineralization of bone is impaired in the absence of vitamin D, giving rise to rickets in infants and osteomalacia in adults. The underlying mechanisms involved in the production of this mineralization defect are still obscure. Calciferol and its metabolites are also involved in bone resorption.

In normal bone, $25\text{-}(OH)D_3$ is the major metabolite present, accounting for over 50 per cent of the total content, while the hormone itself accounts for less than 35 per cent (Barnes and Lawson 1978). Lawson and his colleagues have described two proteins in bone which appear to be able specifically to bind $25\text{-}(OH)D_3$. Autoradiographic studies of rat bone using tritiated $25\text{-}(OH)D_3$ have shown incorporation of radioactivity into hypertrophic cartilage cells of the epiphyseal growth plate, epiphyseal matrix, osteoid, osteoblasts, and osteocytes of metaphyseal bone spicules (Wezeman 1976), i.e. in areas of active mineralization. Weber and his colleagues (Weber, Pons, and Kodicek 1971) divided bones of rachitic chicks, after a dose of labelled cholecalciferol into epiphyseal, metaphyseal, and diaphyseal regions, and studied the uptake of different metabolites. He found $1,25\text{-}(OH)_2D_3$ in the nucleus of bone cells, while $25\text{-}(OH)D_3$ was present in the cytosol. No calciferol metabolites are found in osteoclasts (Barnes and Lawson 1978). On the other hand a specific binding protein for $1,25\text{-}(OH)_2D_3$ has been demonstrated in chick and rat bone cytosol (Kream, Jose, Yamada, and DeLuca 1977).

1.3.3.1. *Bone resorption*

It has been disputed as to whether vitamin D metabolites have any direct effect on bone, or whether the skeletal lesions associated with vitamin D deficiency are secondary to faulty absorption of calcium and phosphate. It is now accepted, however, that both $1,25\text{-}(OH)_2D_3$ and to a lesser extent 25-$(OH)_2D_3$ are involved in bone resorption (Tanaka and DeLuca 1973; Garabedian et al. 1974; Peacock, Gallagher, and Nordin 1974; Reynolds 1974; DeLuca 1974, 1976; Russell, Smith, Walton, Preston, Basson, Henderson, and Norman 1974; Reynolds, Pavlovitch, and Balsan 1976).

In organ culture as little as 65 pmol of $25\text{-}(OH)D_3$ per ml of culture fluid induced measurable bone resorption, whereas 500 times that amount of vitamin D produced no effect. $1,25\text{-}(OH)_2D_3$ works even more rapidly and efficiently (Holick, Schnoes, and DeLuca 1971; Haussler, Boyce, Littledike, and Rasmussen 1971; Raisz et al. 1972; Omdahl and DeLuca 1973; Reynolds 1973). $1,25\text{-}(OH)_2D_3$ in organ culture is approximately 100 times more effective on a weight basis than $25\text{-}OHD_3$ (Reynolds 1973). Further physiological doses of $25\text{-}(OH)D_3$ do not induce bone calcium mobilization in nephrectomized rats, whereas $1,25\text{-}(OH)_2D_3$ is always more effective than $1,24,25\text{-}(OH)_3D_3$ in calcium mobilization.

The relative effectiveness of some D_3 metabolites in inducing bone resorption are shown in Table 9.1. The effect of $1,25\text{-}(OH)_2D_3$ is in some way related to the effect of PTH. Although both hormones enhance calcium mobilization from bone independently in organ culture, conflicting data indicate that $1,25\text{-}(OH)_2D_3$ and PTH may have an interdependent role in the control of bone resorption and calcium mobilization in vivo (Garabedian et al. 1974; Reynolds 1974). The effects of $1,25\text{-}(OH)_2D_3$ in vivo require the presence of PTH, and conversely PTH effects on calcium mobilization are diminished in states of vitamin D deficiency (Fraser, Kooh, and Scriver 1967; Rasmussen and Bordier 1974). On the other hand the fact that PTH stimulates adenyl cyclase activity in bone cell fractions from vitamin-D-deficient rats indicates that PTH has a direct action on bone cells, though the hormone has no effect on calcium mobilization from the bones of such rats (Barnes and Lawson 1978). Barnes and Lawson (1978) consider that the parathyroid hormone independent bone-mobilizing action of $1,25\text{-}(OH)_2D_3$ mainly affects bone phosphate, but that some mobilization of calcium also occurs. Study of the appearance of osteoclasts present on bone surfaces in organ culture following exposure to $1,25\text{-}(OH)_2D_3$ showed no increase in number of osteoclasts, but an increase in the size of the ruffled border and of the clear zone. Of all the resorbing agents examined, only PTH increased the number of osteoclasts (Holtrop, Cox, Clark, Holick, and Anast 1979; Holtrop, King, Cox, and Reit 1979; Holtrop and Raisz 1979).

1.3.3.2. Bone mineralization

Though the defective mineralization of bone and cartilage in osteomalacia and rickets can be cured by the administration of calciferol, there is still uncertainty as to how this is brought about. Various proposals have been made.

1.3.3.2.1. *Action on intestinal absorption and bone resorption increasing Ca and P levels.* It has been suggested that lack of calcification in rickets and osteomalacia may perhaps be dependent upon reduced Ca and P_1 levels in the plasma consequent upon reduced bone mobilization and reduced intestinal absorption. Some experimental evidence to support this proposal is available. For example calcification can be observed in isolated bones from rachitic rats placed in normal serum, but not in serum from rachitic rats (Neuman and Neuman 1958). The infusion of inorganic phosphate into patients with nutritional rickets will result in mineralization though the osteomalacia of chronic renal failure does not respond to large intakes of calcium (Eastwood, Bordier, Clarkson, Tunchot, and de Wardener 1974), while Rasmussen and Bordier (1974) reported that osteomalacia patients only showed an increase in the calcification front after treatment with calciferol and not after phosphate infusion.

More recently Dickson and Kodicek (1979), using a density flotation technique, have shown in the bones of vitamin-D-deficient chicks, that exposure to calciferol metabolites induces the appropriate change from a low density calcified phase corresponding to the ACP phase described by Termine and Posner (1967), to a high density phase corresponding to hydroxyapatite, in the bones. The authors consider this is due to the action of calciferol on the bone-forming cells.

1.3.3.2.2. *Action on defective matrix.* Recently, Barnes and Lawson (1978) have suggested that there may be structural defects in the matrix in rickets and osteomalacia due to lack of calciferol that prevent normal mineralization. Changes in hydroxylation of bone collagen and in the cross links have been reported in the matrix of rickety animals and may be important in mineralization (Barnes and Lawson 1978). Further, Owen and her colleagues (Owen and Triffitt 1976) have noted a decreased retention of α_2HS glycoprotein and albumin in the bone of rabbits deficient in vitamin D. How far this is the cause or the effect of defective mineralization is not at present known. Raisz and his colleagues state that 'Vitamin D appears to be a growth hormone for the skeleton to the extent that in its absence growth as well as mineralization is impaired. However we found that $1,25\text{-}(OH_2)D_3$ inhibited collagen synthesis in organ culture . . . 1,24,25 Trihydroxyvitamin D_3 was also inhibitory . . . 25 hydroxyvitamin D_3 and 24,25 dihydroxyvitamin D_3 had no consistent effect on collagen synthesis.' (Raisz, Maina, Gworek, Dietrich, and Canalis 1978.) Other workers report an increase in proteoglycan synthesis in rachitic bone in response to calciferol (Hjerquist 1964a,b; Howell and Carlson 1965) and an increase in phospholipids (Wuthier 1971). Since the phospholipids associated with mineralization are derived from the matrix vesicles (see p. 88) which appear to be present in normal numbers in rachitic cartilage and since initiation of crystal formation can be induced at these sites, either *in vivo* by intraperitoneal administration of phosphate to vitamin D and phosphate deficient rats, or *in vitro* by incubation of rachitic cartilage in the presence of adequate phosphate and calcium (Anderson and Sajdera 1976), it would appear that synthesis and functioning of phospholipids is not affected by calciferol. It is at present controversial as to whether lack of vitamin D may, in part, be responsible for the high incidence of fractures of the neck of the femur in the elderly (Baker, McDonnell, Peacock, and Nordin 1979; Wootton and Reeve 1979).

1.3.3.2.3. *Importance of 24,25-(OH)$_2$D$_3$*. Until recently it has been assumed that the metabolites concerned in rickets are 25-(OH)D$_3$ or 1,25-(OH)$_2$D$_3$, but recently Ornoy and his colleagues have suggested that consideration should be given to 24,25-(OH)$_2$D$_3$.

When rachitic chicks are exposed to various treatments with metabolites of vitamin D, the presence of 24,25-(OH)$_2$D$_3$ is reported by Ornoy and his colleagues (Ornoy, Goodwin, Noff, and Edelstein 1978) to be essential for healing (see Table 9.1). In young growing chicks a combined treatment with the two renal hydroxylated metabolites of vitamin D was able to prevent the bone changes seen in rickets, and the bones were indistinguishable from those seen in birds treated with cholecalciferol. 1,25-(OH)$_2$D$_3$ alone was unable to prevent the changes characteristic of rickets, in spite of normal levels of calcium and phosphate. The authors suggest that 1,25-(OH)$_2$D$_3$ raises the calcium and phosphate level through its effect on intestinal absorption, while in some way 24,25-(OH)$_2$D$_3$ acts directly on bone to enable mineralization to occur. Its mode of action is not known.

1.3.4. THE PARATHYROID GLAND

The interaction of vitamin D metabolites and the parathyroid gland have already been discussed on p. 147. In addition to the long established interaction between calciferol and parathyroid hormone on calcium transport in the intestine, bone and kidney, the two hormones — one a steroid the other a peptide — interact at the level of the tissues in which they themselves are formed (Wasserman and Comar 1961).

Parsons (1978), having reviewed the experimental evidence, concludes that in some way calciferol is involved in the secretory responses of the parathyroid glands to circulating levels of plasma calcium. It appears unlikely to be the 1,25-(OH)$_2$D$_3$ metabolite that is involved, but it may be the 24,25-(OH)$_2$D$_3$ derivative. On the other hand, chick parathyroid glands contain a calciferol acceptor system capable of binding endogenous or exogenous 1,25-(OH)$_2$D$_3$ to a weight for weight concentration at least 4-fold higher than that in the circulating blood (Henry and Norman 1975).

2. THE PARATHYROID HORMONE (PTH)

In 1909 MacCallum and Voegtlin observed that surgical removal of the parathyroid glands was followed by a profound fall in blood calcium, associated with tetany and convulsions, which could be relieved by calcium administration. In 1925 Collip prepared a stable and physiologically active extract of beef parathyroid glands, which raised the serum calcium level and restored it to normal in parathyroidectomized dogs, so relieving their tetany. In their classic experiments in 1933 Hastings and Huggins carried out replacement transfusions in dogs using blood from which most of the calcium had been removed. Even when half the blood volume was replaced with this calcium depleted blood every 10 minutes it was extremely difficult to lower the blood calcium sufficiently to cause tetany, after the infusion was stopped. McLean in 1957 postulated a feedback mechanism to control secretion of the hormone, hypocalcaemia stimulating its production while hypercalcaemia suppresses it. Potts and his colleagues showed in 1968 that plasma PTH concentration has a linear inverse relationship to plasma calcium over a wide range (Potts, Buckle, Sherwood, Ramberg, Mayer, Kronfeld, Deftos, Care, and Aurbach 1968) (Fig. 9.5).

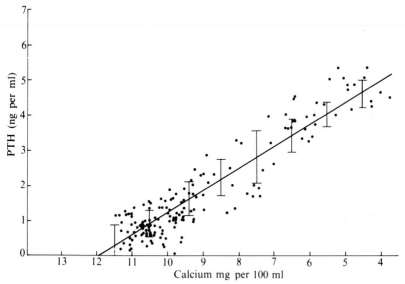

FIG. 9.5. Relationship between concentrations of blood calcium (treated as independent variable) and parathyroid hormone (dependent variable). Linear relationship derived from treating data as a simple regression by the least-squares method. Vertical lines and horizontal bars given standard deviation of observed from predicted hormone concentrations over each interval of linear function. (From Potts *et al.* (1968) by courtesy of authors and publishers.)

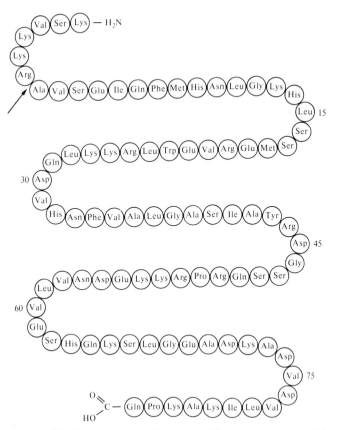

FIG. 9. 6. Structure of bovine proparathyroid hormone. The arrow between positions 6 and 7 shows the site of cleavage of the prohormone to produce PTH itself. (From Russell (1976) by courtesy of author and publishers.)

Today we recognize that calcium homeostasis is maintained by the interaction of a steroid hormone 1,25-$(OH)_2D_3$ and a peptide hormone, the parathyroid hormone. The latter acts both on the kidney and on bone. It probably has no direct effect on the intestinal absorption of calcium.

The possible interaction of vitamin D with the parathyroid gland has already been discussed (see p. 147). Calciferol is probably somehow involved in the secretory responses of the parathyroid gland to circulating levels of plasma calcium (Parsons 1978).

2.1. Chemistry

PTH is a single-chain polypeptide of 84 amino acids, devoid of disulphide linkages, with an amino-terminal and a carboxyl-terminal (see Fig. 9.6). The complete amino acid structure of bovine and porcine parathyroid hormone (PTH) is now known and considerable progress has been made in analysis of the amino-acid sequence of human PTH. In the human molecule, 80 out of 84 residues are known. The human is not greatly different from the bovine form shown, but the sequence of the carboxyl-terminal residue differs in human PTH (Rosenblatt, Segre, Tregear, Shephard, Tyler, and Potts 1978). The limited quantity of human PTH available has led to the use of immuno-assay techniques exclusively, rather than bioassay, to monitor the presence of different fragments in human plasma. Once it is released into the circulation the metabolic fate of PTH is extremely complex (Habener and Potts 1976). It exists in the glands as proparathyroid hormone, a chain with at least 90 amino acids. A further preprò PTH containing 115 amino acids has been isolated (Habener and Potts 1979a).

After secretion, the hormone undergoes further fragmentation into a number of immuno-reactive fragments. The dominant circulating form is a carboxy-terminal fragment, consisting of about two thirds of the intact gland secreted hormone (Canterbury and Reiss 1972; Segré, Habener, Powell, Tregear, and Potts 1972; Rosenblatt et al. 1978). This fragment is inactive. Only the first 29 amino acids, reading from the N-terminal end, are active (Segré, Rosenblatt, Reiner, Mahaffy, and Potts 1979; Rosenblatt et al. 1978; Habener and Potts 1979a). It is not yet clear whether fragments may be secreted from the gland into the blood stream in small amounts, as may the proparathyroid hormone itself.

PTH itself has a short half life. It is cleared from the blood stream within 30 minutes, and possibly within 8 minutes. The rate of disappearance is faster in rats than in dogs (Neuman et al. 1975). Smaller fragments have a longer half life. More recently Neuman and his colleagues (Neuman, Neuman, and Lane 1979) found both PTH and large metabolites were removed at the same rate, reaching a plateau in less than one hour.

Habener and Potts (1976) state 'in order to be active any circulating fragment of endogenous bovine parathyroid hormone must present a fragment from the amino terminal portion of the hormone sequence no shorter at the carboxyl end than residue 27, and no shorter at the amino end than residue 2.'

Using PTH labelled with iodine at amino acid 43, i.e. a region of the molecule *not* required for biological activity, Neuman and his colleagues found (Neuman et al. 1975) that high concentrations of intact bovine hormone and large metabolites occurred rapidly in kidney, liver, and bone in rats, dogs, and chickens. There was no deposition in the intestine. Degradation occurred rapidly in all three target organs. Fresh sera did not degrade the hormone rapidly or extensively. Degradation was rapid in the perfused liver. Working with organ cultures Gaillard and his colleagues (Herrman-Erlee, Gaillard, and Nijweide 1979) conclude there are two classes of PTH receptors in bone; one mediating the cAMP and lactate response, and one mediating the calcium and citrate response. The binding of bPTH 1-34 fragment to its receptor they found less stable than that of the bPTH 1-84 fragment.

2.2. Physiological stimulus to PTH secretion

The major physiological stimulus to secretion of PTH is a fall in ionized calcium (Ca^{2+}) concentration. A rise in plasma Ca^{2+} above normal suppresses PTH secretion.

A positive or negative calcium challenge in normal volunteers is accompanied by changes in the level of the circulating active PTH fragment (Chambers *et al*. 1979). Other ions are less important, but low levels of Mg^{2+} appear to impair the secretion of PTH and this, together with an impaired target organ response, may explain the hypocalcaemia occasionally seen in severe magnesium deficiency in man.

2.3. Effect of PTH on the kidney

The effect of PTH on the kidney is twofold. It controls the excretion of phosphate and calcium, and probably of other ions, and it controls the hydroxylation of $25\text{-}(OH)_2D_3$.

2.3.1. PHOSPHATE AND CALCIUM EXCRETION

Parathyroid hormone controls the excretion of both phosphate and calcium in the urine (Dennis *et al*. 1979). This controlling effect may be modulated by vitamin D metabolites (Parsons 1978; DeLuca 1978) (see p. 117). The first and most characteristic event to follow an injection of PTH is an increased excretion of phosphate. A marked drop in phosphate excretion follows parathyroidectomy. The increased excretion is due to an inhibition of phosphate reabsorption in the proximal convoluted tubules, probably in the latter part (Dennis *et al*. 1979) (see p. 123). PTH also increases the renal resorption of calcium which occurs in both proximal and distal tubules. Dennis and his colleagues (1979) are uncertain as to how far these effects are mediated through cyclic AMP. It is generally agreed, however, that all the effects of PTH on the kidney are mediated through cyclic AMP (see also p. 161). Recently, a physiologically important PTH receptor has been identified in chicken renal plasma membranes using the amino-terminal fragment GPTH 1-34 which activated adenylate cyclase (Nissenson and Arnaud 1979). The effect of PTH on the secretion of phosphate and cyclic AMP is shown in Fig. 9.7 (Chase and Aurbach 1967, 1968).

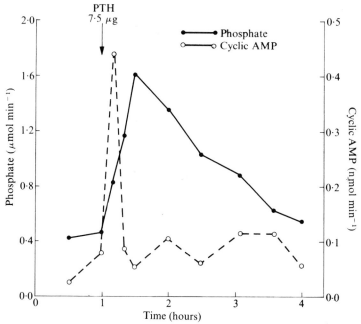

FIG. 9.7. The effect of parathyroid hormone on the excretion of phosphate and cyclic 3′,5′-AMP by a parathyroidectomized rat. Parathyroid hormone (7·5 μg) was injected intravenously over a 2-minute period at the point shown by the arrow. (From Chase and Aurbach (1968) by courtesy of the authors and the publishers.)

2.3.2. CONTROL OF HYDROXYLATION OF 25-(OH)D₃

The vital hydroxylation of 25-OHD₃ to 1,25-(OH₂)D₃ or 1,24,25-(OH)₂D₃ takes place in the kidney under the control of the parathyroid. Parathyroidectomy of rats on a diet low in calcium reduces the production of 1,25-(OH)₂D₃ from 25-(OH)₂D₃ to negligible levels. This is corrected by administration of parathyroid hormone (Fraser and Kodicek 1970, 1973) Garabedian *et al.* 1974; Holick, Kleiner-Bossaler, Schnoes, Kastern, Boyle, and DeLuca 1973; Stanbury, Hill, and Mawer 1973). The proximal convoluted tubules are the site where hydroxylation is thought to occur.

2.4. Effect on bone

The effect of PTH on bone is more complex than was originally thought. Its well recognized action is to increase bone resorption and to raise plasma calcium but there is good evidence that it may also move calcium into bone and increase osteoblastic activity. It has both an anabolic and catabolic effect (Gaillard, Wassenaar, and Wijke-Wheeler 1977). Apart from the chemical and experimental results to be discussed, this response of all bone cells is supported by the characteristic but variable histological picture found in primary hyperparathyroidism (Bordier and Tun Chot 1972).

A single section may show excessive resorption, osteoporosis, and osteitis fibrosa, as well as increased disorderly bone formation and incomplete calcification. Using a synthetic active fragment (1-34) (see p. 153) Gaillard and his colleagues (Gaillard, Wassenaar, and Wijke-Wheeler 1977) have shown that in organ culture a high concentration is catabolic while a low concentration is anabolic (Reeve 1978).

2.4.1. ANABOLIC EFFECT

All observers have noted that the anabolic effect of PTH is shown at low doses, especially if the hormone is given continuously. Parsons and his colleagues noted increased bone formation in dogs given extremely low doses continuously (Parsons, Darly, and Reit 1973; Parsons 1976). They have also reported improvement of osteoporosis in patients given similar treatment (Parsons, Meunier, Neer, and Reeve 1979). Bingham and her colleagues (Bingham, Brazell, and Owen 1969) noted an increase in RNA synthesis in both osteoblasts and preosteoblasts, 24 hours after the administration of parathyroid extract to young rabbits (see Fig. 9.8), while Kalu demonstrated increased matrix formation as shown by increased incorporation of (^{3}H) proline, and increased mineralization after 21 days treatment of thyro-parathyroidectomized rats with 50 units of PTH a day (Kalu, Doyle, Pennock, and Foster 1970). Gaillard and his colleagues (Herrman-Erlee *et al.* 1979) using organ culture techniques, have described, with low doses of bPTH (1-34), an increased maturation of cartilage cells, an increased number of active osteogenic cells, especially inside the primitive marrow cavity, resulting in some cases in heterotopic osteoid formation.

2.4.2. CATABOLIC EFFECT

In a classic paper in 1948 Barnicot described resorption by osteoclasts which occurred round parathyroid tissue grafted into mouse calvaria. Net removal of calcium from bone occurs in response to relatively high doses. Parsons (1976) considers there is very little experimental evidence on the role that PTH-induced osteolysis may play in normal physiology. He suggests that possibly in the face of a low calcium diet and possibly in the early hours of the morning the hormone may be increased in the circulation to prevent plasma calcium from falling.

Parathyroid hormone has at least two effects on calcium mobilization. It

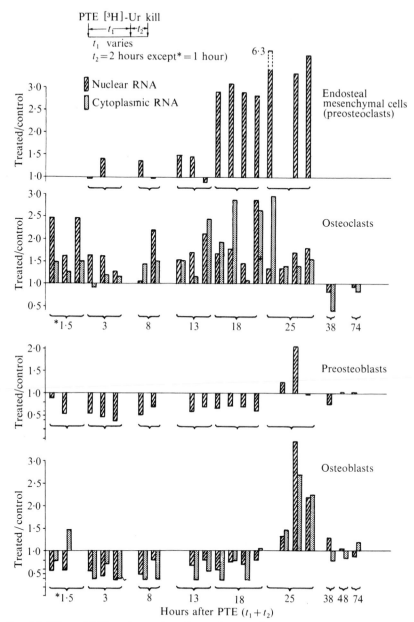

FIG. 9.8. Effect of PTE on the number of osteoclasts on the endosteal surface of young rabbit bone. (From Bingham et al. (1969) by courtesy of the authors and publishers.)

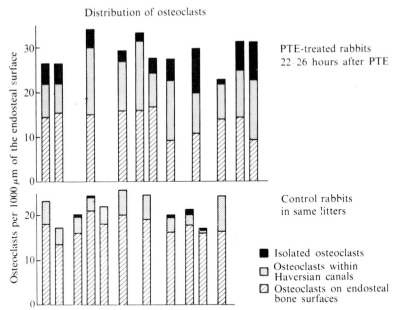

FIG. 9.9. Effects of PTE on incorporation of (^{3}H)uridine in different bone cell types in the mid-shaft of young rabbits. The amount of (^{3}H)uridine incorporated into nuclear and cytoplasmic RNA over a short period of time in different cell types was measured at various times after injection of PTE. Results were compared between PTE-treated and paired control animals in the same litter. Each bar, or pair of bars, in the histogram represents the ratio of the results from each pair of animals. Osteoblasts and preosteoblasts were studied on the periosteal surface and osteoclasts and mesenchyme cells on the endosteal surface of the mid-shaft of the femur of each animal. Results for different cell types from the same animals appear vertically above each other in the histograms. (From Bingham *et al.* (1969) by courtesy of authors and publishers.)

rapidly stimulates the translocation of calcium from bone to extracellular fluid as measured by the use of ^{45}Ca both *in vivo* and in tissue culture and it also promotes an increase both in the number and activity of the cells concerned with resorption. The immediate release of ^{45}Ca is thought by Talmage and his colleagues to be due to the action of the hormone on the osteocytes and lining cells on bone surfaces (see p. 41) leading to the movement of Ca^{2+} from bone fluid to extravascular and hence vascular fluid (Matthews and Martin 1971; Talmage 1970; Talmage and Grubb 1977).

This can be seen within two hours, but at least 24 hours must elapse before there is any histological evidence of increased resorption or an increased number of osteoclasts can be seen microscopically (Raisz and Niemann 1969; Bingham *et al.* 1969; Reynolds and Dingle 1970). In Fig. 9.8 is seen the effect of an injection of parathyroid extract on the number of osteoclasts on the endosteal surface of young rabbits' bones. In Fig. 9.9 are seen the effects of PTH on incorporation of (^{3}H) uridine in different bone cell types in the mid-shaft of young rabbits' femurs (Bingham *et al.* 1969), and in Fig. 9.10

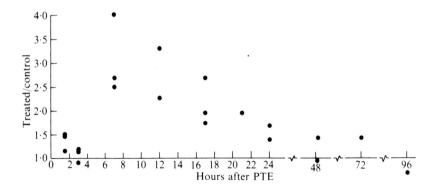

Effect of PTE on cytoplasmic RNA (osteoclasts)

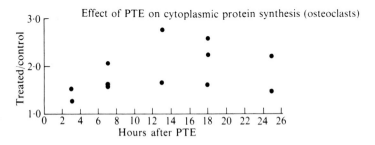

Effect of PTE on cytoplasmic protein synthesis (osteoclasts)

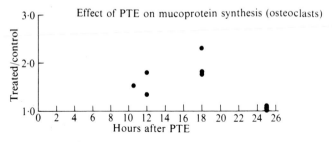

Effect of PTE on mucoprotein synthesis (osteoclasts)

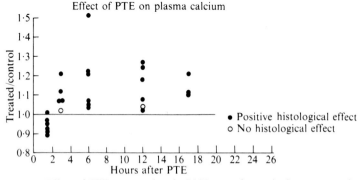

FIG. 9.10. Effect of PTE on cytoplasmic RNA, protein synthesis, mucoprotein synthesis in osteoclasts, and on the plasma calcium in young rabbits. (From Bingham (1968) by courtesy of the author.)

the effect on cytoplasmic RNA, protein synthesis and mucoprotein synthesis in osteoclasts and on the plasma calcium (Bingham 1968).

There is a considerable increase in both isolated osteoclasts and those within Haversian canals. In tissue culture the release of calcium is associated with histological changes in the osteoclasts and greatly increased resorption, which can be seen microscopically (Reynolds and Dingle 1970). Holtrop (Holtrop and Raisz 1979) has recently shown that PTH in organ culture, unlike prostaglandin and 1,25-$(OH_2)D_3$ increases the number of osteoclasts as well as enlarging the 'ruffled' border of existing osteoclasts.

2.4.3. OVERALL EFFECT ON BONE

It would appear likely, though this is difficult to prove experimentally, that PTH through both its anabolic and catabolic actions on bone, together with its action directly on the kidney and indirectly on intestinal absorption, serves under normal conditions to maintain a steady level of calcium in the plasma. The most recent evidence that this may be so comes from an analysis of the effects of administration of diphosphonates in Paget's disease (see p. 111). In this condition there is an unexplained excess of both resorption and apposition of bone. Treatment with diphosphonates results in a decreased action of both osteoblast and osteoclast function associated with a transient increase of circulating PTH (Meunier et al. 1979; Reitsma et al. 1980; van Breukelen et al. 1979; Frijlink et al. 1979).

2.5. Effect of PTH on the intestine

It was thought at one time that PTH had a direct effect on the absorption of calcium in the gut. It is now generally accepted that the intestinal absorption of calcium is controlled by 1,25-$(OH)_2D_3$, so that the effect of PTH can only be described as indirect through its control of hydroxylation of 25-OHD_3. There is no evidence that it exerts any effect directly on the gut (Parsons 1976). DeLuca (1977) has described it as having a modulating effect on intestinal adsorption through its effect on hydroxylation of 25-OHD_3.

2.6. Mode of action

2.6.1. BINDING SITES

It is now generally agreed that PTH does not enter the cell on which it acts but binds to appropriate receptors on the cell membrane. Such receptors have been identified in chicken renal plasma membranes (Nissenson and Arnaud 1979). In the case of bone it is thought that there are different binding sites for the initiation of calcium entry and calcium exit from the cell (see p. 154). Binding of hormone to receptors takes place in the region of

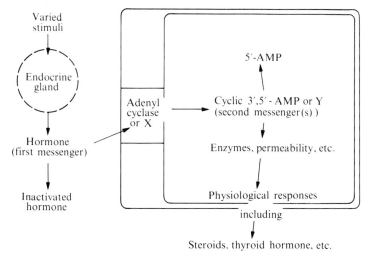

FIG. 9.11. Schematic representation of the second messenger concept. (From Robinson *et al.* (1971) by courtesy of authors and publishers.)

residues 15–30. Activation of the receptor as reflected in the activation of adenyl cyclase also requires the presence of NH_3-terminal amino acids 1-3 (Habener and Potts 1979*b*).

2.6.2. CYCLIC AMP

There is good evidence that the action of PTH on both bone and kidney is mediated through the adenyl cyclase mechanism, first described by Sutherland in 1965 as a mechanism which might explain the action of many hormones (Sutherland, Øye, and Butcher 1965). This mechanism is illustrated diagrammatically in Fig. 9.11. In 1968 Chase and Aurbach showed that the phosphaturic effect of an injection of PTH was preceded by a great increase in the excretion of cyclic AMP, and others have since shown that the phosphaturic effect could be mimicked by cyclic AMP or its dibutyril derivative but not by other nucleotides (Russell, Casey, and Fleisch 1968). At the same time Wells and Lloyd (1968) showed experimentally that drugs known to affect the levels of cyclic AMP in a variety of tissues will alter serum calcium levels. They therefore suggested that the level of cyclic AMP in bone cells determines the rate of mobilization of calcium and secondarily the level of serum calcium. Parathyroid hormone acts, then, as first messenger to increase cyclic AMP in both bone and kidney cells. This hypothesis receives support from the observations of many workers (Murad, Brewer, and Vaughan 1970; Melson, Chase, and Aurbach 1970; Segré *et al.* 1979). The renal cells involved are those in the tubules of the cortex and are quite distinct from those affected by vasopressin (Robison, Butcher, and Sutherland 1971).

The problem of binding to renal receptors, and the release of cyclic AMP has recently been further studied by Potts and his colleagues (Segré *et al.* 1979). Binding in canine renal cortical plasma membrane occurred only with biologically active fragments. Biologically inactive fragments, peptide hormones such as insulin, calcitonin, glucagon, and adrenocortical hormone do not bind significantly. An excellent correlation was found quantitatively between the relative binding affinity of intact hormone and several synthetic PTH agonists and their relative biologic potency in the adenylate cyclase assay using the same membrane preparations. Further, the relative binding efficiency of two synthetic PTH agonists correlated with their relative inhibiting potencies *in vitro*, providing evidence that some PTH analogues bind to the hormone receptor without stimulating adenylate cyclase and that the inhibitory properties of these agonists can be attributed to their affinity for the hormone receptor.

Rasmussen (1972) in his review of the cellular basis of mammalian calcium homeostasis concludes that PTH activates kidney and bone cells by an activation of membrane-bound adenyl cyclase resulting in an increased movement of calcium into these cells. He concludes that the unique features of mammalian extracellular calcium homeostasis lies not in the development of unique or new cellular control systems, but in the highly selective manner in which a common biochemical control device is regulated by specific extracellular messengers in the highly differentiated cells of the mammalian organism. In addition, this view of the control of both cellular and extracellular calcium

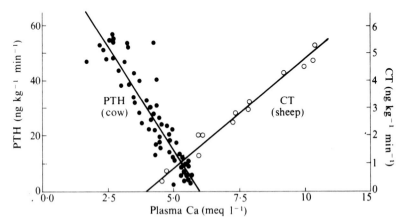

FIG. 9.12. Effect of plasma calcium on secretion rate of parathyroid hormone and calcitonin. (From Copp (1969) by courtesy of author and publisher.)

homeostasis emphasizes that the concentration of this ion is of critical importance in regulating both key extra- and intracellular, or more correctly cytosolic, systems and that changes in its concentration within the cell cytosol are an important means of regulating cell function.

3. CALCITONIN

In 1961 Copp demonstrated in a series of elegant experiments that in dogs there was a plasma calcium lowering hormone – calcitonin – as well as a hormone that raised plasma calcium, PTH, which was already well known (Copp, Cheney, and Davidson 1961; Copp 1963).

The opposing action of the two hormones is well illustrated in Fig. 9.12. It is now known, at least in sheep and cows, that as the plasma calcium rises for any reason above its normal level, the level of calcitonin in the plasma rises, and as the plasma calcium falls the level of PTH rises. The secretion rate of calcitonin, measured by bioassay of thyroid blood in the pig is proportional to the blood calcium concentration (Care, Cooper, Duncan, and Orimo 1968; Care, Bruce, Boelkins, Kenny, Conaway, and Anast 1971).

For many years it was disputed as to whether calcitonin played any role in human calcium homeostasis, though it was recognized as important in many mammals and in fish. It was often spoken of as a vestigial hormone. Improved methods of analysis, however, using a sensitive bioassay technique, indicate that calcitonin probably plays a part in protecting the skeleton in man from excessive osteoclastic resorption (Hillyard, Cooke, Coombes, Evans, and MacIntyre 1977; Hillyard, Stevenson, and MacIntyre 1978; Stevenson, Hillyard, MacIntyre, Cooper, and Whitehead 1979).

3.1. Origin of calcitonin

Calcitonin is formed by the cells of the ultimobranchial body, which is clearly defined in embryonic life but becomes incorporated in very different ways in the organs of the neck during development in different species. In the original experiments in dogs, Copp and his colleagues perfused the isolated parathyroid–thyroid complex and concluded the new hormone came from the parathyroid gland. In 1963, however, Hirsch, Gauthier, and Munson, using the rat, demonstrated a hypocalcaemic factor in the thyroid gland which they called thyrocalcitonin. In 1964, proof that calcitonin, the calcium-lowering hormone, originated in the thyroid came from the separate perfusion of the thyroid and parathyroid glands of the goat, a procedure which cannot be applied in dogs (Foster, MacIntyre, and Pearse 1964). It is now agreed that calcitonin and thyrocalcitonin are one and the same and that in mammals the hormone arises in the C cells of the thyroid gland. These cells are distinct from the follicular cells which produce thyroxine. They were first recognized as the source of calcitonin in 1964 by Foster, MacIntyre, and Pearse, and have now been found in the thyroid gland of a large number of mammals including the dormouse, dog, rat, guinea pig, cow, hamster, bat, goat, cat, bear, ox, horse, sheep, rabbit, and monkey as well as man (Anast and Conaway 1972). In lower vertebrates, fishes, birds, reptiles, and amphibians the ultimobronchial bodies remain distinct structures separate from the thyroid gland, and they are the source of calcitonin.

The C cells share certain characteristics with other cells producing polypeptide hormones. These characteristics include a high content of glycerophosphate dehydrogenase and cholinesterase and the ability to synthesize and concentrate 5-hydroxytryptamine. They are part of the APUD cell series derived embryologically from the neural crest (Pearse and Polak 1972). In Fig. 9.13 is shown a specially stained preparation of a guinea-pig thyroid showing the C cells in relation to the follicular cells. C cells have been found in man in both the thymus and the parathyroid, and these tissues show calcitonin activity (Foster, Byfield, and Gudmundsson 1972). A preliminary report from Deftos and his colleagues (Deftos, Catherwood, Bone, Watkins, Guillemia, and Parthemore 1979) claims to have isolated calcitonin from the pituitary in a number of divergent mammalian and submammalian animal species.

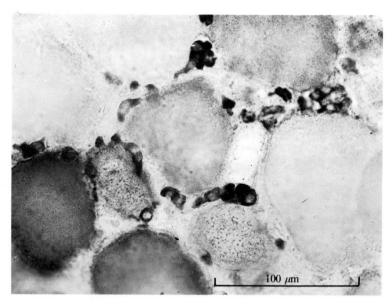

FIG. 9.13. Guinea pig thyroid. Frozen section fixed in Pearson's fixation and reacted with butyrylthiocholine (Koelle's method) to show cholinesterase. The enzyme (black) is present exclusively in the cytoplasm of the C cells. This illustration shows the normal appearance and (maximal) concentration of C cells in the gland. (From Pearse (1968) by courtesy of author and publishers.)

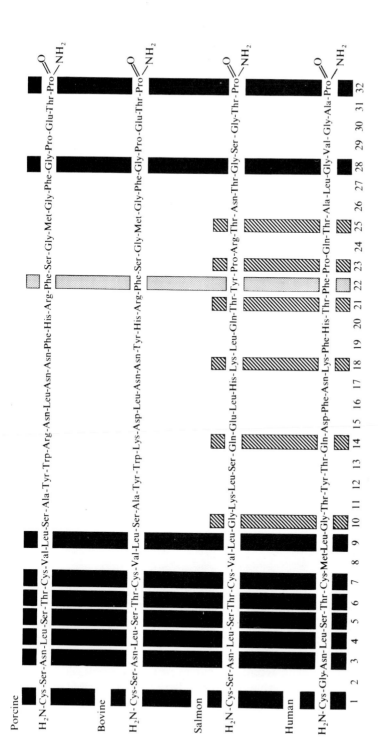

FIG. 9.14. Amino-acid sequences of porcine, bovine, salmon, and human calcitonin. Solid bars indicate common amino acids. (From Potts and Deftos (1974), reproduced through the courtesy of the National Academy of Sciences, US.)

3.2. Chemistry

Pure calcitonin was first isolated from pig thyroid in 1968 (Potts *et al.* 1968; Franz, Rozenthaler, Zelinder, Doepfner, Huguerin, and Guttman 1968; Kahnt, Riniker, MacIntyre, and Neher 1968). It is a straight-chain peptide containing 32 amino-acid residues with a disulphide bridge between cysteine residues in positions 1 and 7. Human calcitonin has also been isolated and synthesized, as has that of the ox and the salmon (Copp 1972). The amino-acid sequences of porcine, bovine, human, and salmon calcitonin are shown in Fig. 9.14. All the calcitonins so far isolated have the same basic structure containing 32 amino acids with a seven-membered disulphide ring at the NH_2-terminus and prolinamide at the COOH-terminus. There is also an aromatic amino acid (tyrosine or phenylaline) at position 22 and glycine at position 28. The differences in the intermediate amino acids are considerable between porcine, salmon, and human calcitonin. The entire molecule appears to be essential, since removal of the amide group at the COOH-terminus or shortening the chain by a single amino acid appears to result in almost complete loss of biological activity (Potts and Deftos 1974). Since only nine residues, seven of these situated within the first nine amino-acid residues, are common to the amino-acid sequences of calcitonin in all species so far known, it suggests that this region of the molecule must be intimately related to biological activity.

Salmon calcitonin is 30–50 times as active in the rat and possibly 100–200 times more active in the human (Neer, Parsons, Krane, Deftos, Shields, Copp, and Potts 1969) than the mammalian calcitonins, all of which appear to have the same biological activity (Copp 1972). Human calcitonin is readily isolated from medullary carcinoma of the thyroid. This tumour may contain 5000 times more calcitonin than normal tissue per unit of weight (Cunlitte, Hall, Hudgson, Gudmundsson, Williams, Galante, Black, Johnston, Shuster, Joplin, Woodhouse, and MacIntyre 1968).

3.3. Plasma levels

Calcitonin in peripheral plasma or in tissues is heterogeneous. This heterogeneity accounts in part for the different values hitherto reported for normal levels (Deftos, Roos, Bronzert, and Parthemore 1975; Singer and Habener 1974; Jullienne, Calmettes, Raulais, Milhaud, and Moukhtar 1978). Recently more satisfactory techniques have been reported (Hillyard *et al.* 1977; Parthemore and Deftos 1978).

Calcitonin levels, with recent techniques of measurement, in 55 normal adult men show a mean value of 24 pg/ml ± 18 pg with a range of < 10–75 pg/ml (Parthemore and Deftos 1978). In women the levels are twenty-five per cent less and often indetectable. During pregnancy and lactation or administration of oestrogen progestagin contraceptive pills, however, the

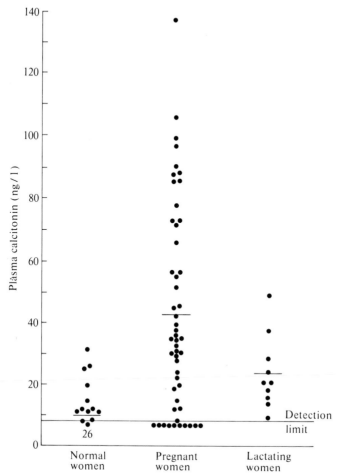

FIG. 9.15. Plasma-calcitonin levels in normal, pregnant and lactating women. Horizontal bars are group means. Plasma calcitonin levels were significantly higher in pregnant and lactating women than in normal women ($p < 0.001$). (From Hillyard *et al.* (1978) courtesy of authors and publishers.)

level equals or exceeds male concentrations (Hillyard *et al.* 1978) (see Fig. 9.15). Indeed it has been suggested that protection of the vertebral skeleton may provide a physiological role for calcitonin (Stevenson *et al.* 1979) insuring that more calcitonin circulates at times of increased calcium need.

Normal calcitonin levels show a circadian variation with a peak around midday and they respond to known stimuli for calcitonin release, i.e. perfusion of calcium, pentagastrin and glucagon (Deftos, Powell, Parthemore, and Potts 1973). They do not respond to oral calcium or food (Hillyard *et al.*

1977; Parthemore and Deftos 1978). Extremely high levels are found in cancers affecting the C cells of the thyroid gland, thyroid medullary carcinoma, without any change in the blood calcium level (see p. 166). The level is also raised in a substantial proportion of common neoplasms. It has indeed been suggested that an elevated calcitonin may be useful as a tumour marker.

3.4. Action

Calcitonin when ingested exerts an immediate effect on bone cells and a less understood effect on the kidney. Immunohistochemical techniques have localized receptors for calcitonin in both bone and kidney cells (Rao, Heersche, Sturtridge, and Marchuk 1979).

3.4.1. BONE

Calcitonin is far more effective in young than in old animals and in children rather than adults, since sensitivity to calcitonin is related to rates of bone turnover. In young animals, a fall in the level of both plasma calcium and phosphate is the most obvious effect of injecting calcitonin. The greatest effect occurs between 30 minutes and 3 hours. The response is also obtained in parathyroidectomized rats. It cannot therefore be explained solely on the basis of suppression of parathyroid action. It also occurs in eviscerated and nephrectomized rats without any change in the calcium content of soft tissues, so it is reasonable to assume that its primary action is on bone.

3.4.1.1. *Resorption*

There is ample experimental evidence that calcitonin exerts a direction action on bone resorption. This was first proposed by Milhaud and his colleagues (Milhaud, Moukhtar, Bourichon, and Perault 1965) on the basis of isotope studies in rats. Rats also show a diminished excretion of hydroxyproline following calcitonin injection, presumably due to diminished collagen destruction (Martin, Robinson, and MacIntyre 1966; Aer 1968). Radiographic and histological examination of the vertebrae of parathyroidectomized rats given calcitonin showed a decreased number of osteoclast in early experiments (Foster, Doyle, Bordier, and Matrajt 1966). Recent histological studies both in tissue culture and *in vivo* preparations have shown not only a decrease in numbers but changes in the character both of the osteocytes and the osteoclasts (Holtrop, Raisz, and Simmons 1974; Holtrop, King, Cox, and Reit 1979; Norimatsu, Vander Weil, and Talmage 1979). Evidence that this action on bone is a direct one was elegantly demonstrated by MacIntyre, Parsons, and Robinson (1967). In the isolated tibia of the cat perfused with blood from its own carotid connected to the popliteal artery via a pump, infusion of porcine calcitonin causes an arteriovenous difference in calcium concentration of up to 5 per cent, corresponding to net retention of calcium in bone. When taken in conjunction with the determination of calcium clearance in the tibia the effect is of the right order of magnitude to account for the hypocalcaemic action of calcitonin in the whole animal. Whalen and his colleagues have described changes in the bones of young growing rats in whom an excess of calcitonin was induced either by chronic administration of calcitonin, or parathyroidectomy, or both (Whalen, Krook, Nunez, Pennock, and Doyle 1973).

Tissue culture experiments tell the same story (Reynolds 1972, 1974). Calcitonin blocks resorption *in vitro*, whether induced by PTH (Friedman and Raisz 1965; Raisz and Niemann 1969; Reynolds and Dingle 1970), or by vitamin A (Reynolds 1968), or by $25\text{-}OHD_3$ and $1,25\text{-}(OH)_2D_3$ (Trummel, Raisz, Blunt, and DeLuca 1969). There is no clear-cut evidence from tissue culture experiments as to whether the influence of calcitonin on resorption affects both mineral and matrix. Anast and Conaway (1972), having reviewed the evidence, conclude that *in vitro* the resorption of both matrix and mineral is inhibited by calcitonin. Reynolds and Dingle (1970) conclude that calcitonin prevents the differentiation of new osteoclasts and decreases the effectiveness of existing osteoclasts. Vitamin A, like PTH, causes an increased release of acid proteases from embryonic rat calvaria grown in tissue culture; however, calcitonin does not inhibit the increased release of acid hydrolases in response to vitamin A even though bone resorption is prevented (Reynolds 1968). Reynolds (1972) has more recently suggested that calcitonin may be involved in the control of the activity of a collagenase, but that in the very young bone used in tissue culture the picture is obscured by large pools of collagen precursor masking any effect of calcitonin on mature mineralized collagen.

3.4.1.1.1. *Escape phenomenon*. In his study of the effects of calcitonin on bones in tissue culture Raisz and his colleagues (Raisz, Au, Friedman, and Nieman 1967) described what they called 'the escape phenomenon', i.e. the transient nature of the inhibitory effect of calcitonin on bone resorption. A similar effect has been described *in vivo* in rats by Messer and Copp (1974) and by Cooper (Cooper, Bolman, Linehan, and Wells 1978). Rats injected with calcitonin once a day, for weeks or months, responded daily with a short period of hypocalcaemia, but if the calcitonin was injected continuously for long periods by a series of minipumps ensuring a high blood level of calcitonin, hypocalcaemia was not maintained. It is noteworthy that patients with C cell carcinomas do not have hypocalcaemia. This escape phenomena has been studied by Tashjian and his colleagues (1978) using tissue culture of rats calvaria. They conclude that it is due to long-term occupancy of the appropriate binding sites and a very high affinity hormone-binding site complex, and is not due to loss of biological activity of calcitonin or to generation of peptide fragments. Escape was detectable 16 hours after their

THE PHYSIOLOGY OF BONE

experiment started and was complete within 24 hours. Loss of activity was reversible if the bone was placed in a calcitonin free medium.

3.4.1.2. *Apposition*

It has been suggested that calcitonin may increase bone formation in patients with Paget's disease receiving long-term treatment with calcitonin (Doyle, Pennock, Greenberg, Joplin, and MacIntyre 1974; Doyle, Woodhouse, Glen, Joplin, and MacIntyre 1974). There is no other evidence that calcitonin affects bone growth.

3.4.2. KIDNEY

Despite numerous studies suggesting that calcitonin has an effect on renal secretion of calcium, sodium, magnesium, and phosphate the question whether endogenous calcitonin has an important direct effect on the kidney under physiological conditions remains to be clarified (Cochran, Peacock, Sachs, and Nordin 1970; Bijvoet, Sluysveer, Vries, and Koppen 1971; Keeler; Walker, and Copp 1970; Foster *et al.* 1972). Russell (1976) states 'that large doses of calcitonin increase the renal excretion of calcium, sodium and phosphate and alter the soft tissue distribution of these ions. In man the renal effects can probably be considered pharmacological'. He gives no further evidence. Since calcitonin binds to renal tissue and elevates cyclic AMP concentrations (Heersche, Marcus, and Aurbach 1974), and since the receptors that bind the calcitonin differ from those for PTH or vasopressin which also increase AMP in the kidney, it is likely that the hormone has some effect on renal tubular transport but all workers agree that further work is needed to confirm and clarify the position.

Heynen and his colleagues (Heynen, Kanis, Oliver, Ledingham, and Russell 1976) have suggested that endogenous calcitonin protects against renal bone disease. They propose that a possible factor in the pathogenesis of renal bone disease is a failure to secrete calcitonin in adequate amounts. They found that concentrations of endogenous calcitonin were lower in patients on dialysis with bone disease than in those without bone disease, while in some patients without bone disease the calcitonin levels were high. This hypothesis awaits confirmation.

3.5. Factors that effect plasma calcitonin levels other than calcium

3.5.1. GASTROINTESTINAL PEPTIDES

Much of the work on factors that control the secretion of calcitonin has been done on the pig since in this animal the thyroid and parathyroid gland are anatomically separate. This means that the thyroid gland can be manipulated and thyroid venous blood completely collected without disturbing the function of the parathyroid gland (Cooper *et al.* 1978). Care and his colleagues (1968, 1971) found that there was no increase in blood calcium after feeding calcium but an increased secretion of calcitonin. This increase proved to be due to increased secretion of gastrin, a gastrointestinal peptide (Cooper, Schwesinger, Mahgoub, and Ontjes 1971). There is now good experimental evidence that in the pig gastrin is a calcitonin secretagogue and that together with blood calcium it may normally stimulate calcitonin release following feeding. There is no satisfactory evidence as yet that gastrin is effective in other species (Cooper *et al.* 1978) but, nevertheless, in the rat feeding leads to calcitonin release even when the blood calcium level is subnormal (Talmage, Doppett, and Cooper 1975). Baby rats secrete large amounts of calcitonin when they are suckling (Cooper, Obie, Toverud, and Munson 1977) and their lactating mothers release large amounts when they eat (Toverud and Munson 1976). Talmage has recently suggested that perhaps an important physiological function of calcitonin is temporarily to store calcium obtained during feeding in bone-fluid, for use during the fasting periods between meals (Talmage and Vander Wiel 1979). In man, it has been found, that though some patients with medullary thyroid carcinoma respond to an injection of pentagastrin alone, the best results are achieved with a combination of pentagastrin and calcium.

3.5.2. INTERACTION WITH OTHER HORMONES

3.5.2.1. *Parathyroid hormone*

Cooper and his colleagues (1978) consider that PTH can indirectly effect calcitonin release since they consider they have experimental evidence that PTH, as well as blood calcium, can stimulate release of gastrin. This PTH-induced release, they suggest, can be inhibited by calcitonin.

3.5.2.2. *Somatostatin*

(A microhormone with widespread inhibitory action on release of pituitary hormones.) Again Cooper suggests that somatostatin can inhibit or largely reverse a hypergastrinemia induced by calcium or acetylcholine or PTH.

3.6. Clinical use

3.6.1. PAGET'S DISEASE

There is good evidence from many clinics that calcitonin given over several years will give relief from bone pain and induce both radiological, histological and biochemical improvement in Paget's disease of bone, a condition characterized by both excessive resorption and apposition. Analysis of the glyco-proteins of the matrix shows a lower content of α_2HS glycoprotein (Ashton, Höhling, and Triffitt 1976; Chakravorty 1979) than is found in a normal bone. Human or synthetic human calcitonin is preferable to porcine or bovine hormone in treatment since both the latter may act as an antigen (DeRose, Singer, Anramides, Flores, Dziadiw, Bakder, and Wallach 1974; Chakravorty 1979). Potts and his colleagues report the development of antibodies in 50 per cent of 21 patients with Paget's disease treated with sal-mon calcitonin.

Hosking and his colleagues (Hosking *et al.* 1976) in 1976 reported great clinical success with a combination of synthetic human calcitonin and low doses of ethane-1 hydroxy-1, 1-diphosphonate (EHDP). Whether this com-bination will prove more successful than the use of diphosphonates alone (see p. 111) is not yet known.

3.6.2. HYPERCALCAEMIA

Calcitonin is reported to be useful in treating certain forms of hypercalcaemia, namely, that associated with disseminated malignant disease (Foster, Joplin, MacIntyre, Melvin, and Slack 1966); hyperthyroidism (Bijvoet, Sluys Veer, and Jansen 1968); hyperparathyroidism (West, Joffe, Sinclair, and O'Riordan 1971); idiopathic hypercalcaemia of infancy (Milhaud and Job 1966); and vitamin D intoxication in both children and adults (West *et al.* 1971).

3.6.3. IDIOPATHIC OSTEOPOROSIS

Reports of treatment with calcitonin in osteoporosis are conflicting (Foster *et al.* 1972). Experimental conditions like osteoporosis induced in rats by administration of vitamin A (Matrajt, Tun-Chot, Bordier, and Hioco 1971), or in cats by feeding calcium-deficient diets alone (Jowsey 1969) are prevented if calcitonin is given at the same time. In man, reports of short-term studies are encouraging (Hioco, Bordier, Miravet, Denys, and Tun-Chot 1970; Milhaud, Calmettes, Jullienne, Tharaud, Bloch-Michel, Cavaillon, Colin, and Moukhtar 1972), but long-term studies are still awaited.

10. Some Biological Factors in Skeletal Homeostasis

DEVELOPMENT, growth, and maintenance of the skeleton as a whole is controlled by a large and ever growing number of complex interacting factors arising in both the hypothalamus and the endocrine glands. These factors interact with one another and with their target organs by a variety of feedback mechanisms. Any discussion of the mechanisms involved must recognize that the simple study of the effects of any one hormone, such as oestrogen, on a single bone in organ culture may give most misleading results. Oestrogen for instance has no effect on an organ culture of a growing bone, yet through its effect on 1-hydroxylase in the kidney it may exert a powerful effect on the skeleton (Castillo *et al.* 1977) (see p. 194).

There are a group of hormones circulating in the blood stream that appear to influence skeletal growth and development in the skeleton as a whole. These include growth hormone, the thyroid hormones, the sex hormones, and the glucocorticoids.

1. SKELETAL GROWTH

1.1. Height and weight

Many different tables of height and weight of the growing 'normal' child have been determined showing the variation with age and sex and the deviations from the mean that may be expected. Such a curve for normal boys is shown in Fig. 10.1. This gives the mean figure and the values for 1 and 2 standard deviations round the mean. Appropriate curves for girls are also available.

These curves allow for what is known as the adolescent spurt, a remarkable sudden increase in height and weight associated with the development of secondary characteristics in both girls and boys at puberty (Fig. 10.2). No such sudden growth spurt is recognized in other species.

The data in the chart are composite from a number of children whose adolescence spurts did not coincide in time. As a result, the sharpness of the individual spurts is smoothed out, and the magnitude decreased. Consequently, when plotting growth (height and weight) curves for an individual child undergoing the sharp adolescent spurt the curves will jump to a higher 'channel'. For this reason, in the standard curves for height and weight,

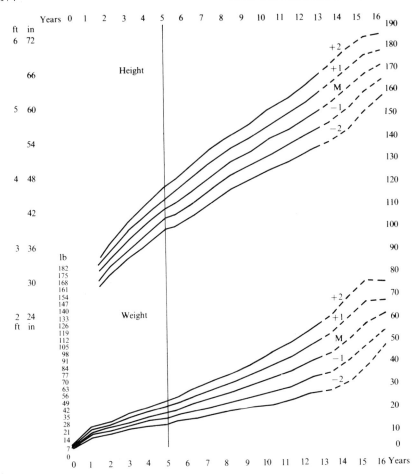

Fig. 10.1. Height and weight chart for boys. This particular chart was constructed from data from the Oxford Child Health Survey and the London County Council report on the heights and weights of school pupils in the county of London in 1954. M = mean figure. Standard deviations are shown as + and − on either side.

continuous lines have been replaced by dotted lines from the age when the adolescence spurt is likely to start. In order to compare growth with other parameters, such as mental development, for instance, height is often expressed in terms of 'height-age'. Thus, if a child is said to have a height-age of 4 years, it is meant that he has the mean height of a 4-year-old.

1.2. The velocity of growth

It is also important to measure the velocity of growth. Mean constant height

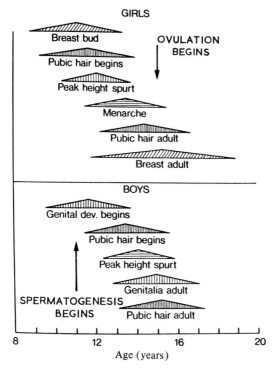

FIG. 10.2. Sequence of pubertal changes in boys and girls. (From Short (1976) by courtesy of author and publishers.)

velocity curves for boys and girls are shown in Fig. 10.3 (Tanner, Whitehouse, Hughes, and Carter 1976; Tanner, Whitehouse, Murubini, and Resele 1976). The absolute value of peak height velocity varies from one child to another. Marshall (Marshall 1978) found a mean value of 10·3 cm/yr with a standard variation of 1·54 cm/yr in 49 healthy boys. For girls, the average peak velocity was 9 cm/yr with a standard deviation of 1·03 cm/yr. For girls the mean age at peak height velocity was 12·14 ± 0·14 yr with a standard deviation of 0·88 years. The mean for boys was 14·06 ± 0·14 years with a standard deviation of 0·92 years.

1.3. The adolescent spurt

Tanner and his colleagues give the take-off point for the growth spurt for girls as 10·3 years and for boys 12 years (Tanner, Whitehouse, Hughes, and Carter 1976; Tanner, Whitehouse, Marubini, and Resele 1976). Mean constant height curves for girls and boys are shown in Fig. 10.4. The higher height

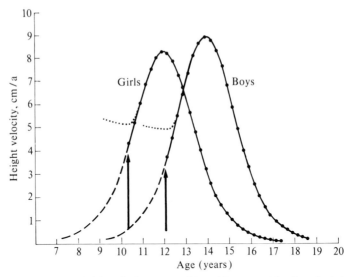

FIG. 10.3. Mean-constant height velocity curves, girls and boys, resulting from logistic fit. The arrows indicate take-off points. Dotted lines are empirical means prior to take-off +0·5 yr. (From Tanner *et al.* (1976*b*) by courtesy of authors and publishers.)

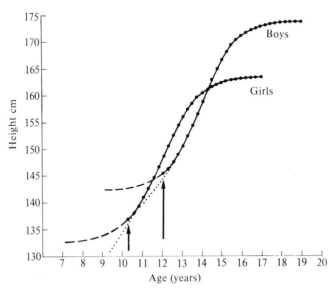

FIG. 10.4. Mean-constant height curves, girls and boys, resulting from logistic fit. The arrows indicate take-off points, girls at 10·3, boys 12·0 years. Dotted lines are empirical means prior to take-off + 0·5 yr. (From Tanner *et al.* (1976*b*) by courtesy of authors and publishers.)

attained in the boys, Tanner attributes to their later start of the spurt which gives them nearly two years longer growing time than the girls.

Boys grow a mean of 28 cm between take-off and cessation of the spurt, while girls only grow a mean of 25 cm (Short 1980). Thus, two-thirds of the mean height difference of 10 cm between adult men and women is accounted for by the delayed onset of the height spurt in boys, and one third by its increased magnitude.

1.3.1. THE SEX HORMONES

Before considering the factors involved in the adolescent growth spurt something must be said about the sex hormones. It has not yet been demonstrated that these hormones play any important part in general body growth before puberty (Winter 1978). The gonads, and to a lesser extent the adrenals, synthesize several sex hormones. The ultimate concentration in serum of these steroids at any point in time depends upon their respective rates of gonadal and adrenal secretion plus the effects of peripheral interconversion, binding to serum protein and varying rates of metabolism and excretion (Winter 1978).

The principal circulating androgen in adult man is testosterone, 95 per cent of which is secreted by the Leydig cells of the testes (Baird, Horton, Longcope, and Tait 1969). Some oestradiol is also secreted by the testes but most is derived by peripheral conversion from testosterone. Androgen secretion in the male is primarily under the influence of the pituitary lutenizing hormone (LH) mediated via hypothalamic neurosecretion of, LH, releasing hormone.

In adult women the major sex hormone is estradiol which is secreted by the ovary. Most of the circulating testosterone in women is derived from peripheral conversion of androstenedione which is secreted by both ovaries and adrenals (Baird et al. 1969).

In the circulation, the majority of the sex steroids are bound either to albumin or to specific high affinity binding globulins. Except in the first few days of life, the level of binding of sex steroids remains relatively unchanged during childhood and puberty (Radfar, Ansusingha, and Kenny 1976). In target organs the circulating steroid becomes bound to specific cytoplasmic receptor proteins. For discussion of the effects of oestrogen and testosterone see pages 192, 193.

1.3.2. FACTORS RESPONSIBLE FOR THE ADOLESCENT GROWTH SPURT

The factors responsible for the adolescent growth spurt are clearly complicated. Some attempt to analyse them has recently been made by Short (Short 1980). His analysis does not attempt to reach a cellular level. The part played by the cells of bone and cartilage is not defined. The growth of antlers might prove a possible model. The antler is composed of true bone formed by ossification of a cartilaginous primordium that develops at its growing tips in a process that is intermediate between intramembranous and endochondral ossification (see p. 91). The rate of antler growth can be spectacular in the larger species of deer. In the North American elk for example the maximum growth rate is 2·75 cm/day (Goss 1970). Antlers are cast and regrown every year. Casting occurs in response to falling levels of testosterone, which is said to activate osteoclasts at the base of the antler pedicle where the living bone of the skull is united with the dead bone of the 'hard horn' antler. Small doses of testosterone can prevent this casting from taking place. Since testicular activity waxes and wanes during the year in response to changing photoperiods it is this seasonal testicular regression that normally produces casting of the antlers. The same effect can be achieved by castrating a male deer in 'hard horning' when antler casting will occur a few weeks later (Lincoln, Youngson, and Short 1970). Following casting, new antlers begin to grow from the pedicle stump almost at once, at a time when blood testosterone level is low: as growth proceeds the testosterone level is rising. Short concludes, that at what might be called a macroscopic level 'growth hormone is essential for normal growth even though the effect may be largely a permissive one under normal circumstances. It is the pubertal increase in testicular testosterone secretion that is responsible for first initiating and ultimately terminating the peak height spurt in normal bones' (Short 1980).

All those who have worked with growth-hormone-deficient boys consider that growth at puberty requires continuous treatment with both growth hormone and testosterone (Tanner, Whitehouse, Hughes, and Carter 1976; Tanner, Whitehouse, Marabini, and Resele 1976; Aynsley-Green, Zachmann, and Prader 1976; Preece and Tanner 1977) which should be maintained till adult height is achieved. In girls it appears probable that the steadily rising oestrogen secretion at the ages of 8–10 initially stimulates long bone growth and then induces epiphyseal fusion and cessation of growth (Brown, Harrison, and Smith 1978). While accepting that oestrogens alone can regulate normal bone growth, Short raises the question (Short 1980) whether androgens may not also be involved and whether there may not be important synergistic effects between the two hormones in stimulating or inhibiting bone growth, the androgens in the case of females being derived both from the ovary and adrenals. Short concludes that oestrogen is the prime mover in the growth spurt in girls. He further emphasizes that it must be remembered that a steroid can exhibit both stimulatory and inhibitory effects on bone growth depending on the dose.

1.4. Skeletal proportions

The ratio of the upper and lower segments of the body measured from the symphysis pubis is of particular importance. At birth this ratio is approxi-

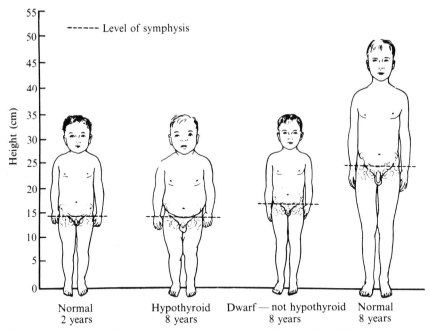

FIG. 10.5. The figures of normal boys, 2 years and 8 years old respectively, illustrate the change in the ratio of upper and lower skeletal segments measured from the symphysis pubis. At birth the ratio is 1·7/1·0 and at 10 years 1·0/1·0. The hypothyroid dwarf having the height of a 2-year-old retains the infantile proportions of 2 years. Dwarfs of pituitary or primordial type, however, attain the more mature proportions of their chronological age. (From Wilkins and Fleischmann (1941) by courtesy of authors and publishers.)

mately 1·7/1. The legs grow more rapidly than the trunk, so that by the age of 10–11 years the segments are approximately equal. Wilkins (1965) considers that the upper/lower ratio should be compared not only with the average ratio for a child of the same age and sex, but also with the ratio of the average child having the same height as shown in Fig. 10.5. This ratio is disturbed in certain types of dwarfism.

1.5. Osseous development or 'bone age'

The appearance and subsequent development of the various epiphyseal centres of ossification normally follow a fairly definite pattern and time schedule. There is no absolute 'normal', and a number of difference reference tables are available. It is important to use one reference table only in studying any particular patient or group of patients and, if it is impractical to obtain radiographs of all joints, to obtain an average bone age, to restrict examination to the same joint. Wilkins' (1965) advice to obtain pictures of all joints can hardly be recommended when the possible radiation dose is considered.

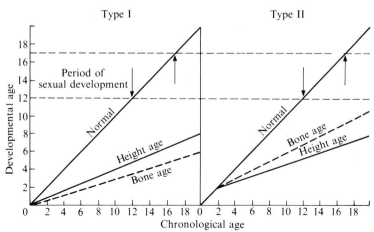

FIG. 10.6. Patterns of growth and development (see text). (From Wilkins (1965) by courtesy of author and publishers.)

1.6. Maturation of the features and naso-orbital configuration

There are no satisfactory measurements or norms for the changes that occur in naso-orbital configuration, but those with clinical experience are able to recognize departures from the normal pattern.

In Fig. 10.6 are seen two different patterns of growth and development illustrating differences in 'height-age' and 'bone-age'. For the purpose of the charts it is assumed that the 'average' time for the onset of puberty is 12 years and that sexual development is complete at 17 years. The average period of adolescent development is seen between the two arrows. Neither Type 1 nor Type 2 reaches sexual development within the period of life seen on the charts. Type 1 is the usual pattern seen in hypothyroidism and in some cases of hypopituitary dwarfism. The rate of osseous development is retarded to an even greater degree than the rate of growth. Type 2 is found in other cases of hypopituitary dwarfism. The rate of osseous development is relatively less retarded than that of growth but lags below the normal.

Marshall (1978) gives some information on changes in individual bones at different ages.

2. FACTORS AFFECTING BONE GROWTH AND DEVELOPMENT OTHER THAN HORMONES

In any discussion of the effect of hormones upon skeletal growth and development, it must be remembered that a variety of external factors are also involved in causing disturbances and abnormalities, such as diet, disease, maternal care, and prenatal influences (Prader, Tanner, and Harnack 1963). The lines of arrested bone growth associated with period of infection are easily recognized in radiographs. The stunting seen in emotionally deprived and neglected children, even though they are adequately fed, is well documented though unexplained. Such children show a normal response of growth hormone to hypoglycaemia (Kaplan, Abrams, Bell, Conte, and Grumbach 1968). There are also genetic effects which may act through hormone abnormalities or through inborn errors of metabolism.

3. HORMONES THAT AFFECT SKELETAL GROWTH

3.1. Growth hormone —Somatotropin

Growth hormone or somatotropin is synthesized by certain cells in the pituitary gland itself. Synthesis and release into the blood stream is, however, controlled by complicated factors present in the hypophysiotrophic area of the hypothalamus or an even higher location in the central nervous system (Rona and Tanner 1977).

The hormone is present in the human pituitary gland in much higher concentration than other pituitary hormones. The average gland contains 5 mg of HGH, which is about 1 per cent of its whole weight. This does not appear to vary with age or sex in adults.

3.1.1. CHEMISTRY

Human growth hormone is a single chain polypeptide of 191 amino acids with two intrachain disulphide bridges (Niall, Hogan, Tregear, Segre, Hwang, and Friesen 1973). Its structure is unique. Endogenous growth hormone exists in plasma in two, or possibly more, discrete forms which may differ in biological properties. At times of high secretion at least one fraction which is capable of reacting in radioimmunoassay lacks biological activity (Sneid, Jacobs, Weldon, Trivedi, and Daughaday 1975).

3.1.2. SECRETION

Many and varied stimuli, such as exercise, stress, sleep, ingestion of protein, a fall in the circulating level of glucose or free fatty acids, or administration of arginine, glucagon, vasopressin or L-dopa will all cause a rise in growth hormone secretion in healthy individuals (Winter 1978). These stimuli appear to act through neural mechanisms, with final control of pituitary synthesis and release of the hormone being mediated by an as yet unidentified hypothalamic growth-hormone releasing factor, spoken of as GHRF. Further growth hormone release is influenced by a hypothalamic release-inhibiting hormone called somatostatin, which also acts to inhibit secretion of thyroid stimulating hormone (TSH) glucagon and insulin (Winter 1978).

3.1.3. SOMATOMEDINS

It now seems probable that growth hormone exerts its action through the production in the liver, and possibly to a small extent in the kidney, of a family of growth-hormone-induced small peptides, known as somatomedins. They act collectively to promote synthesis of DNA, RNA and protein in cartilage and to stimulate the incorporation of sulphur into cartilage gluco-saminoglycans (Daughaday, Hall, Raben, Salmon, Van den Brande, and Van Wyk 1972). Their stimulatory effects are offset in part by circulating somatomedin inhibitors and the net biological activity of somatomedins in plasma thus reflect a balance between both sets of factors (Phillips and Vassipoulou-Sellin 1980).

Labelled growth hormone shows early localization, chiefly in liver, kidney, and adrenal zona glomerulosa in the rat and not at all in cartilage or muscle (Mayberry, van den Brande, van Wyk, and Wadell 1971). Somatomedins are produced in isolated perfused rat livers and possibly kidney slices in a medium containing growth hormone (McConaghy 1972). They are usually now isolated from large volumes of plasma or serum (Phillips and Vassipoulou-Sellin 1980). When somatomedin was first isolated it was called sulphation factor because its first demonstrated action was to increase the uptake of radioactive sulphate by cartilage of hypophysectomized rats (Salmon and Daughaday 1957) growth hormone itself having no such effect *in vitro*.

The somatomedins produce effects very similar to those of insulin, acting to stimulate glucose or amino acid transport and to promote glucose oxidation and lipid synthesis (Clemmons, Hintz, Underwood, and Van Wyk 1974). Indeed somatomedin appears capable of binding to insulin receptors on adipocytes, chondrocytes and hepatocyte membranes. Van Wyk and his colleagues (Van Wyk, Underwood, Baseman, Hintz, Clemmons, and Marshall 1975), however, consider it likely that another set of 'growth' receptors exist on many cells which are responsive to smaller amounts of somatomedin and are primarily responsible for its growth-promoting effects. The somatomedins circulate in plasma bound to larger carrier proteins, the synthesis of which also appears to be growth hormone dependent (Cohen and Nissley 1976). None of these peptides, however, can substitute entirely for serum in the maintenance of *in vitro* cell growth (Chochinov and Daughaday 1976).

3.1.4. BLOOD LEVELS

Basal concentrations of growth hormone in serum from children or adults range from less than 1 to 5 ng/ml. It is secreted in intermittent bursts, largely during early sleep (Winter 1978). Very high concentrations are found in the new-born but these decline to basal levels within a few weeks. Plasma somatomedin levels are low at birth. During infancy growth hormone plays an important role in the maintenance of normoglycemia during fasting but it may not become essential for normal growth until some time during the first year of life. Some children with congenital growth-hormone deficiency may not show an impairment of growth velocity until they are 1 or 2 years old.

Control of normal levels of growth-hormone is probably exercised by a decrease of blood somatomedin, at least in children (Tanner 1972). Growth-hormone levels are high in kwashiokor (Plimstone, Becker, and Hanson 1971; Godard and Zahnd 1971). Also in favour of this feedback mechanism is the high concentration of growth hormone in children who are unable to secrete somatomedin because of an inherited defect. Tanner suggests that somatomedin alters the sensitivity of the hypothalamic GHRF site and thus serves to modulate its response to a variety of short-term stimuli (Tanner 1972).

Somatomedin C. Somatomedin C (partially purified), when added to the culture media in which rat calvaria were placed in a chemically defined medium with the addition of bovine albumin, stimulated collagen synthesis to the same extent as insulin (Raisz, Canalis, Dietrich, Kream, and Gworek 1978). When the two agents were given together they did not produce an additive effect. In the case of cartilage, somatomedin has been reported as more potent than insulin. Raisz and his colleagues (Raisz, Canalis, Dietrich, Kream, and Gworek 1978) suggest it is possible that the osteoblast receptor is an insulin receptor and that in the case of bone the somatomedin preparation was acting with non-suppressible insulin-like activity.

3.1.5. GROWTH-HORMONE DEFICIENCY

Growth-hormone deficiency may be total or partial and may occur as an isolated deficiency or in association with deficiency of other pituitary hormones, i.e. thyroid-stimulating hormone (TSH), adreno-cortical tropic hormone (ACTH), or gonadotrophins. Rona and Tanner (1977), who made a survey of the children in England with known growth-hormone deficiency, concluded it was a disorder, or group of disorders, for which they could find no definite cause. They consider that though originally it was thought to be a disorder of the pituitary gland itself, it now usually follows degeneration of the hypophysiotrophic area of the hypothalamus, or of higher locations in the central nervous system. The reason for the degeneration is unknown. In proven cases of deficiency the response to treatment is satisfactory.

Those who have worked with growth-hormone-deficient boys, as already discussed on p. 183, agree that treatment should be continuous, rather than given intermittently, and that it should be accompanied by testosterone during the period of the adolescent spurt (Tanner, Whitehouse, Hughes, and Carter 1976; Tanner, Whitehouse, Marubini, and Resele 1976; Aynsley-Green et al. 1976; Preece and Tanner 1977).

In some socially deprived children, growth is absent and so is growth hormone. The reasons for this are not known. They recover when moved to better surroundings but do not respond to HGH administration if left in the defective home conditions (Tanner 1972).

3.1.5.1. *The pituitary dwarf*

Deficiency of growth hormone in childhood results in pituitary dwarfism. Characteristically, the pituitary dwarf shows less retardation of osseous development than of growth, but is far behind the normal in both. Before birth, and in early infancy, deficiency of pituitary function does not impair growth. The diagnosis is unequivocally established only by radioimmuno-assay and failure to cause a rise in plasma growth-hormone with appropriate tests. African pigmies are genetic dwarfs. They have no deficiency in immuno-logically active growth hormone and do not respond to injected growth hormone. It is thought that there must be some unexplained failure of end organ responsiveness (Merimée, Lillicrap, and Rabinowitz 1965; Merimée, Hall, Rabinowitz, McKusick, and Rimoin 1968).

3.1.5.2. *Somatomedin deficiency*

There are a few patients, resembling children who are seriously deficient in growth hormone, whose levels of the hormone are normal or even high. The syndrome is due to an autosomal recessive gene. They have been shown to suffer from somatomedin deficiency and do not grow when given growth hormone (Tanner 1972).

3.1.6. GROWTH HORMONE, SOMATOTROPIN, EXCESS

Excessive secretion of somatotropin is usually due to an eosinophil adenoma of the adenohypophysis. If it occurs in a child the result is gigantism; if in an adult acromegaly.

3.1.6.1. *Pituitary gigantism*

Excess of somatotropin in a child results in acceleration of growth. Heights in excess of 8 feet may be reached. If the excess secretion continues, the changes of acromegaly are seen.

3.1.6.2. *Acromegaly*

Though acromegaly may be associated with a tumour of the pituitary, it is now thought that it usually starts as a disruption of the hypothalamic control, with chronically elevated levels of growth hormone (Lawrence, Goldfine, and Kirsteins 1970) and, in the acute stage, of somatomedin (Cryer and Daughaday 1969).

There is general coarsening of the facial features due to an increase of connective tissue, for example thickening of the lips. Increased cartilaginous growth results in enlargement of the ears and nose. The growth of the mandible causes a jutting jaw and alveolar bone growth causes the teeth to separate. Enlargement of the frontal and maxillary sinuses results in a prominent brow and long face. There is broadening and enlargement of hands and feet due to periosteal overgrowth and thickening again of connective tissue. There is excessive sweating and parenthesis of the hands and feet. There is not at present agreement as to whether acromegalics show increased secretion of growth hormone during sleep, as occurs in normals (Carlson, Gillin, Gorden, and Snyder 1972; Halse and Gordeladze 1978).

Metabolic changes. Total urinary hydroxyproline excretion is usually increased (Jasin, Fink, Wise, and Ziff 1962; Halse and Gordeladze 1978). After successful treatment with bromocriptine, a long-acting dopamine antagonist, this increased hydroxyproline excretion is reduced, if not abolished. Halse and Gordeladze (1978) could find no change in the bone obtained by iliac puncture and question whether the increased hydroxyproline came from bone or soft-tissue collagen. The soft-tissue swellings, presumably due to change in connective tissue, so prominent a feature of acromegaly, were also reduced by bromocriptine treatment. The same workers were able to demonstrate a fall in serum GH level associated with the reduction in hydroxyproline excretion. Bromocriptine raises growth-hormone levels in normal subjects but lowers them in acromegalics (Wass, Thorner, Morris, Rees, and Mason 1977).

The calcium balance is negative, and the phosphorus balance may be negative. Urinary calcium excretion is increased. Studies with ^{47}Ca reported by Bell and Bartter (1967) gave evidence of greatly increased bone-resorption rate and calcium accretion rate. These authors draw attention to the fact that there is often a negative phosphorus balance in acromegaly, while short-term experiments giving growth hormone to normal subjects may induce a positive balance. This difference emphasizes the danger of interpreting findings in clinical disease on the basis of short-term metabolic studies.

3.1.7. INTERACTION WITH OTHER HORMONES

There is interaction between growth hormone and other hormones but the whole pattern of interaction is somewhat confused.

3.1.7.1. *Thyroid*

Since both growth hormone and thyroid-stimulating hormone (TSH) arise in the anterior pituitary it is not surprising that they both affect skeletal homeostasis, particularly skeletal growth. The normal proportions of calcified cartilage to primary spongiosa in the metaphysis are maintained only when both human growth hormone and thyroid hormones are present. While the effects of these two hormones are difficult to separate, growth hormone sustains the rate of growth of the bones in length, while thyroxine controls differentiation and maturation of chondrogenic and osteogenic tissues. Treatment of hypophysectomized rats with only thyroxine, produces rapid premature closure of epiphyseal lines. Treatment of thyroidectomized rats with growth hormone not only produces rapid proliferation of epiphyseal cartilage, but the cells fail to hypertrophy and there is no further development of calcified tissue. The production rate of growth hormone is much lower than normal in hypothyroidism and higher than normal in hyperthyroidism. Hypothyroidism is associated with decreased synthesis, storage, and release of growth-hormone (Glick, Roth, Yalow, and Berson 1965).

Growth hormone may depress the uptake of radioiodine by the thyroid, in patients with hypopituitarism and it may lower serum thyrotropin (Root, Rosenfield, Bangiovanni, and Everlein 1973; Root, Snyder, Rezvani, Digeorge, and Utiger 1973). Wilkinson (Wilkinson, Anderson, and Smart 1972) reports a case of iodide-induced hypothyroidism and dwarfism which, on correction of the hypothyroidism at the age of 24 years, grew 23 cm in height and underwent puberty, while the growth-hormone response to hypoglycaemia was also restored.

3.1.7.2. *Corticosteroids*

In general, corticosteroids inhibit growth-hormone response, especially to insulin hypoglycaemia. The effect depends to some extent on dose and duration of treatment. Patients with Cushing's syndrome are often unresponsive to hypoglycaemia, whereas patients with Addison's disease may show increased responses to insulin hypoglycaemia. ACTH, on the other hand, can stimulate release of growth hormone and responsiveness to insulin hypoglycaemia (Catt 1970). It is essential to remember this inhibiting effect of the corticosteroids on growth hormone when treating children with cortisol, as for instance in asthmatics.

3.1.7.3 *Parathyroid hormone*

Suppression of parathyroid function is not a feature of acromegaly (Halse 1979).

3.2. Insulin

The question as to whether insulin is a hormone necessary for human growth, is raised by some workers in view of the insulin-like actions of somatomedin. The position at the moment is far from clear (Winter 1978).

In organ culture using rat calvaria maintained in a chemical defined medium containing bovine serum albumin, the addition of insulin was found by Raisz and his colleagues (Raisz, Canalis, Dietrich, Kream, and Gworek 1978) to produce a substantial increase in labelled proline incorporation and total collagen content. The total amount of new collagen deposited was 128 μg/bone, compared to 78 μg/bone in the controls. Morphologically, the bone showed numerous plump morphologically normal osteoblasts and an increase in new matrix, which was deposited in an orderly manner on the old bone surface. Raisz concludes there is some factor, not yet identified, other than insulin or somatomedin, in serum that affects bone growth. McIntyre (1978) suggests that insulin increases plasma $1,25\text{-}(OH)_2D_3$ in diabetic rats and so has an effect on bone.

3.3. Glucagon

Glucagon is a polypeptide hormone secreted by the α cells of the islets of Langerhans. There is no satisfactory evidence to implicate it in bone physiology. It has been said to have a slight lowering effect on serum levels of calcium and phosphate (Kalu, Hillyard, and Foster 1972). In rats the effect of PTH in increasing urinary hydroxyproline excretion is increased by simultaneous administration of glucagon. Rats treated with glucagon for 12 days excrete less hydroxyproline in their urine than controls. In both intact and thyroparathyroidectomized rats, glucagon decreases incorporation of (^{3}H) proline into bone. Similar results are obtained in nephrectomized rats. It has been suggested that glucagon can inhibit bone resorption and possibly bone formation (Kalu *et al.* 1972). Though glucagon has no proven effect on bone, a delicate balance between the plasma concentrations of insulin and glucagon appears to be necessary for the regulation of metabolism. Disturbance of this balance may well have effects on bone growth.

3.4. Prolactin

Since the chemical structure of human prolactin is very like that of human growth hormone, the question has been raised as to whether it acts as a growth factor. There is no good evidence that it does so. Acromegalic patients often show an increased secretion of prolactin. McIntyre (1978) has suggested that prolactin acts through somatomedin as a growth factor.

3.5. Thyroid hormones

Lack or excess of the thyroid hormones, thyroxine and tri-iodothyrine, has an effect on both the growing and mature skeleton. The concentration of these metabolic hormones in the blood is controlled by an adenohypophyseal hormone, thyrotropin (thyroid-stimulating hormone TSH). In the blood the two hormones are transported mostly bound to certain plasma proteins. Thyroxine is mainly bound to thyroxine-binding protein TBG and in part to thyroxine-binding prealbumin and albumin. Tri-iodothyrinine is less avidly bound, principally to prealbumin and albumin. The active components are the unbound fractions, which are approximately 0·024 per cent of the total thyroxine and 0·5 per cent of the total tri-iodothyrinine.

3.5.1. MODE OF ACTION

The thyroid hormones have many actions but the primary one is a calorigenic (increased oxygen consumption) effect on many, if not all, tissues, possibly through an effect on intracellular oxidative phosphorylation (Lee and Laycock 1978). A deficiency of thyroid hormones results in a general retardation of growth and organ maturation with a striking reduction in the rates of cell division in all proliferating tissues (Greenberg, Najjar, and Blizzard 1974). Replacement with thyroxine is followed by enhanced protein synthesis and a recovery in statural growth. Both thyroxine and triiodothyronine can stimulate cell growth in tissue culture but excessive amounts inhibit growth. Oppenheimer (1973) thinks he has evidence for an effect of thyroid hormones directly upon mitochondria concerned with energy metabolism and thermogenesis.

It can only be concluded that the thyroid hormones are essential for all cell growth and maintenance, but the precise cellular mechanisms by which they act are still not clearly understood.

3.5.2. EFFECT ON GROWTH AND DEVELOPMENT

As far as the skeleton is concerned, in broad terms it may be said that thyroid hormones affect osteogenesis while growth hormone affects chondrogenesis. The exact relationship between these hormones is still obscure. Hypothyroidism in man reduces or delays the expected peak elevation in plasma growth-hormone following insulin-induced hypoglycaemia. Further, the pituitary content of growth hormone in hypothyroid rats is much reduced. Both of these abnormalities are restored to normal with thyroid hormone.

Normal growth and development cannot occur in the absence of the thyroid gland.

In prenatal life, after the thyroid gland has become functional, thyroxine or triiodothyronine or both are essential for differentiation and maturation of foetal tissue, particularly the central nervous system and the skeleton. There is no evidence that the thyroid hormone is required before the foetal thyroid develops (Greenberg et al. 1974).

3.5.3. DEFICIENCY OF THYROID HORMONES

3.5.3.1. *The thyroid dwarf or cretin*

Long-standing hypothyroidism dating from birth or very early childhood, if not treated, results in the most severe forms of dwarfism seen. The child remains infantile in build (see Fig. 10.5), having a ratio of upper/lower skeletal segments, as measured from the symphysis pubis, more commensurate with his height than with his age, and thereby differing from the growth-hormone-deficient dwarf. There is also a failure of development of the nasal–orbital contours and retardation of osseous development or bone age. Delay in ossification of the epiphyses may occur in other conditions, for instance, in pituitary dwarfs having no thyroid deficiency, in some children stunted from nutritional causes, and in cases of delayed adolescence; but it does not, in such cases, respond to thyroid treatment (Wilkins 1965). As well as delay in ossification there may be abnormal epiphyseal ossification. This lesion has been called epiphyseal dysgenesis, and appears to be a specific manifestation of hypothyroidism. The secondary centre of ossification normally first shows in the radiograph as a single small shadow which enlarges in a regular fashion. In the cretin or hypothyroid child, months or even years may elapse before it is first seen, then simultaneously and over a large area of cartilaginous epiphyses there appear multiple small areas of ossification giving the classical picture of the 'stippled' epiphysis (Collins 1966).

The effects of replacement therapy with thyroid hormones depend on the age at which the deficiency occurred and how soon the treatment is begun.

At post-mortem the cortex of the long bones may be greatly thickened and the marrow cavity replaced by thick bony trabeculae lined with osteoblasts but poor in osteoclasts. The excess of bone may be so great as to simulate osteopetrosis (Schmidt 1962; Silverman and Currarino 1960). Soft tissues may calcify.

Wilkins (1965) reports finding hypercalcaemia in some cretinous infants, which was corrected by thyroid treatment. He attributes this to an impaired rate of calcium deposition in bone, with the possibility of an increased absorption from the gut as a contributory factor.

3.5.3.2. *Hypothyroidism or myxoedema*

Deficiency of circulating thyroid hormone may be due to primary thyroid disease, or secondarily, to reduced TSH from the adenohypophysis.

There are no striking effects on the skeleton in adults from deficiency of thyroid hormones. The plasma calcium and phosphorus are usually normal and the plasma alkaline phosphatase is low, though some patients may have hypercalcaemia (Lowe, Bird, and Thomas 1962). Heaney and Whedon (1958) have found a low rate of bone-formation by kinetic analysis. Detenbeck and

Jowsey (1969) have noted the same using microradiographic techniques in dogs following thyroidectomy. Some of these patients have dense bones and some have nephrocalcinosis. Nephrocalcinosis has been reproduced experimentally in the rat made hypothyroid at birth (Royer and Mathieu 1962). An abnormal retention of calcium has been reported (Krane, Brownell, Stanbury, and Corrigan 1956).

3.5.3.3. 'Pituitary' hypothyroidism

Thyrotropin is usually the third adenohypophyseal hormone to be affected in hypopituitarism being preceded by decreased gonadotrophin and somatotrophin. There are no recognized skeletal effects at present reported.

3.5.4. EXCESS OF THYROID HORMONES

Thyrotoxicosis. Excess of thyroid hormones is rare in children. Hyperthyroidism is associated with an acceleration of both growth and osseous development.

Effect on adults. Thyrotoxicosis is nearly always due to disease of the thyroid gland itself. Hyperthyroidism induced by ectopic secretion of TSH is exceedingly rare.

In adults with an excess of circulating thyroid hormones considerable changes are noted both in calcium metabolism and in bone histology. The severe changes first noted by Von Recklinghausen in 1891 are now rarely seen because of early diagnosis and treatment of hyperthyroidism.

The histological, biochemical, and radiological changes seen today are probably all dependent upon the finding of Mundy and his colleagues (1976) using an organ culture technique, that both thyroxine and triiodothyronine when added to the culture medium at concentrations approaching those which occur in thyrotoxicosis will stimulate bone resorption by osteoclasts.

3.5.4.1. Histological changes

The main feature of the histological change depends on an increased rate of bone turnover. There is increased osteoclastic activity which is responsible for the thinning of bone trabeculae and increased porosity of cortical bone; fibrous tissue being laid down in these newly created spaces (Adams and Jowsey 1967). Jowsey using histological, in conjunction with biochemical studies, describes osteoporosis characterized by increased bone-resorption and normal or increased bone-formation (Adams and Jowsey 1967; Adams, Jowsey, Kelly, Riggs, Kinney, and Jones 1967). This agrees with the findings of Krane and his colleagues (Krane *et al.* 1956) using ^{45}Ca and the technique of isotope dilution. They conclude that bone-formation as well as bone-destruction are proceeding at increased rates in thyrotoxicosis.

3.5.4.2. *Radiographic changes*

The overall picture is indistinguishable from that associated with primary or secondary osteoporosis (Smith, Fraser, and Wilson 1973). X-rays of the second metacarpal bones show thinning of the cortices compared with normal controls. There may be decreased density of the spine with or without crush fractures. The severity of the changes depends to some extent on sex and age, also the length of time the hyperthyroidism has gone untreated.

3.5.4.3. *Biochemical changes*

The majority of patients have plasma calcium and phosphorus levels within the normal range though the mean calcium level tends to be higher than that found in normal subjects. Plasma phosphorus is also reported to be higher than average though within the normal range. Urinary calcium is frequently raised and tubular reabsorption of phosphorus is also raised (Smith *et al.* 1973). Faecal calcium is also often raised and may be higher than the dietary intake. The calcium balance is usually negative and not affected by vitamin D (Smith *et al.* 1973).

There is a further group of patients where hyperthyroidism is associated with hypercalcaemia. They have been reviewed by Parfitt and Dent (1970), who consider the hypercalcaemia may be associated with hyperparathyroidism either as a manifestation of associated primary hyperparathyroidism or as a direct complication. In the first case they consider the association is genuine but the cause unknown. It is rare. In the second case successful treatment of hyperthyroidism invariably lowers plasma calcium to normal. They suggest eight theories to explain the hypercalcaemia which occurs as a direct complication, none of which they consider satisfactory: (a) accelerated bone turnover with immobilization; (b) accelerated bone turnover with reduced renal clearance of calcium; (c) adrenal insufficiency; (d) concomitant primary hyperparathyroidism; (e) increased parathyroid hormone secretion without structural changes; (f) potentiation of parathyroid hormone action; (g) calcitonin deficiency; (h) potentiation of vitamin D action.

3.6. The sex hormones

Something has already been said about the sex hormones in discussing the growth spurt (p. 177). The characteristic female sex hormones are spoken of as oestrogens and are largely secreted by the ovary. The characteristic male hormones, spoken of as androgens, are largely secreted by the testes. Small amounts of both are also secreted by the adrenal cortex (Lee and Laycock 1978). It must, however, always be remembered that androgens are found in female serum and oestrogens in male serum, and both act synergistically in either sex throughout life (see p. 177). It would seem that the sex hormones are produced in small amounts during childhood but do not appear to influence growth to any dramatic extent until puberty when as already discussed (p. 177) they are the basis for the adolescent growth spurt, the related changes in body composition, the appearance of secondary sexual characteristics (see Fig. 10.2) and eventual epiphyseal fusion (Short 1980). They continue to affect the skeleton throughout life though less dramatically.

3.6.1. THE ANDROGENS

Androgen production in the male is primarily under the control of the pituitary luteinizing hormone (LH). Follicle stimulating hormone (FSA) may have a synergistic role in steroidogenesis but its major actions are upon testicular growth and spermatogenesis. Control of these pituitary gonadotropins is mediated by the hypothalamic neurosecretory factor LH–RH. In adult men the principal circulating androgen is testosterone, 95 per cent of which is secreted by the testis (Baird et al. 1969). Less than 5 per cent is produced by the adrenals. Short (1980) suggests that when oestrogen excretion starts to rise in girls at the age of 9–10, ovarian androgen secretion may also rise.

3.6.1.1. *Testosterone*

Testosterone is responsible for the development of secondary sex characteristics and for the growth and development of the skeleton which occurs at puberty (see p. 177). Treatment of children with growth hormone deficiency requires, not only growth hormone, but continuous testosterone (see p. 183). Short (1980) has postulated a 'double threshold' effect of testosterone on bone growth, namely that high blood levels may stimulate bone growth, while a fall in level results in cessation of growth. He illustrates his argument in part by an analysis of antler growth and shedding. 'Not only does testosterone inhibit the osteoclastic activity that leads to antler casting but small amounts are essential for normal antler growth and development and large amounts convert the living velvet antler into the dead bone of the "hard horn" antler.' He concludes that it is the pubertal increase in testicular testosterone secretion that is responsible for first initiating and ultimately terminating the peak height spurt in normal boys.

3.6.1.2. *Excessive androgen secretion*

In precocious puberty the increased androgen secretion accelerates growth and somatic development, including skeletal maturation. This may result in tall stature in children but short adult height (Styne and Grumbach 1978). Zachmann and his colleagues (Zachmann, Ferrandez, Murset, Gnehm, and Prader 1976) conclude that adult height in 'tall boys' (only rarely due to pituitary disorders (pituitary adenoma, homocystinuria, Klinefelter's syndrome, and others) may best be treated by testosterone started in early puberty and that the suppressing effects on pituitary and testicular function are fully reversible. The effect, they consider, is on growth velocity and is exclusively due to the anabolic effect on bone of testosterone, while the effect of oestrogen in 'tall girls' is due to an inhibitory effect on somatomedin, which reduces growth velocity, and secondarily to an increased secretion of androgen, possibly through the adrenals, which accelerates bone age.

3.6.1.3. *Site of action of testosterone*

These observations on the effect of testosterone on bone growth suggest it must act on osteoblasts and chondroblasts, the cells responsible for growth in length and width of bones. On the other hand Raisz and his colleagues have shown that testosterone has no effect on bone in organ culture (Raisz, Canalis, Dietrich, Kream, and Gworek 1978). Recent work from DeLuca's group (see p. 144) suggest that androgens exert some influence on bone by affecting $24,25\text{-}(OH_2)D_3$ in the kidney. There is clearly much work to be done.

3.6.2. THE OESTROGENS

The oestrogens are largely synthesized in the ovary, the major oestrogen is oestradiol, the other two being oestrone and 17 β oestradiol: a little is produced in the testis and a little by peripheral conversion from circulating testosterone. The corpus luteum, the fetaplacental unit, and the adrenal cortex also produce a little.

3.6.2.1. *Effects in animals (other than man)*

The growth spurt does not occur in animals, it appears to be peculiar, at least in its marked form, to man. However, the effects of oestrogen on growing mice is striking (Silberburg and Silberburg 1971). The reason for this is not clear except that perhaps pregnancies, particularly in laboratory mice, are frequent and therefore the demands on the skeleton for calcium are large. This oestrogen effect on the turnover of bone in the mouse skeleton may well account for the greater frequency of cancers in the skeleton of female mice following injection of bone-seeking radionuclides than in male mice (Nilsson 1973).

3.6.2.2. *Effects in birds*

Recent studies have thrown considerable light on the effects of oestrogen in birds (Tanaka *et al.* 1976; Castillo *et al.* 1977). Oestrogen is probably responsible for the remarkable changes in calcium metabolism during the egg-laying cycle. As much as 1 g of calcium is incorporated into the egg shell within 1 day as the female reaches maturity. This is associated with an increased absorption of calcium, in serum calcium and in medullary bone. At the same time a phosphoprotein for transport of calcium is formed in the liver, and there is increased oestrogen in the plasma and in the urine. The egg-laying female quail or chicken has been found also to have high levels of 25-$(OH)D_3$-1-hydroxylase in the kidney. A similar high level can be induced in the male bird following administration of oestradiol, but though there is an associated rise in plasma calcium, no calcium is retained in increased medullary bone. If the male is castrated no rise in the 1-hydroxylase occurs unless testosterone is also given. Clearly androgen as well as oestrogen is required to produce the increase in 1-hydroxylase, another example of the synergistic action of the two sex hormones. While oestradiol stimulates the production of 1-hydroxylase in the female bird it suppresses the production of 24-hydroxylase. Homogenates from the male quail kidney on the other hand appear to convert 25-$(OH)D_3$ to 24,25-$(OH_2)D_3$. The mechanism, or indeed significance, of the synergism between these two sex hormones in stimulating 1-hydroxylase is not known (Castillo et $al.$ 1977). Other hormones such as FSH (follicle-stimulating-hormone) cortisone, testosterone, and progesterone even at high dose levels of oestradiol produce little or no change in 1-hydroxylase though testosterone appeared to suppress 24-hydroxy-vitamin D hydroxylase.

The stimulation of 1-hydroxylase in birds by oestrogen is greater than that produced by PTH and since the effect of the two hormones is additive it suggests that they may well function by a different mechanism (Castillo et $al.$ 1977).

3.6.2.3. *Effects in man*

3.6.2.3.1. *Normal bone.* The experiments just described on the effects of oestrogen on calcium metabolism in birds, indicating that these effects were mediated through the hydroxylation of 25-$(OH)D_3$ in the kidney, at once suggest that oestrogen might have similar effects in man. The evidence that this is so is discussed below in connection with studies of osteoporosis.

3.6.2.3.2. *Osteoporosis.* Osteoporosis is a disorder characterized by reduction in the quantity and the structural bony material per unit volume of bone as an organ. There are no recognized significant abnormalities in the bony material that remains. It may affect all the bones of the body (Heaney 1976b) though the axial skeleton is more severely affected than the long bones.

A decrease in bone mass may occur in a variety of circumstances. The most controversial form of osteoporosis is that associated with ageing, and in women both after the menopause and after oophorectomy. Osteoporosis is found much more rarely in young people, though a form spoken of as idiopathic osteoporosis does occur in younger people. It is also present in severe form in hypercortisonism, whether this is idiopathic, as in Cushing's syndrome, or induced by cortisone therapy (p. 200), and in hyperthyroidism (p. 190).

3.6.2.3.2.1. *Osteoporosis associated with aging.* The literature covering what one may call idiopathic osteoporosis is immense, and until recently unrewarding. No attempt is made to review it here. It is generally agreed that there is a general loss of bone in both men and women as they age. What has been questioned is whether a pathological loss of bone can be distinguished from this normal loss (Dunnill *et al.* 1967; Sissons *et al.* 1967). Morgan and his colleagues (Newton-John and Morgan 1968, 1970; Morgan 1973) consider that there are considerable normal variations in the amount of bone in any skeleton when growth stops, therefore there will be considerable variations in the amount of bone lost in the process of aging, and the thinner bones found in some people in old age are simply due to the fact that they began with less bone. Nordin and his colleagues, on the other hand, consider that there is a group of patients, especially women after the menopause, whose osteoporosis associated with crush-fracture of the spine is pathological (Gallagher, Aaron, Horseman, Marshall, Wilkinson, and Nordin 1973; Saville 1973). Gallagher and his colleagues have stated that however osteoporosis may be defined and whatever the contribution of aging or other cause may be, there is an unmistakeable osteoporotic syndrome characterized by vertebral crush-fractures, with or without biconcavity, which occurs predominantly in post-menopausal women (Gallagher *et al.* 1973).

Calcium metabolism in the aging and in osteoporosis

Early studies using either radiocalcium absorption or metabolic balance techniques have uniformly found that intestinal calcium absorption decreases with aging in both sexes, particularly when over 70 years of age (Nordin, Wilkinson, Marshall, Gallagher, Williams, and Peacock 1976). All studies, with one exception (Avioli, McDonald, and Lee 1965), have shown that osteoporotic patients have low calcium absorption compared with age-matched controls.

Recently Gallagher and his colleagues (Gallagher *et al.* 1979a,b) have attempted to analyse the effects of vitamin D metabolites on calcium absorption in normal ageing subjects and osteoporotic patients. They conclude on the basis of extensive experimental observations that inadequate metabolism of 25-OHD_3 to $1,25\text{-(OH)}_2\text{D}_3$ contributes significantly to decreased calcium absorption in both osteoporotics and elderly subjects. In patients with osteoporosis they suggest that this abnormality could result from a decrease in factors that normally stimulate $1,25\text{-(OH)}_2\text{D}_3$ production such as the decreased parathyroid hormone secretion and the increased serum phosphate they were able to demonstrate. In elderly subjects they are unable to exclude a primary abnormality in metabolism of 25-(OH)D to 1,25-(OH)$_2$ analogous to that seen in ageing rats.

3.6.2.3.2.2. *Osteoporosis associated with the menopause.* Since osteoporosis whether mild or severe, is so often associated with the menopause and is found in young women after oophorectomy, it has been attributed, at least in women, to lack of oestrogen and has for over 30 years been treated with oestrogen with what Heaney has described as 'unscientific enthusiasm among the protagonists in the oestrogen controversy' (Heaney 1976*b*).

Pincus and his colleagues in 1955 stated that both oestrogen and androgen levels were low in menopausal women. More recently in a group of women with vertebral compression fractures associated with post-menopausal osteoporosis, Riggs (Riggs, Ryan, Wahner, Jiang, and Mattox 1973) found plasma testosterone, oestrogen, and gonadotropin levels were not significantly different from those in age-matched controls and concluded that these observations did not support the suggestion that women, in whom clinically apparent osteoporosis develops at the menopause, have a greater post-menopausal decline in sex hormones.

Manolagas and his colleagues (Manolagas, Anderson, and Lindsay 1979) have described their observations that women who lost bone rapidly after oophorectomy had a significantly higher urinary cortisol excretion and a paradoxically diminished cortical response to corticotropin than women with a slow bone loss. They suggest that cortisol by its catabolic effect may be a significant factor in causing osteoporosis.

3.6.2.3.2.3. *Treatment. Oestrogen.* The literature covering the treatment of osteoporosis with oestrogen is both extensive and inconclusive (Heaney 1976*b*; Nachtigall, Nachtigall, Nachtigall, and Beckman 1979). It is not reviewed here. The most recent case control study suggests it may be preventive (Hutchinson, Polansky, and Feinstein 1979).

1,25-(OH)$_2$D$_3$ Since the powerful effect of oestrogen on the metabolism of vitamin D was demonstrated by DeLuca and his colleagues (see p. 194), several reports of successful treatment of osteoporosis with 1,25-(OH)$_2$D$_3$ have appeared (Gallagher, Riggs, Fisman, Arnaud, and DeLuca 1976; DeLuca 1977; Lindholm, Sevastikoglo, and Lindgren 1978; Gallagher, Riggs, Johnson, and DeLuca 1979; Haas, Dambacher, Lauffenburger, Lammle, and Olam 1979; Lindgren and Lindholm 1979).

3.6.2.3.2.4. *Idiopathic osteoporosis in young age groups.* A recent study of the solubility and synthetic rate of bone collagen from a group of patients who were neither post-menopausal nor senile, but who had a history of severe spontaneous compression fractures, has indicated that abnormalities in the biosynthetic stages of bone matrix formation were present, and it is suggested that these patients represent a variant of normalcaemic hyperthyroidism (Henneman, Pak, Bartter, Lifschitz, and Sanzenbacher 1972). No assay of plasma PTH was made.

Bordier and his colleagues (Bordier, Miravet, and Hioco 1973) have analysed their findings in what appear to be a similar group of young patients with compression fractures and conclude that the critical feature of the disease is a decreased capacity to replace the amount of tissue removed by osteo-clastic resorption, i.e. to some failure of osteoblast activity. They do not think the parathyroid gland is involved.

3.7. The adrenocortical steroids

As far as the skeleton is concerned, the glucocorticoids, particularly cortisol, are the most important of the steroid hormones secreted by the adrenal cortex. Reports of the effect of the corticosteroids on skeletal tissue are often con-fusing and conflicting. One reason for this is that workers have used very different dose levels (Parsons 1978) and worked under conditions where it has not been possible to know the concentrations reaching the cells. It also makes a considerable difference whether water-soluble or insoluble deriva-tives are used in organ culture. Further, it is important to know just what corticosteroid is used. Cortisol, for instance, inhibits the growth of femora from 9-day-old chick embryos, but tetrahydrocortisol and 11 β-hydroxy-androstenedione (a metabolite of cortisol), are without effect (Murota, Endo, Tamaoki 1967; Murota, Shikita, and Tamaoki 1966).

Normal glucocorticoid secretion is essential for survival but it does not appear to be a major factor in normal human growth though excess of adreno-cortical steroids, whether due to therapeutic administration or to excess endogenous production, produce severe changes in both bone and cartilage.

3.7.1. CORTISOL

Cortisol is the major glucocorticoid in man. Of the total cortisol in serum, roughly 10 per cent, is available for metabolic effect, while the rest is bound to corticosteroid-binding globulin and other serum proteins, largely albumin. In target tissues it binds to specific cytoplasmic receptors. (Feldman, Oziak, Koehler, and Stern 1975.) This hormone receptor complex is then transplanted to the nucleus to initiate synthesis of new messenger RNA which in turn codes for the proteins that give rise to the hormone's metabolic effect (Winter 1978).

3.7.1.1. *Effect on skeletal homeostasis*

3.7.1.1.1. *Bone growth*. In organ culture, using foetal rat bones, Raisz and his colleagues (Raisz, Canalis, Dietrich, Kream, and Gworek 1978) found that glucocorticoids produced an unusual dual effect. There was an initial stimulation followed by inhibition of both collagen and non-collagen protein synthesis. This confirms the earlier observations of Jee (Jee, Park, Roberts, Blackwood, and Kenner 1970) that prolonged glucocorticoid treatment prevented replication and differentiation of osteoblast precursors. There was an inhibiting effect on protein RNA and DNA synthesis at extremely low concentrations, which Raisz (Raisz, Canalis, Dietrich, Kream, and Gworek 1978) suggests may be a mechanism by which bone growth can be regulated physiologically. Prockop and his colleagues (1979) state that glucocorticoids, which inhibit collagen synthesis at somewhat lower concentrations than those at which they inhibit synthesis of other proteins, decrease the hydroxylases and glycosyltransferases in a parallel fashion.

3.7.1.1.2. *Bone resorption*. It is now clear that the steroids exert an inhibitory effect on the metabolism of prostaglandins. In the case of bone, as indicated in discussing the mechanism of resorption (see p. 51), it is known that resorption, associated with the presence of secondary malignant deposits and myeloma, is dependent upon an excessive production of prostaglandin E_2 by the local macrophages. The effect of administered cortisone in reducing the hypercalcaemia dependent upon excessive resorption may well be due to its known effect on prostaglandin synthesis rather than to any direct effect on bone cells.

3.7.1.1.3. *Effect on calcium absorption*. In 1968 Norman reviewed the evidence which suggested that in some way cortisone antagonizes or partially inhibits the action of vitamin D in promoting calcium absorption. It has been suggested (Favus, Kimberg, Millar, and Gershon 1973) that this is due to hormone-related biochemical alterations in the mucosal cell containing the transport mechanism. The hormone has no effect on the synthesis of the vitamin-D-dependent intestinal calcium-binding protein.

3.7.1.1.4. *Cartilage*. Cortisone inhibits the longitudinal growth of the appendicular skeleton through interference with the normal metabolic changes that occur in cartilage matrix (Chapter 4, p. 88). The epiphyseal cartilage of animals injected with cortisol is thinner than normal, with few hypertrophic cells, and in rats there is failure to resorb the spicules of highly calcified cartilage in the metaphysis. This results in a dense appearance of the bones in radiographs. Elegant experimental work from Fell and her co-workers has shown that cortisone exerts these effects by stabilizing lysosomal membranes, thus preventing the release of acid hydrolases, particularly cathepsin D, which are needed in normal cartilage matrix metabolism (Chapter 11, p. 210). This effect of cortisone on lysosomal membranes can be antagonized by vitamin A, which acts to release the hydrolases by attacking the lipoproteins of the lysosome membrane (Chapter 11, p. 202) (Thomas 1956; Fell and Thomas 1961; Dingle, Fell, and Lucy 1966; Barrett, Sledge, and Dingle 1966; Weston, Barrett, and Dingle 1969).

3.7.1.2. *Therapeutic administration of cortisol*

3.7.1.2.1. *Effect on growth*. Steroid therapy is now used for a variety of conditions in both children and adults. In children particularly the risks of severe interference with growth when steroids are given continuously for asthma or nephrosis, for instance, must not be forgotten (Preece 1976). In Fig. 10.7 is shown the height velocity chart of a boy with hypercortisolism due to an adrenal adenoma. Note the catch-up growth which followed removal of the tumour.

It is not at present clear to what extent this inhibition of growth represents solely a direct action of glucocorticoids upon growing cartilage or to what degree suppression of growth hormone secretion and antagonism of its effects may contribute.

In adults excess administration of cortisol for treatment of a variety of conditions may give rise to the symptoms associated with Cushing's syndrome, particularly swelling of the face and bone pain dependent on osteoporosis.

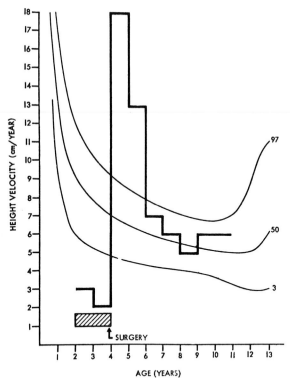

FIG. 10.7. Height velocity chart of a boy with hypercortisolism due to an adrenal adenoma. Note the catch-up growth which followed removal of the neoplasm. (From Winter (1978) by courtesy of author and publishers.)

3.7.1.3. *Cushing's syndrome*

Cushing's syndrome, in which there is an excess secretion of cortisol, is rare in children and more common in women than men. It may be due to a tumour in the adrenal or the pituitary or therapeutic administration of cortisol. The characteristic skeletal lesion, osteoporosis (see p. 199), may result in collapse of vertebrae, kyphosis, and spontaneous fracture. There may be severe bone pain. The serum alkaline phosphatase is either normal or elevated. The blood calcium is normal but there may be hypophosphataemia. Long-term therapy with Bromocriptine may result in a fall in plasma ACTH in pituitary-dependent Cushing's syndrome, but plasma cortisols are unaltered (Kennedy, Sheridan, and Montgomery 1978).

11. The Vitamins

MELLANBY in 1945 described vitamins A and D as 'The David and Jonathan of Nutrition. Although their functions are different, they are both concerned with the building maintenance of bone structure'. Today vitamin D is regarded as a hormone essential to calcium homeostasis and is discussed elsewhere (Chapter 9, p. 139). Vitamins A and C are essential to different aspects of bone and cartilage metabolism and something is known of the mechanism of their action. Vitamin K is now recognized as playing an important role in the synthesis of a matrix glycoprotein–osteocalcin (see p. 74). It is still not clear that vitamin E has any essential role in either skeletal or mineral homeostasis.

1. VITAMIN A

1.1. Chemistry

Vitamin A is a generic term that includes all compounds with the biological activity of retinol. It is carried in the plasma, by a specific protein known as retinol-binding protein (RBP), where it exists as holo-RBP, i.e. a 1 : 1 molar complex with retinol. Apo-RBP is free of retinol. Holo-RBP in plasma, binds very tightly to specific cell surface receptors which recognize the protein moiety of RBP. During the transport process across the cell plasma membrane only the retinol is internalized. Within cells vitamin A is always associated with cellular proteins or lipid rich structures. Some common metabolic reactions of retinol are esterification, oxidation to retinaldehyde, isomerization, conjugation with glucuronic acid, and phosphorylation. Retinaldehyde is oxidized to retinoic acid, which is much used experimentally. No metabolite has yet been found with activity greater than that of the vitamin itself (DeLuca, Glover, Heller, Olson, and Underwood 1977). Retinoic acid can replace retinol in maintaining growth but not in reproduction or vision.

1.2. Effects of vitamin A

Both an excess or deficiency of vitamin A have important effects on the skeleton. It was originally shown by Moore and his colleagues (Moore, Huffman, and Duncan 1935) in cattle, and by Mellanby (1944–5), in puppies, that the extensive nervous lesions occurring when the animals were fed a vitamin A deficient diet were due to bony overgrowth causing compression of nerves where they left the skull or spinal canal. Bones of the skull, unrelated to nerves, were also found to be thickened, as were those of the pelvis, while the marrow cavity of the long bones was reduced. The overall picture was one of failure of remodelling associated with continued growth, particularly on periosteal surfaces. If vitamin A was fed to the deficient puppies, normal osteoblastic and osteoclastic activity was restored. Mellanby concluded that the vitamin affected both osteoblasts and osteoclasts. Excess of vitamin also has a remarkable effect on endochondral ossification. Fell and Mellanby (1950, 1952) found that, if vitamin A was added to the culture medium surrounding a chick or mouse limb bone-rudiment, extensive resorption of bone occurred with great disturbance of epiphyseal cartilage growth.

The early observations of Mellanby have been confirmed by more recent studies using both chick, mouse, and embryonic human bone in organ culture (Rajan 1969; Rajan and Hopkins 1970; Reynolds 1972). Such organ and tissue culture experiments have shown that vitamin A (retinol) added to the culture medium in which long bones are grown results in (a) great changes in the region of the epiphyseal cartilage as evidenced by loss of metachromatic staining; and (b) rapid increase in bone resorption.

1.2.1. EFFECT ON CARTILAGE

It has long been clear that vitamin A exerts a marked effect on cartilage. Excess of vitamin A is known to produce severe birth defects, especially in the limbs. This is not a general growth inhibition since the whole foetus is not involved. Kochhar (1977) using retinoic acid found that esposure of a mouse limb bud in culture inhibited chondrogenesis in certain areas and that only brief exposure was needed. Cell death was highest eighteen hours after treatment. Cells that survived were unable to grow at normal rates and their biosynthetic capabilities were altered, large areas of cartilage not being replaced by bone.

Early experiments indicated that there was a severe disturbance of the metabolism of mucopolysaccharides of cartilage, produced by both a deficiency (Dziewiatkowsky 1954; Pasternak 1968) or an excess of vitamin A (Fell and Mellanby 1950; Fell, Mellanby and Pelc 1956). Fell and Thomas (1960, 1961) first showed in tissue culture studies that, both *in vivo* and *in vitro*, enzymes such as papain mimicked the effects of vitamin A on cartilage in certain respects but not in others. They suggested that the changes in cartilage seen in experimental hypervitaminosis A may be the result of activation of a proteolytic enzyme with properties similar to papain. That a lysosomal cathepsin might be the enzyme concerned was supported by finding that cartilage extract had a proteolytic activity with a pH optimum of 3 (Lucy, Dingle, and Fell 1961). Further work has shown that the basic effect of vitamin A on cartilage matrix results from the vitamin's action in releasing lysosomal enzymes, particularly cathepsin D, by altering the permeability of lysosomal membranes (Weston, Barrett, and Dingle 1969). The release of cathepsin D results in the intra- and extra-cellular degradation of the glyco-protein element of the organic matrix.

Such release can be blocked if an antiserum to cathepsin D is added to the culture medium. The antiserum has no inhibiting effect on other lysosomal hydrolases or proteolytic enzymes (Weston *et al.* 1969). It is now concluded by Dingle and his colleagues that cathepsin D is the major enzyme respon-sible for the degradation of chondromucoprotein, both in normal remodelling and growth and in vitamin A excess (see p. 202). Woessner (1973*a,b*) disputes this, however, and considers that the enzyme involved is probably not cathep-sin D itself but a protease, not yet identified, which is present as an impurity. Using human foetal long bones Rajan (Rajan 1969; Rajan and Hopkins 1970) has produced the same effects with vitamin A as Fell and her colleagues using mouse- and chick-embryo bones. Reynolds (1972) has suggested, on the basis of preliminary experiments, that calcitonin may prevent, at least partially, the effects of vitamin A on the resorption of cartilaginous human digits in organ culture.

1.2.2. EFFECT ON BONE

There is experimental evidence to suggest that vitamin A has more than one effect on bone. It causes resorption and is also implicated in glycosamino-glycan metabolisms.

1.2.2.1. *Resorption*

As long ago as 1948 Barnicot (Barnicot 1948*b*) showed that small fragments of crystalline vitamin A acetate attached to endocranial surfaces of pieces of parietal bone from the skulls of mice about 1-week old, and then thrust into the central hemisphere of littermates, caused areas of resorption. This resorptive activity of vitamin A has since been confirmed, both in long bones from embryonic mice (Raisz 1965) and in postnatal mouse calvaria in culture (Reynolds 1968). Reynolds describes typical areas of resorption associated with an increased number of multinucleated osteoclasts. He considers that the vitamin first stimulates the activity of existing osteoclasts and subsequently stimulates the differentiation of progenitor cells to increase the number of osteoclasts (Reynolds and Dingle 1970). The same workers also noted a loss of recognizable osteocytes in rat but not in mouse calvaria; and the osteo-blasts assumed a fibroblastic character, a picture they described as similar to that seen with PTH. Reynolds is, however, doubtful of the effect of the vitamin on osteocytes (Reynolds 1972). He suggested in 1968 that calcitonin may block the demineralizing activity of vitamin A without affecting the release of acid hydrolases (Chapter 9). He now considers that calcitonin may be involved in the control of the activity of a collagenase (Reynolds 1972), whose activity is distinct from that of the lysosomal enzymes released by vitamin A, thus accounting for the fact that such hydrolases are still present when calcitonin (CT) is added to a mouse calvaria tissue-culture media rich in vitamin A.

1.2.2.2. *Glycosaminoglycan metabolism*

Harris (1977) has recently reported that lack of dietary vitamin A increased the amount of sulphur present in the glycosaminoglycan fraction of guinea-pig bone and suggested that vitamin A may critically influence the degree of calcification achieved by affecting glycosaminoglycan metabolism in the relevant cells.

1.2.3. OTHER EXPLANATIONS OF MODE OF ACTION OF VITAMIN A

Kistler (1978) does not agree that vitamin A acts by releasing lysosomal enzymes and has produced rather confused experimental evidence that the vitamin inhibits RNA and protein synthesis.

Chertow and his colleagues (Chertow, Buschmann, and Henderson 1975; Chertow, Williams, Norris, Baker, and Hargis 1977) consider that vitamin A stimulates PTH secretion and that this may account for some of the effects of excess vitamin A. *In vitro* they found retinol stimulates hormone secretion, possibly through modification of cell or cell organelle membranes, since the effect was inhibited by vitamin E and hydrocortisone. *In vivo* when given to healthy men, as vitamin A palmitate, they found a rise in serum PTH and possibly in calcium.

1.2.4. LONG-TERM INGESTION OF EXCESS VITAMIN A IN MAN

Frame and his colleagues have described three interesting cases who had for several years taken an excess of vitamin A. The outstanding findings were hypercalcaemia associated with bone resorption and periosteal calcification (Frame, Jackson, Reynolds, and Umphrey 1974).

2. VITAMIN C

Vitamin C is concerned both in the synthesis of collagen and of glycosamino-glycans (Kodicek 1965).

2.1. Scurvy

It has long been recognized that in scurvy, a disease due to lack of vitamin C, there is impaired formation of bone and the failure of bone repair after injury. The cortex of the long bones shows thinning and increased fragility. The epiphyseal zones are fragile and irregular. In the diaphysis the trabeculae are thin without osteoid seams and without an osteoclastic reaction. In children, the most characteristic changes are in the epiphysis; the cartilage cells continue to multiply in columns and the matrix calcifies forming a fragile brittle network which breaks and is responsible for the characteristic X-ray picture, giving the scorbutic band or Trummerfeld. There may be complete failure of osteoid formation, osteoblasts are few, and connective tissue fibroblasts appear to predominate. The osteoclasts are less affected. Subperiosteal haemorrhages are common.

2.2. Effects on collagen and glycosaminoglycans

There seems little doubt that the abnormalities seen in scurvy are attributable to impaired formation of matrix, particularly the impaired synthesis of collagen. Working with cartilaginous limb bone-rudiments from embryonic chicks in culture it has been shown that the addition of ascorbic acid to a chemically defined medium greatly increases the collagen synthesis and eliminates excessive hydration of the cortex (Reynolds 1972). The minimum concentration of ascorbic acid necessary to prevent the excessive hydration usually observed in bone-rudiments growing *in vitro* is $50 \mu g \, ml^{-1}$. A higher level of $80 \mu g \, ml^{-1}$ was the minimum dose required for maximum synthesis (Reynolds 1967). The action of ascorbic acid appears extremely specific. Dehydroascorbic acid failed to prevent the hydration and did not promote collagen synthesis. Isoascorbic acid was about one-third as active as an equal dose of ascorbic acid in promoting collagen synthesis (Reynolds 1967).

The important part played by ascorbic acid in collagen synthesis is discussed in detail by Gould (1960, 1968, 1970). It is thought that both the *in vitro* and the clinical effects of ascorbic-acid deficiency are the direct consequence of an impairment of hydroxylation of collagen proline and lysine where ascorbic acid is required as a reducing co-factor (Prockop *et al.* 1979; Barnes 1973). Levene and his colleagues (Levene and Bates 1976; Levene, Ockleford, and Barber 1977) who have studied collagen synthesis is cultured 3T6 fibroblasts, found that the fibres laid down lack the banding pattern typical of collagen. This effect they consider may be obscured *in vivo* by secondary effects.

Hajek and Solursh (1977) have recently studied the effect of ascorbic acid on chick-embryo sternal chondrocytes in cell culture. They found at the end of four days there was a 58 per cent increase in the number of cells and

35 per cent increase in protein. Collagen was increased by 116 per cent and the incorporation of ^{35}S was also accelerated. Though the number of cells was increased, the size and protein content of individual cells was reduced. This effect on both collagen and glycosaminoglycan synthesis is consistent, they consider, with Dorfman's original suggestion that it is 'co-regulated'. The mechanism of action on sulphate incorporation is not understood (Schwartz and Adamy 1977). Lack of vitamin C depresses the incorporation of glucose into galactosamine in granulation tissue in healing wounds. Histochemical staining suggests that acid mucopolysaccharides are reduced and replaced by neutral mucopolysaccharide material (Kodicek 1965).

3. VITAMIN K

Vitamin K is essential for the biosynthesis of a group of calcium-binding proteins, some of which are present in plasma and others in different tissues such as kidney and liver. The vitamin functions as a co-factor for an enzyme that carboxylates peptide-bound glutamyl residues and converts them to γ-carboxyglutamyl residues. Such residues are powerful Ca^{2+} binders. Their importance was first recognized as a factor in prothrombin synthesis. As Hauschka has said 'prothrombin is the first example of a protein in which specific binding sites, in this case for calcium, are generated enzymatically'. In 1975 Hauschka and his colleagues (Hauschka, Lian, and Gallop 1975) isolated from bone a small protein rich in vitamin-K-dependent calcium-binding amino acid γ-carboxyglutamate (Gla) which they called osteocalcin (see p. 74). Though the physiological role of osteocalcin is still uncertain (Reddy and Suttie 1979) the fact that, after collagen, it is the next most abundant protein in bone, suggests that vitamin K is important in bone matrix metabolism. For further discussion of this exciting and expanding field of bone physiology the proceedings of a recent symposium should be consulted (Suttie 1979).

4. VITAMIN E

There is little evidence that vitamin E (tocopherols) has any effect on the skeleton. It has recently been reported, with no supporting evidence, that monkeys severely deficient in tocopherol have exhibited skeletal dystrophy and marrow failure (DeLuca et al. 1977). It has been suggested that vitamin E might be concerned in the formation of collagen cross-links. Rao and Bose (1971) described how the simultaneous administration, daily, of both β-aminopropionitrile and a relatively high dose of vitamin E (3 mg per animal) to rats fed on vitamin-E-deficient diet, afforded some protection against the lathyric changes induced in rats by the nitrile alone. Brown, Button, and Smith (1967) observed slight changes in collagen solubility and in the rate of formation and stability of gels of collagen from vitamin-E-deficient rats and therefore suggested there might be some defect in the formation of cross-links.

12. Enzymes in Bone and Cartilage

No attempt will be made in this chapter to review the literature covering the enzymes in bone and cartilage. It is extensive and somewhat confused. Far more is known about the catabolic enzymes than about those concerned in anabolic processes.

It is now recognized that enzyme antagonists—notably α_2 macroglobulin —exist in serum and synovial fluid, to many of the powerful enzymes involved in matrix degradation (Starkey and Barrett 1977). Failure to recognize the existence of such antagonists may have been responsible in the past for inability to demonstrate the presence of an enzyme in experiments using tissue and cell culture techniques. It is also accepted that certain powerful enzymes are not necessarily stored in the cell but are freshly synthesized on demand. Further, many enzymes are dependent on the presence of different metals and it is becoming increasingly recognized that a deficiency of one of the trace metals present in bone may result in severe general, as well as skeletal, abnormalities (see p. 100).

One of the many questions that arise is, do the enzymes that degrade the macromolecules and those that synthesize the macromolecules of bone and cartilage matrix exist in the same cell? This question is particularly important in the case of cartilage where the only cell seems to be the chondrocyte that is apparently concerned with both the synthesis and degradation of matrix. In the case of bone these functions appear to be separate; the osteoblast synthesizes the matrix, the osteoclast and perhaps other mononuclear cells (see p. 100) resorbs the matrix.

1. THE ACID AND ALKALINE PHOSPHATASES

Vaes and his colleagues (Vaes 1973; Lieberherr, Vreven, and Vaes 1973; Vreven, Lieberherr, and Vaes 1973) have reviewed the character and distribution of the acid and alkaline phosphatases. They conclude that there are three distinct acid phosphatases (acid β-glycerophosphatase, phosphoprotein phosphatase, and acid inorganic pyrophosphatase) and probably one alkaline phosphatase found in bone. In subcellular fractions of bone homogenates, the highest specific activity of alkaline inorganic pyrophosphatase and other alkaline phosphatase activities was found in the 'microsomal fraction'. The acid hydrolases were found in the light mitochondrial fraction. In cytoplasmic extracts of bone the various acid phosphatases occur in latent form to the extent of 50–60 per cent of their activity. They can be unmasked by a series of treatments which suggest they are present in lysosomes. As Vaes says, the precise cytological nature of the material bearing the alkaline phosphatase in bone cells remains to be elucidated.

In earlier papers Vaes (1968a,b) gives an account of the acid hydrolases released into the culture media under the influence of PTH (see p. 49).

Something has already been said about the importance of the phosphatases in calcification mechanisms, particularly in relation to their presence in matrix vesicles (p. 88).

2. ENZYMES CONCERNED WITH MATRIX DEGRADATION

Dingle (1973b) has divided the enzymes concerned with matrix turnover into five groups here discussed. He suggests two stages in matrix breakdown. In the first stage, the initial cleavage of both the major macromolecules, i.e. collagen and proteoglycans, he considers is proteolytic and extracellular. Such cleavage may facilitate diffusion and perhaps alter the interaction of the matrix molecules with the cell surface, allowing endocytic activity to take place. Complete breakdown of collagen and proteoglycan then takes place within the lysosomes, which contain both peptidases and sulphatases.

2.1. Acid proteinases

Both cathepsin D and cathepsin E are functionally related to pepsin.

2.1.1. CATHEPSIN D

This enzyme has been completely purified for several species (Barrett 1972). Cathepsins from different organs within the same species are immunologically identical but do not cross-react between species. Cathepsin D has a molecular weight of about 45 000 and does not require activation. The most recent work suggests it has no action on collagen (Burleigh et al. 1974) contrary to earlier experiments (Morrison 1970). It has, however, an important effect on cartilage. When acting on purified proteoglycan or on whole cartilage, cathepsin D has a pH optimum of 5·0, which is similar to that found for the autolytic degradation of human and animal cartilage by endogenous enzymes. Tissue culture experiments indicate a cleavage of each proteoglycan molecule at perhaps 2–4 places along the polypeptide back-bone, without evidence of degradation of the polysaccharide side-chains, though there may be some enzymic desulphation. This means that only a very limited proteolytic attack is necessary to cause extensive damage to the integrity of the tissue. Cathepsin D has been shown by immunocytochemical techniques to be present in lysosomes within the cell, but may also be demonstrated extracellularly in those regions where matrix degradation is taking place (Dingle 1973b). This has been demonstrated in cartilage and in the bones of young chicks where cartilage is in process of being replaced by bone mineral.

Dingle (1973a) has described a further protease, which he calls cathepsin F, that is specific for cartilage proteoglycans, is active up to pH 7, and membrane-bound.

2.1.2. CATHEPSIN E

This enzyme has been isolated from bone marrow (Lapresle 1971) and though it has a similar mode of action to cathepsin D it is immunologically distinct (Weston 1969). Dingle (1973a) suggests it has a role in the formation of the marrow cavity and may have a part to play in the intravacuolar digestion of protein-containing material.

2.1.3. CATHEPSIN A

Cathepsin A is found in both rabbit-ear cartilage and monkey articular cartilage (Ali and Evans 1973).

2.1.4. CATHEPSIN C

Cathepsin C is present in rabbit-ear cartilage (Ali and Evans 1973).

2.2. The thiol proteinases

2.2.1. CATHEPSIN B_1

This cathepsin, has recently been recognized to have an important role in the degradation of collagen. Though much of the work has been done on the cathepsin isolated from liver it is known to be present in bone and cartilage.

It may well be the major agent in intracellular breakdown of collagen. Burleigh and her colleagues have shown, using several different assay systems, that the reactive products from cathepsin B_1 degradation at pH 3–5 differ from the cleavage products resulting from the action of neutral collagenase (see p. 211) (Burleigh et al. 1974).

The initial action is cleavage of the non-helical region of collagen containing the cross-link. The enzyme also attacks the helical region, rapidly degrading it to low-molecular-weight peptides. Its action is completely inhibited by the plasma protein α_2 macroglobulin. This cathepsin also degrades isolated proteoglycans and adult human cartilage, the optimum pH being 3–5, but more activity was shown towards a neutral pH than with cathepsin D. The enzyme is known to have a lysosomal localization, but it is not known whether it is also released in the same extracellular sites as cathepsin D (Dingle 1973a).

2.3. The neutral proteinases

This rather heterogeneous group contains plasmin, the collagenases, and enzymes capable of cartilage proteoglycan degradation, the glycoprotein-degrading enzymes (SPGases).

2.3.1. COLLAGENASES

Lazarus (1973) defines collagenases as enzymes capable of degrading native collagen fibrils under physiological conditions of temperature and pH; or as enzymes which cleave native collagen molecules in solution through the characteristic helical part of the molecule. This definition precludes enzymes such as trypsin and pronase being designated collagenases, since they effect a limited digestion of an end of the native collagen molecule. This characteristic cleavage takes place at 25 °C, and serves only as a criterion for identification of these enzymes. At 35 °C highly purified collagenase, readily degrades native collagen in solution, gelatin-insoluble collagen, and collagen fibrils to small peptides (Werb and Burleigh 1974).

The first vertebrate collagenase was discovered in tadpole tail tissues in primary culture by Gross and Lapiere (1962). Previous attempts to find collagenase in tissue homogenates had failed, probably because of inhibitors in the tissues. Another reason was that the enzyme can bind, after release from cells, to insoluble fibrillar substrate in both active and latent form. More than 30 collagenases from different mammalian tissues have been described (Harris and Cartwright 1977). Their similarities are more striking than their differences. They are active in the presence of certain metal ions and are inhibited completely by chealting agents. It is probable that Zn^{2+} may be an integral component of mammalian collagenase and that Ca^{2+} is essential for their activity. The enzyme can only be extracted, if at all, from tissues in small quantities. The only exception is the polymorphonuclear leucocyte which contains collagenase in specific granules (Murphy, Reynolds, Bretz, and Baggiolini 1977), but this enzyme differs from the collagenase of connective tissue. There has been considerable discussion as to whether latent collagenase is present as a pro-enzyme awaiting activation by proteinases or is an enzyme inhibitor complex formed by active collagenase combined with inhibitors (Reynolds, Murphy, Sellers, and Cartwright 1977; Harris and Cartwright 1977). The serum proteins, α_2 macroglobulin and β_1 anticollagenase, are well recognized inhibitors and others have been isolated from a number of tissues (Reynolds *et al.* 1977). Reynolds and his colleagues favour the latter hypothesis for which they have produced experimental evidence. They consider that the relative concentrations of active enzyme and inhibitor determine the sites and extent to which collagen resorption takes place, and that collagenase is synthesized under the control of specific stimuli such as hormones (Harris and Cartwright 1977), prostaglandins (Robinson, Tashjian, and Levene 1975), or lymphokines (Wahl, Wahl, Mergenhagen, and Martin 1975). They suggest that active collagenase is secreted by cells and that experimentally observed latent collagenase represents complexes formed extracellularly between active enzyme and a tissue inhibitor, which they have identified and partially characterized in rabbit bone (Sellers and Reynolds 1977).

Collagenase, however, can no longer be thought of as the only enzyme concerned in the physiological degradation of collagen, though as Burleigh says 'It is probably the most important enzyme initiating the degradation'. She considers that the activity of crude lysosomal enzyme preparations against collagen, that are reported, can be attributed at least in part to the thiol proteinases, particularly cathepsin B, with possible contributions from 'collagenolytic cathepsin'. Other thiol proteinases such as papain can also degrade collagen. She also lists the serine proteinase, and granulocyte elastases as capable of degrading native collagen and the metallo proteinases (Burleigh 1977). Such enzymes probably act on the collagen molecule rather differently to the collagenases, possibly by attacking the inter- and intra-molecular cross links. It is not yet clear whether these other proteinases contribute to the degradation of collagen by acting synergistically with the collagenase system or by providing a complete alternative route of degradation.

2.3.2. NEUTRAL METALLO-PROTEINASES

Rabbit bones in culture produce specific collagenase and neutral metal proteinase activity in latent forms that can be activated by either 4-amino-phenylmercuric acetate or trypsin. The metal proteinase activity has been resolved into two enzymes, distinct from collagenase, that degrade gelatin and cartilage proteoglycans (Sellers, Reynolds, and Meikle 1978). Reynolds and his colleagues suggest 'it seems likely that rabbit bones synthesize and secrete neutral metallo-proteinases, whose activities are under common control and which together are capable of completely degrading the extracellular matrix.' They do not commit themselves as to which cell performs the synthesis. Is it the osteoclast or associated macrophages?

2.4. Glycosidases

Lysozyme is known to occur in cartilage. Hyaluronidase has been described in the bones of young rats localized in lysosomes. Dingle (1973b) is doubtful whether either of these enzymes are important, at least, in the initial stages of matrix breakdown.

2.5. Miscellaneous enzymes

In this group Dingle (1973a) includes the peptidases and sulphatases. Several are present in skeletal tissue lysosomes. They may play a part in the completion of the breakdown of the matrix molecules in the vacuolar system.

It is perhaps of significance that most of the matrix-degrading enzymes have a relatively low molecular weight, probably below 50000. This is a rough limit to the material that can readily diffuse through cartilage matrix. It is possible to show that the enzymes, which are produced locally, can diffuse from the cell to their substrate; the inhibitors in serum, on the other hand, with higher molecular weights, cannot reach the enzymes until the latter either diffuse out of the matrix or until the matrix is sufficiently degraded to allow the large molecule to diffuse in (Dingle 1973a).

3. PART PLAYED BY SOFT TISSUE ADJACENT TO BONE OR CARTILAGE

The clinical problems of joint disease whether rheumatic or osteoarthritic in origin have stimulated intensive study of the underlying joint pathology. The possible part played by synovial membrane and synovial fluid has been much investigated.

Fell and her colleagues (Fell and Barrett 1973; Poole, Barrett, and Fell 1973) have shown in the case of articular cartilage that under certain pathological conditions (a) the cells of adjacent soft tissue, synovium, or marrow may release an enzyme or enzymes into the adjacent articular cartilage and this process is stimulated by a non-lytic cellular reaction with antibody in the presence of compliment; (b) the cartilage matrix is degraded and its permeability increased so that it can no longer exclude immunoglobulins and compliment from the tissue; (c) antibodies and compliment then gain direct access to the chondrocytes, the surfaces of which become the site of an antigen–antibody reaction; (d) if the reaction is not too severe the chondrocytes are stimulated to increased synthesis and secretion of lysosomal enzymes which contribute to the disintegration of the matrix. More recent work (Fell 1978; Fell and Jubb 1977) has indicated that synovial membrane affects the cartilage in two ways: by a direct action on the matrix and by an indirect action mediated through living chondrocytes. The significance of these observations is discussed by Dingle (Dingle 1979; Dingle, Saklatuala, Hembry, Tyler, Fell, and Jubb 1979).

Bibliography

ADAMS, P. H. and JOWSEY, J. (1967). Bone and mineral metabolism in hyperthyroidism: an experimental study. *Endocrinology* **81,** 735–40.

—— JOWSEY, J., KELLY, P. J., RIGGS, B. L., KINNEY, V. R., and JONES, J. D. (1967). Effects of hyperthyroidism on bone and mineral metabolism in man. *Q. Jl Med.* **36,** 1–15.

AER, J. (1968). Effect of thyrocalcitonin on urinary hydroxyproline and calcium in rats. *Endocrinology* **83,** 379–80.

AIKAWA, J. K. (1978). Biochemistry and physiology of magnesium. *Wld. Rev. Nutr. Diet* **28,** 112–42.

ALFREY, A. C., MILLER, N. L., and TROW, R. (1974). Effect of age and magnesium depletion on bone magnesium pools in rats. *J. clin. Invest.* **54,** 1074–81.

ALI, S. Y. (1976). Analysis of matrix vesicles and their role in the calcification of epiphyseal cartilage. *Fedn Proc., Fedn Am. Socs exp. Biol.* **35,** 135–42.

—— and EVANS, S. (1973). Enzymic degradation of cartilage in osteoarthritis. *Fedn Proc., Fedn Am. Socs exp. Biol.* **32,** 1494–8.

—— SAJDERA, S. W., and ANDERSON, H. C. (1970). Isolation and characterisation of calcifying matrix vesicles from epiphyseal cartilage. *Proc. natn. Acad. Sci. USA* **67,** 1513–20.

—— WISBY, A., and GRAY, J. C. (1978). Electron probe analysis of cross sections of epiphyseal cartilage. *Metab. Bone Dis. and Rel. Res.* **1,** 97–103.

—— —— EVANS, L., and CRAIG-GRAY, J. (1977). The sequence of calcium and phosphorus accumulation by matrix vesicles. *Calc. Tiss. Res.* **22,** suppl. 490–3.

ALLISON, A. C. (1978). Macrophage activation and non specific immunity. *Int. Rev. exp. Path.* **18,** 303–46.

ANAST, C. S. and CONAWAY, H. H. (1972). Review. Calcitonin. *Clin. Orthop.* **84,** 207–62.

ANDERSON, D. W. (1960). Studies of the lymphatic pathways of bone and bone marrow. *J. Bone Jt Surg.* **42A,** 716–17.

ANDERSON, H. C. (1968). Vesicles in the matrix of epiphyseal cartilage; fine structure, distribution and association with calcification. In *Proceedings of the 4th European Regional Conference on Electron Microscopy* (ed. D. S. Bocciarelli) p. 437. Poliglotta Vaticana, Roma.

—— (1969). Vesicles associated with the calcification in the matrix of epiphyseal cartilage. *J. Cell Biol.* **41,** 59–72.

—— (1973). Calcium accumulating vesicles in the intercellular matrix of bone. In *Hard tissue growth repair and remineralization* pp. 213–46. Ciba Foundation Symposium 11 (N S). Elsevier–Excerpta Medica–North Holland Associated Science Publishers, Amsterdam.

—— (1976). Matrix vesicle calcification: Introduction. *Fedn Proc.* **35,** 105–8.

—— (1978). Introduction to the second conference on matrix vesicle calcification. *Metab. Bone Dis. and Rel. Res.* **1,** 83–7.

—— and SAJDERA, S. W. (1976). Calcification of rachitic cartilage to study matrix vesicle function. *Fedn Proc.* **35**, 148–53.

ANDERSON, J., EMERY, E. W., MCALLISTER, J. M., and OSBORN, S. B. (1956). The metabolism of a therapeutic dose of ^{45}Ca in a case of multiple myeloma. *Clin. Sci.* **15**, 567–85.

ANDERSON, J. C., LABEDZ, R. I., and KEWLEY, M: A. (1977). The effect of bovine tendon glycoprotein on the formation of fibrils from collagen solutions. *Biochem. J.* **167**, 345–51.

ANDREWS, A. T. DE B. and HERRING, G. M. (1965). Further studies on bone sialoproteins. *Biochim. biophys. Acta* **101**, 239–41.

—— —— and KENT, P. W. (1967). Some studies on the composition of bovine cortical bone sialoprotein. *Biochem. J.* **104**, 705–15.

ARMSTRONG, W. D. and SINGER, L. (1956). *In vitro* uptake and exchange of bone citrate. In *Ciba Foundation Symposium on Bone Structure and Metabolism* (ed. G. E. W. Wolstenholme and C. M. O'Connor) pp. 103–13. J. and A. Churchill Ltd., London.

ASH, P., LOUTIT, J. F., and TOWNSEND, K. M. S. (1980a). Osteoclasts derived from haematopoietic stem cells. *Nature, Lond.* **283**, 669–70.

—— —— —— (1980b). Giant lysosomes, a cytoplasmic marker in osteoclasts of beige mice. *J. Path.* **130**, 237–45.

ASHTON, B. A., HERRING, G. M., OWEN, M., and TRIFFITT, J. T. (1971). Studies on the non-collagenous proteins of bone. *Israel J. med. Sci.* **7**, 409–11.

ASHTON, B. A., HÖHLING, H. J., and TRIFFITT, J. T. (1976). Plasma proteins present in human cortical bone: Enrichment of the α_2HS-glycoprotein. *Calc. Tiss. Res.* **22**, 27–33.

—— TRIFFITT, J. T., and HERRING, G. M. (1974). Isolation and partial characterization of a glycoprotein from bovine cortical bone. *Eur. J. Biochem.* **45**, 525–33.

AUBERT, J. P. and MILHAUD, G. (1960). Méthode de mesure des principales voies du métabolisme calcique chez l'homme. *Biochim. biophys. Acta* **39**, 122–39.

AVIOLI, L. V. (1969). Absorption and metabolism of vitamin D_3 in man. *Am. J. clin. Nutr.* **22**, 437–46.

—— and HADDAD, J. Q. (1973). Vitamin D: current concepts. *Metabolism* **22**, 507–31.

—— MCDONALD, J. E., and LEE, S. W. (1965). The influence of age on the intestinal absorption of ^{47}Ca in women and its relation to ^{47}Ca absorption in post menopausal osteoporosis. *J. Clin. Invest.* **44**, 1970–7.

AYNSLEY-GREEN, A., ZACHMANN, M., and PRADER, A. (1976). Interrelation of the therapeutic effects of growth hormone and testosterone on growth in hypopituitarism. *J. Paediat.* **89**, 992–9.

BACKWINKEL, K. D. and DIDDAMS, J. A. (1970). Hemangiopericytoma. Report of a case and comprehensive review of the literature. *Cancer* **25**, 896–901.

BAIRD, D. T., HORTON, R., LONGCOPE, C., and TAIT, J. F. (1969). Steroid dynamics under steady-state conditions. *Recent Prog. horm. Res.* **25**, 611–56.

BAKER, M. R., MCDONNELL, H., PEACOCK, M., and NORDIN, B. E. C. (1979). Plasma 25-hydroxy-Vitamin D concentrations in patients with fractures of the femoral neck. *Br. med. J.* **i**, 589.

BALLET, J. J. and GRISCELLI, C. (1978). Lymphoid cell transplantation in human osteopetrosis. In *Mechanisms of localized bone loss* (ed. J. E. Horton, T. M. Tarpley, and W. F. Davis) pp. 399–414. Information Retrieval, Arlington, Va.

BANKS, W. J. (1974). The ossification process of the developing antler. *Calc. Tiss. Res.* **14**, 257–74.

BARNES, D. W. H., BISHOP, M., HARRISON, G. E., and SUTTON, A. (1961). Comparison of the plasma concentration and urinary excretion of strontium and calcium in man. *Int. J. radiat. Biol.* **3**, 637–46.

BARNES, M. J. (1973). Biochemistry of collagens from mineralized tissues. In *Hard tissue growth repair and remineralization* pp. 247–61. Ciba Foundation Symposium 11 (NS). Elsevier–Excerpta Medica–North Holland–Associated Science Publishers, Amsterdam.

—— and LAWSON, D. E. M. (1978). Biochemistry of bone in relation to the function of Vitamin D. In *Vitamin D* (ed. D. E. M. Lawson) pp. 267–302. Academic Press, London.

BARNICOT, N. A. (1948a). The local action of the parathyroid and other tissues on bone in intracerebral grafts. *J. Anat.* **82**, 233–48.

—— (1948b). Local action of calciferol and vitamin A on bone. *Nature, Lond.* **162**, 848–9.

BARRETT, A. J. (1972). Lysosomal enzymes. In *Lysosomes: a laboratory handbook*, (ed. J. T. Dingle) pp. 46–135. North Holland, Amsterdam.

—— SLEDGE, C. B., and DINGLE, J. T. (1966). Effect of cortisol on the synthesis of chondroitin sulphate by embryonic cartilage. *Nature, Lond.* **211**, 83–4.

BASSETT, C. A. L. (1971). Biophysical principles affecting bone structure. In *The biochemistry and physiology of bone* (ed. G. H. Bourne) (2nd edn) Vol. 3, pp. 1–76. Academic Press, New York.

—— PAWLUK, R. J., and PILLA, A. A. (1974). Acceleration of fracture repair by electromagnetic fields. A surgically non-invasive method. *Ann. N.Y. Acad. Sci.* **238**, 242–62.

BAUD, C. A. (1968). Submicroscopic structure and functional aspect of the osteocyte. *Clin. Orthop.* **56**, 227–36.

—— and BOIVIN, G. (1978). Effect of hormones on osteocyte function and perilacunar wall structure. *Clin. Orthop.* **136**, 270–81.

BAUER, G. C. H., CARLSSON, A., and LINDQUIST, B. (1955). Evaluation of accretion, resorption and exchange reactions in the skeleton. *Kgl. Fysiograf. Sallskap. Lund Förh.* **25**, 1.

—— —— —— (1961). Metabolism and homeostatic function of bone. In *Mineral metabolism* (ed. C. L. Comar and F. Bronner) Vol. 1, Part B, pp. 609–76. Academic Press, New York.

BAYLINK, D. and WERGEDAL, J. (1971). Bone formation and resorption by osteocytes. In *Cellular mechanisms for calcium transfer and homeostasis* (ed. G. Nichols and R. H. Wasserman) pp. 257–286. Academic Press, New York.

—— —— and THOMPSON, E. (1972). Loss of protein polysaccharides at sites where bone mineralization is initiated. *J. Histochem. Cytochem.* **20**, 279–92.

BECKER, R. D., BASSETT, C. A., and BACHMAN, C. H. (1964). Bioelectrical factors controlling bone structure. In *Bone biodynamics* (ed. H. M. Frost) pp. 209–32. Little-Brown, Boston.

—— SPADARO, J. H., and BERG, E. W. (1968). The trace elements of human bone. *J. Bone Jt Surg.* **50A**, 326–34.

BEDDOE, A. H. (1978). A quantitative study of the structure of trabecular bone in man, rhesus monkey, beagle, and miniature pig. *Calc. Tiss. Res.* **25**, 273–81.

BÉLANGER, L. F. (1971). Osteocytic resorption. In *The biochemistry and physiology of bone* (ed. G. F. Bourne), (2nd edn) Vol. 3, pp. 239–70. Academic Press, New York.

—— ROBICHON, J., MIGICOVSKY, B. B., COPP, D. H., and VINCENT, J. (1963). Resorption without osteoclasts (osteolysis). In *Mechanisms of hard tissue destruction* (ed. R. F. Sognnaes) pp. 531–6. Publication No. 75. American Association for the Advancement of Science, Washington, DC.

BELL, N. H. and BARTTER, F. C. (1967). Studies of ^{47}Ca metabolism in acromegaly. *J. clin. Endocr. Metalb.* **27**, 178–84.

BELL, P. A. (1978). The chemistry of the Vitamins D. In *Vitamin D* (ed. D. E. M. Lawson) pp. 1–50. Academic Press, London.

BENNETT, B. G. (1972). Global ^{90}Sr fallout and its occurrence in diet and man. In *Biomedical implications of radiostrontium exposure* (ed. M. Goldman and L. K. Bustad) pp. 17–30. Conf. 710201 US Atomic Energy Commission, Office of Information Services.

BERNARD, B. DE, FURLAN, G., STAGNI, N., VITTUR, F., and ZANETTI, M. (1976). Role of a Ca^{2+} binding glycoprotein in the calcification process. *Calc. Tiss. Res.* **22**, suppl. 191–6.

—— STAGNI, N., VITTUR, F., and ZANETTI, M. (1977). Role of Ca^{2+} binding glycoprotein in the process of calcification. In *Calcium binding proteins and calcium function* (ed. R. H. Wasserman, R. A. Corradino, E. Carafoli, R. H. Kretsinger, D. H. Maclennan, and F. L. Siegel) pp. 428–31. North Holland, New York.

BERNARD, G. W. (1978). Ultrastructure localization of alkaline phosphatase in initial intramembranous osteogenesis. *Clin. Orthop.* **135**, 218–28.

—— and PEASE, D. C. (1969). An electron microscopic study of initial intramembranous osteogenesis. *Am. J. Anat.* **125**, 271–90.

BIJVOET, O. L. M. and SLUYS VEER, J. VAN DER (1968). The homeostasis of plasma calcium and phosphate. *Folia med. neerl.* **11**, 161–78.

—— —— and JANSEN, A. P. (1968). Effects of calcitonin on patients with Paget's disease, thyrotoxicosis or hypercalcaemia. *Lancet* **i**, 876–81.

—— —— VRIES, H. R. DE, KOPPEN, A. T. J. VAN. (1971). Natriuretic effects of calcitonin in man. *New Engl. J. Med.* **284**, 681–8.

BINGHAM, P., BRAZELL, I., and OWEN, M. (1969). The effect of parathyroid extract (PTE) on ribonucleic acid (RNA) and protein synthesis in bone and on the level of calcium in the serum. *J. Endocr.* **45**, 387–400.

BINGHAM, P. J. (1968). Study of the cells of the osteogenic connective tissue using autoradiographic techniques. D.Phil. Thesis, Oxford.

BISHOP, M., HARRISON, G. E., RAYMOND, W. H. A., and SUTTON, A. (1960). Excretion and retention of radioactive strontium in normal men following a single intravenous injection. *Int. J. radiat. Biol.* **2**, 125–42.

BLACKWOOD, H. J. J. (1966). Growth of the mandibular condyle of the rat studied with tritiated thymidine. *Archs oral Biol.* **11**, 493–500.

BLAND, M. R., LOUTIT, J. F., and SANSOM, J. M. (1974). Histochemical phosphatases and metachromasia in murine tumours induced by bone seeking radionuclides. *Br. J. Cancer* **29**, 206–22.

BLUMENTHAL, N. C., POSNER, A. S., SILVERMAN, L. D., and ROSENBERG, L. C. (1979). Effects of proteoglycans on *in vitro* hydroxyapatite formation. *Calcif. Tiss. Intl* **27**, 75–82.

BONUCCI, E. (1971). The locus of initial calcification in cartilage and bone. *Clin. Orthop.* **78**, 108–39.

BORDIER, P. J., MIRAVET, L., and HIOCO, D. (1973). Young adult osteoporosis. *Clin. Endocr. Met.* **2**, 277–92.

—— and TUN CHOT, S. (1972). Quantitative histology of metabolic bone disease. *Clin. Endocr. Met.* **1**, 197–215.

BORLE, A. B. (1973). Calcium metabolism at the cellular level. *Fedn Proc.* **32**, 1944–50.

BOSKEY, A. L. (1978). The role of calcium–phospholipid–phosphate complexes in tissue mineralization. *Metab. Bone Dis. and Rel. Res.* **1**, 137–42.

—— and POSNER, A. S. (1976). Extraction of a calcium phospholipid-phosphate complex from bone. *Calc. Tiss. Res.* **19**, 273–83.

—— GOLDBERG, M. R., and POSNER, A. S. (1978). Calcium phospholipid phosphate

complexes in mineralizing tissue. *Proc. Soc. exp. Biol. Med.* **157**, 588–91.
—— —— —— (1979). Effect of diphosphonates on hydroxyapatite formation induced by calcium phosphate complexes. *Calcif. Tissue Int.* **27**, 83–8.

BRAND, J. S., CUSHING, J., and HEFLEY, T. (1979). Potassium, sodium and intracellular fluid space of cells from bone. *Calcif. Tiss. Int.* **29**, 119–25.

BRAUTBAR, N., LEE, D. B. N., COBURN, J. W., and KLEEMAN, C. R. (1979). Influence of dietary magnesium in experimental phosphate depletion : bone and soft tissue mineral changes. *Am. J. Phys.* **237**, 2 E 152–7.

BRIGHTON, C. T. (1977). Bioelectrical effects on bone and cartilage. *Clin. Orthop.* **124**, 2–4.

BROMMAGE, R. and NEUMAN, W. F. (1979). Passive accumulation of magnesium, sodium and potassium by chick calvaria. *Calcif. Tiss. Int.* **28**, 57–63.

BROOKES, M. (1971). *The blood supply of bone.* Butterworths, London.

BROWN, E. D., CHAN, W., and SMITH, J. C. (1978). Bone mineralization during a developing zinc deficiency. *Proc. Soc. exp. Biol. Med.* **157**, 211–14.

BROWN, J. B., HARRISON, P., and SMITH, M. A. (1978). Oestrogen and pregnanediol excretion through childhood menarche and first ovulation. *J. Biosoc. Sci. Suppl.* **5**, 43–62.

BROWN, R. G., BUTTON, G. M., and SMITH, J. T. (1967). Effect of vitamin E deficiency on collagen metabolism in the rat's skin. *J. Nutr.* **91**, 99–106.

BRYANT, F. J. and LOUTIT, J. F. (1963–4). The entry of strontium 90 into human bone. *Proc. R. Soc.* **B159**, 449–65.

BULLAMORE, J. R., GALLAGHER, J. C., WILKINSON, R., NORDIN, B. E. C., and MARSHALL, D. H. (1970). Effect of age on calcium absorption. *Lancet* **ii**, 535–7.

BULUSU, L., HODGKINSON, A., NORDIN, B. E. C., and PEACOCK, M. (1970). Urinary excretion of calcium and creatinine in relation to age and body weight in normal subjects and patients with renal calculus. *Clin. Sci.* **38**, 601–12.

BURCKHARD, J., HAVEZ, R., and DAUTREVAUX, M. (1966). Étude des proteins et glyco-proteides de l'os compact du lapin. *Bull. Soc. Chim. biol.* **48**, 851–61.

BURKHARDT, R. (1970). *Bone marrow and bone tissue.* Springer-Verlag, Heidelberg.

BURKINSHAW, L., MARSHALL, D. H., OXBY, C. B., SPIERS, F. W., NORDIN, B. E. C., and YOUNG, M. M. (1969). Bone turnover model based on a continuously expanding exchangeable calcium pool. *Nature, Lond.* **222**, 146–8.

BURLEIGH, M. C. (1977). Degradation of collagen by non specific proteinases. In *Proteinases of mammalian cells and tissues* (ed. A. J. Barrett) pp. 285–309. North Holland, Amsterdam.

—— BARRETT, A. J., and LAZARUS, G. S. (1974). Cathepsin B, a lysosomal enzyme that degrades native collagen. *Biochem. J.* **137**, 387–98.

BYGRAVE, F. L. (1978). Mitochondria and the control of intracellular calcium. *Biol. Rev.* **53**, 43–79.

CAMERON, D. A. (1972). The ultrastructure of bone. In *The biochemistry and physiology of bone* (ed. G. H. Bourne) (2nd edn) Vol. 1, pp. 191–236. Academic Press, New York.

CAMPO, R. D. and TOURTELLOTTE, C. D. (1967). The composition of bovine cartilage and bone. *Biochim. biophys. Acta* **141**, 614–24.

CANNEIRO, J. and LEBLOND, C. P. (1959). Role of osteoblasts and odontoblasts in secreting the collagen of bone and dentine as shown by autoradiography in mice given labelled glycine. *Expl. Cell Res.* **18**, 291–300.

CANTERBURY, J. M. and REISS, E. (1972). Multiple immune reactive molecular forms of parathyroid hormone in human serum. *Proc. Soc. exp. Biol. Med.* **140**, 1393–8.

CARE, A. D., COOPER, C. W., DUNCAN, T., and ORIMO, H. (1968). A study of thyrocalcitonin secretion by direct measurement of *in vivo* secretion rate in pigs. *Endocrinology* **83**, 161–9.

—— BRUCE, J. B., BOELKINS, J., KENNY, A. D., CONAWAY, H., and ANAST, C. S. (1971). Role of pancreozymin–cholecystokinin and structurally related compounds as calcitonin secretagogues. *Endrocrinology* **89**, 262–71.

CARLSON, H. E., GILLIN, J. C., GORDEN, P., and SNYDER, F. (1972). Absence of sleep related growth hormone peaks in aged normal subjects and in acromegaly. *J. clin. Endocr. Metab.* **34**, 1102–5.

CARR, T. E. F., HARRISON, G. E., and NOLAN, J. (1973). The long-term excretion and retention of an intravenous dose of Ca^{45} in two healthy men. *Calc. Tiss. Res.* **12**, 217–26.

CASTILLO, L., TANAKA, Y., and DELUCA, H. F. (1975). The mobilization of bone mineral by 1,25-dihydroxy vitamin D_3 in hypophosphatemic rats. *Endocrinology* **97**, 995–9.

—— —— and SUNDE, M. L. (1977). The stimulation of 25-hydroxy vitamin D_3-1-α-hydroxylase by oestrogen. *Arch. biochem. Biophys.* **179**, 211–17.

CATT, K. J. (1970). Growth hormone. *Lancet* **i**, 933–9.

—— HARWOOD, J. P., AGUILERA, G., and DUFAU, M. L. (1979). Hormonal regulation of peptide receptors and target cell responses. *Nature, Lond.* **280**, 109–16.

CECIL, R. N. A. and ANDERSON, H. C. (1978). Freeze-fracture studies of matrix vesicle calcification in epiphyseal growth plate. *Metab. Bone Dis. and Rel. Res.* **1**, 89–95.

CHAKRAVORTY, N. K. (1979). Treatment of Paget's disease of bone. *Gerontology* **25**, 151–8.

CHALMERS, J., BARCLAY, A., DAVISON, A. M., MACLEOD, D. A. D., and WILLIAMS, D. A. (1969). Quantitative measurements of osteoid in health and disease. *Clin. Orthop.* **63**, 196–209.

CHALMERS, T. M., DAVIE, M. W., HUNTER, J. O., SZAZ, K. F., PELC, B., and KODICEK, E. (1973). 1-α-hydroxy cholecalciferol as a substitute for the kidney hormone 1,25-dihydroxycholecalciferol in chronic renal failure. *Lancet* **ii**, 696–9.

CHAMBERS, D. J., TULLY, G., RAFFERTY, B., ZANELLI, J. M., CHAYNEN, J., and PARSONS, J. A. (1979). Acute increase and decrease of biologically active circulating human parathyroid hormone (bioPTH) induced by positive and negative calcium challenges within the physiological role. *Calcif. Tiss. Int.* **27**, suppl. 22, p. A6.

CHAMBERS, T. J. (1978). Multinucleate giant cells. *J. Path.* **126**, 125–48.

—— (1979). Phagocytosis and trypsin-resistant glass adhesion by osteoclasts in culture. *J. Path.* **127**, 55–60.

—— (1980). The cellular basis of bone resorption. *Clin. Orthop.* (In press.)

—— and LOUTIT, J. F. (1979). A functional assessment of macrophages from osteopetrotic mice. *J. Path.* **129**, 57–63.

CHAN, S. H. and METCALF, D. (1972). Local production of colony stimulating factor within the bone marrow: Role of non-haematopoietic cells. *Blood* **40**, 646–53.

CHASE, L. R. and AURBACH, G. D. (1967). Parathyroid function and the renal excretion of 3'5' adenylic acid. *Proc. natn. Acad. Sci. USA* **58**, 518–25.

—— —— (1968). Cyclic AMP and the mechanism of action of parathyroid hormone. In *Parathyroid hormone and thyrocalcitonin (calcitonin)* (ed. R. V. Talmage and L. F. Belanger) pp. 247–57. International Congress Series No. 159, Excerpta Medica, Amsterdam.

CHEN, T. C., CASTILLO, L., KORYCKA-DAHL, M., and DELUCA, H. F. (1974). Role of vitamin D metabolites in phosphate transport of rat intestine. *J. Nutr.* **104**, 1056–60.

CHERTOW, B. S., BUSCHMANN, R. J., and HENDERSON, W. J. (1975). Subcellular mechanisms of parathyroid hormone secretion: ultrastructural changes in response to calcium, vitamin A, vinblastine, and cytochalasin B. *Lab. Invest.* **32**, 190–200.

—— WILLIAMS, G. A., NORRIS, R. M., BAKER, G. R., and HARGIS, G. K. (1977). Vitamin A stimulation of parathyroid hormone; interactions with calcium, hydrocortisone, and vitamin E in bovine parathyroid tissues and effects of vitamin A in man. *Eur. J. clin. Invest.* **7**, 307–14.

CHIPPERFIELD, A. R. (1970). Unpublished results.

—— and TAYLOR, D. M. (1968). Binding of plutonium and americium in bone glycoprotein. *Nature, Lond.* **219**, 609–10.

CHOCHINOV, R. and DAUGHADAY, W. H. (1976). Current concepts of somatomedin and other biologically related growth factors. *Diabetes* **25**, 994–1004.

CLAUS-WALKER, J., SINGH, J., LEACH, C. S., HATTON, D. V., HUBERT, C. W., and FERRANTE, N. D. (1977). The urinary excretion of collagen degradation products by quadroplegic patients and during weightlessness. *J. Bone Jt Surg.* **59A**, 209–17.

CLEMMONS, D. R., HINTZ, R. L., UNDERWOOD, L. E., and VAN WYK, J. J. (1974). Common mechanism of action of somatomedin and insulin on fat cells. *Israel J. med. Sci.* **10**, 1254–62.

COBURN, J. W., HARTENBOWER, D. L., and MASSRY, S. G. (1973). Intestinal absorption of calcium and the effect of renal insufficiency. *Kidney Int.* **4**, 96–104.

COCCIA, P. F., KRIVIT, W., CERVENKA, J., CLAWSON, C., KERSEY, J. H., KIM, T. H., NESBIT, M. E., RAMSAY, N. K. C., WARKENTIN, P. I., TEITELBAUM, S. L., KAHN, A. J., and BROWN, D. M. (1980). Successful bone-marrow transplantation for infantile malignant osteopetrosis. *N. Engl. J. Med.* **302**, 701–8.

COCHRAN, M., PEACOCK, M., SACHS, G., and NORDIN, B. E. C. (1970). Renal effects of calcitonin. *Br. med. J.* **1**, 135–7.

COHEN, K. L. and NISSLEY, S. P. (1976). The serum half-life of somatomedin activity. Evidence for growth hormone dependence. *Acta Endocrinol. (Kbh)* **83**, 243–8.

COHN, S. H., BOZZO, S. R., JESSEPH, J. E., CONSTANTINIDES, C., HUENE, D. R., and GUSMANO, E. A. (1965). Formulation and testing of a compartmental model for calcium metabolism in man. *Radiat. Res.* **26**, 319–33.

COLLINS, D. H. (prepared for publication by Dodge, O. G.) (1966). *Pathology of Bone.* Butterworths, London.

COLLIP, J. B. (1925). The extraction of a parathyroid hormone which will prevent or control parathyroid tetany and which regulates the level of blood calcium. *J. biol. Chem.* **63**, 395–438.

CONCEICAO, S. C., WEIGTMAN, D., SMITH, P. A., LUNO, J., WARD, M. K., and KERR, D. N. S. (1978). Serum ionised calcium concentration: measurement versus calculation. *Br. med. J* **i**, 1103.

COOPER, C. W., OBIE, J. F., TOVERUD, S. V., and MUNSON, P. L. (1977). Elevated serum calcitonin and serum calcium during suckling in the baby rat. *Endocrinology* **101**, 1657–64.

—— SCHWESINGER, W. H., MAHGOUB, A. M., and ONTJES, D. A. (1971). Thyrocalcitonin, stimulation of secretion by pentagastrin. *Science N.Y.* **172**, 1238–40.

COOPER, G. W., BOLMAN, III, R. M., LINEHAN, W. M., and WELLS, S. A. Jr. (1978). Interrelationship between calcium, calcemic hormones and gastrointestinal hormones. *Recent Prog. Horm. Res.* **34**, 259–83.

COPP, D. H. (1969). Endocrine control of calcium homeostasis. *J. Endocr.* **43**, 137–61.

—— (1972). Calcitonin. In *The biochemistry and physiology of bone* (ed. G. H. Bourne) (2nd edn) Vol. 2, pp. 337–56. Academic Press, New York.

—— CHENEY, B., and DAVIDSON, A. G. F. (1961). Evidence for a new parathyroid hormone which lowers blood calcium. *Proc. Can. Fed. biol. Soc.* **4**, 17.

CRYER, P. E. and DAUGHADAY, W. H. (1969). Regulation of growth hormone secretion in acromegaly. *J. clin. Endocrinol. Metab.* **29**, 386–93.

CUNLIFFE, W. J., HALL, R., HUDGSON, P., GUDMUNDSSON, T. V., WILLIAMS, E. D., GALANTE, L., BLACK, M. M., JOHNSTON, I. D. A., SHUSTER, S., JOPLIN, G. F., WOOD-HOUSE, N. J. Y., and MACINTYRE, I. (1968). A calcitonin-secreting thyroid carcinoma. *Lancet* ii, 63–6.

DAUGHADAY, W. H., HALL, K., RABEN, M., SALMON, W. D. Jr., VAN DEN BRANDE, J. L., and VAN WYK, J. J. (1972). Somatomedin : a proposed designation for the 'sulphation factor'. *Nature, Lond.* **235**, 107.

DAVIES, R. E., KORNBERG, H. L., and WILSON, G. M. (1952). The determination of sodium in bone. *Biochem. J.* **52**, XV.

DAVIS, R. H., MORGAN, D. B., and RIVLIN, R. S. (1970). The excretion of calcium in the urine and its relation to calcium intake, sex and age. *Clin. Sci.* **39**, 1–12.

DEFTOS, L. J., POWELL, D., PARTHEMORE, J. G., and POTTS, J. T. Jr. (1973). Secretion of calcitonin in hypocalcemic states in man. *J. clin. Invest.* **52**, 3109–14.

—— ROOS, B. A., BRONZERT, D., and PARTHEMORE, J. G. (1975). Immunochemical heterogeneity of calcitonin in plasma. *J. clin. endocr. Metab.* **40**, 409–12.

—— CATHERWOOD, B. D., BONE, H. G., WATKINS, W., GUILLEMIN, R., and PARTHEMORE, J. G. (1979). Calcitonin in the pituitary. *Calcif. Tiss., Int. Suppl.* **27**, No. 35, p. A9.

DELUCA, H. F. (1972). Parathyroid hormone as a trophic hormone for 1,25-dihydroxy-vitamin D_3, the metabolically active form of vitamin D. *New Engl. J. Med.* **287**, 250–1.

—— (1974). Vitamin D. *Am. J. Med.* **57**, 1–12.

—— (1976). Recent advances in our understanding of the vitamin D endocrine system. *J. Lab. clin. Med.* **87**, 7–26.

—— (1977). Vitamin D metabolism. *Clin. Endocr., Suppl.* **7**, 1–17.

—— (1978). Vitamin D and calcium transport. *Ann. N.Y. acad. Sci.* **307**, 356–75.

DELUCA, L. M., GLOVER, J., HELLER, J., OLSON, J. A., and UNDERWOOD, B. (1977). Recent advances in the metabolism and function of vitamin A and their relationship to applied nutrition. Report of the International A consultative group.

DENNIS, V. W., STEAD, W. W., and MYERS, J. L. (1979). Renal handling of phosphate and calcium. *Ann. Rev. Physiol.* **41**, 257–71.

DEPORTER, D. A. (1979). The possible role of the fibroblast in granuloma-induced bone resorption in the rat. *J. Path.* **127**, 61–4.

DEROSE, J., SINGER, F. R., AURAMIDES, A., FLORES, H., DZIADIW, R., BAKDER, R. K., and WALLACH, S. (1974). Response of Paget's disease to porcine and salmon calci-tonin. *Am. J. Med.* **56**, 858–66.

DETENBECK, L. C. and JOWSEY, J. (1969). The effect of thyroidectomy and parathyroidec-tomy in the remodelling of bone defects in adult dogs. *Clin. Orthop.* **65**, 199–202.

DIAMOND, A. G. and NEUMAN, W. F. (1979). Macromolecular inhibitors of calcium phosphate precipitation in bone. In *Vitamin K metabolism and vitamin K dependent proteins* (ed. J. W. Suttie) pp. 259–62. University Park Press, Baltimore.

DICKSON, I. R. and KODICEK, E. (1979). Effect of vitamin D deficiency on bone formation in the chick. *Biochem. J.* **182**, 429–35.

—— POOLE, A. R., and VEIS, A. (1975). Localization of plasma α_2HS glycoprotein in mineralising human bone. *Nature, Lond.* **256**, 430–2.

DINGLE, J. T. (1973*a*). Lysosomal enzymes in skeletal tissues. In *Hard tissue growth, repair and remineralization* pp. 295–313. Ciba Foundation Symposium II (NS). Elsevier–Excerpta Medica–North Holland–Associated Science Publishers, Amster-dam.

—— (1973*b*). The role of lysosomal enzymes in skeletal tissues. *J. Bone Jt Surg.* **55B**, 87–95.

—— (1979). Recent studies on the control of joint damage: the contribution of the Strangeways Research Laboratory. *Ann. Rheum. Dis.* **38**, 201–14.

—— FELL, H. B., and LUCY, J. A. (1966). Synthesis of connective tissue components. The effect of retinol and hydrocortisone on cultured limb bone rudiments. *Biochem. J.* **98**, 173–81.

—— SAKLATVALA, J., HEMBRY, R., TYLER, J., FELL, H. B., and JUBB, R. (1979). A cartilage catabolic factor from synovium. *Biochem. J.* **184**, 177–80.

DIRKS, J. H. and QUAMME, G. A. (1978). Renal handling of magnesium. *Adv. Exp. Med. Biol.* **103**, 51–69.

DIXON, M. and WEBB, E. C. (1964). *Enzymes.* (2nd edn). Longmans Green, London.

DIXON, T. F. and PERKINS, H. R. (1952). Citric acid and bone metabolism. *Biochem. J.* **52**, 260–5.

—— —— (1956). Citric acid and bone. In *The biochemistry and physiology of bone* (ed. G. H. Bourne) pp. 309–23. Academic Press, New York.

DOLPHIN, G. W. and EVE, I. S. (1963). The metabolism of strontium in adult humans. *Phys. med. Biol.* **8**, 193–203.

DOMINGUEZ, J. H. and RAISZ, L. G. (1979). Effect of changing hydrogen ion, carbonic acid and bicarbonate concentration on bone resorption in vitro. *Calcif. Tiss., Int.* **29**, 7–13.

DORFMAN, A., PEI-LEE, HO, STROM, C. M., VERTEL, B. M., and UPHOLT, W. B. (1977). The differentiation of cartilage. *Adv. Pathobiol.* **6**, 104–23.

DOTY, S. B. and SCHOFIELD, B. H. (1971). Metabolic and structural changes within osteocytes of rat bone. In *Calcium, parathyroid hormone and calcitonin* (ed. R. V. Talmage and P. L. Munson) pp. 353–64. Excerpta Medica, Amsterdam.

—— —— (1972). Electron microscopic localization of hydrolytic enzymes in osteoclasts. *Histochem. J.* **4**, 245–58.

DOYLE, F., PENNOCK, J., GREENBERG, P. B., JOPLIN, G. F., and MACINTYRE, I. (1974). Radiological evidence of a dose-related response to long-term treatment of Paget's disease with human calcitonin. *Br. J. Radiol.* **47**, 1–8.

—— WOODHOUSE, N. J. Y., GLEN, A. C. A., JOPLIN, G. F., and MACINTYRE, I. (1974). Healing of the bones in juvenile Paget's disease treated by human calcitonin. *Br. J. Radiol.* **47**, 9–15.

DRESCHER, D. and DELUCA, H. F. (1971). Possible precursor of vitamin D stimulated calcium binding protein in rats. *Biochem.* **10**, 2308–12.

DREZNER, M. K. and HARRELSON, J. M. (1979). Newer knowledge of vitamin D and its metabolites in health and disease. *Clin. Orthop.* **139**, 206–31.

DUNNILL, M. S., ANDERSON, J. A., and WHITEHEAD, R. (1967). Quantitative histological studies on age changes in bone. *J. path. Bact.* **94**, 275–91.

DZIEWIATKOWSKI, D. D. (1954). Vitamin A and endochondral ossification in the rat as indicated by the use of ^{35}S and ^{32}P. *J. exp. Med.* **100**, 10–24.

EANES, E. D. and POSNER, A. S. (1965). Kinetics and mechanism of conversion of non-crystalline calcium phosphate to crystalline hydroxy apatite. *Trans. N.Y. Acad. Sci.* **28**, 233–41.

—— —— (1967). X-ray scattering study of bone apatite. In *Proceedings of the conference on small angle X-ray scattering* (ed. H. Brumberger) pp. 493–501. Gordon and Breach, New York.

—— —— (1970). Structure and chemistry of bone mineral. In *Biological calcification* (ed. H. Schraer) pp. 1–26. North-Holland, Amsterdam.

—— TERMINE, J. D., and NYLEN, M. U. (1973). An electron microscope study of the formation of amorphous calcium phosphate and its transformation to crystalline apatite. *Calc. Tiss. Res.* **12**, 143–58.

EARNSHAW, M. (1979). Personal communication.

EASTOE, J. E. (1955). The amino acid composition of mammalian collagen and gelatin. *Biochem. J.* **61**, 589–600.

—— (1961). The chemical composition of bone. In *Biochemists' handbook* (ed. C. Long) pp. 715–20. Van Nostrand, Princeton, NJ.

—— and EASTOE, B. (1954). The organic constituents of mammalian compact bone. *Biochem. J.* **57**, 453–9.

EASTWOOD, J. B., BORDIER, P. J., CLARKSON, E. M., TUNCHOT, D. E., and DE WARDENER, H. E. (1974). The contrasting effects on bone histology of vitamin D and of calcium carbonate in the osteomalacia of chronic renal failure. *Clin. Sci., Mol. Med.* **47**, 23–42.

EDELMAN, I. S., JAMES, A. H., BADEN, H., and MOORE, F. D. (1954). Electrolyte composition of bone and the penetration of radiosodium and deuterium oxide into dog and human bone. *J. clin. Invest.* **33**, 122–31.

ELLSASSER, J. C., FARNHAM, J. E., and MARSHALL, J. H. (1969). Comparative kinetics and autoradiography of ^{45}Ca and ^{133}Ba in ten year old beagle dogs. *J. Bone Jt Surg.* **51A**, 1397–1412.

EVANS, R. D., KEANE, A. T., KOLENKOW, R. J., NEAL, W. R., and SHANAHAN, M. M. (1969). Radiogenic tumours in the radium and mesothorium cases studied at M.I.T. In *Delayed effects of bone-seeking radio-nuclides* (ed. C. W. Mays, W. S. S. Jee, R. D. Lloyd, B. J. Stover, J. H. Dougherty, and G. N. Taylor) pp. 157–94. University of Utah Press.

FACCINI, J. M. (1969). Fluoride and bone. *Calc. Tiss. Res.* **3**, 1–16.

—— and CARE, A. D. (1965). Effect of sodium fluoride on the ultrastructure of the parathyroid glands of the sheep. *Nature, Lond.* **207**, 1399–1401.

FAVUS, M. J., KIMBERG, D. V., MILLAR, G. N., and GERSHON, E. (1973). Effect of cortisone administration on the metabolism and localization of 25-hydroxycholecalciferol in the rat. *J. clin. Invest.* **52**, 1328–35.

FELDMAN, D., DZIAK, R., KOEHLER, R., and STERN, P. (1975). Cytoplasmic glucocorticoid binding proteins in bone cells. *Endocrinology* **96**, 29–36.

FELL, H. (1956). Skeletal development in tissue culture. In *The biochemistry and physiology of bone* (ed. G. H. Bourne) (1st edn) pp. 401–41. Academic Press, New York.

FELL, H. B. (1978). Synoviocytes. *J. clin. Path. Suppl.* **17**, 14–24.

—— and BARRETT, M. E. J. (1973). The role of soft connective tissue in the breakdown of pig articular cartilage cultivated in the presence of complement-sufficient antiserum to pig erythrocytes. i. Histological changes. *Int. Archs Allergy appl. Immun.* **44**, 441–68.

—— and JUBB, R. W. (1977). The effect of synovial tissue on the breakdown of articular cartilage in organ culture. *Arthritis Rheum.* **20**, 1359–71.

—— and MELLANBY, E. (1950). Effect of hypervitaminosis A on foetal mouse bones cultivated *in vitro*. *Br. med. J.* **ii**, 535–9.

—— —— (1952). The effect of hypervitaminosis A on embryonic limb bones cultured in vitro. *J. Physiol., Lond.* **116**, 320–49.

—— and THOMAS, L. (1960). Comparison of the effects of papain and vitamin A on cartilage. ii. The effect on organ culture of embryonic skeletal tissue. *J. exp. Med.* **111**, 719–43.

—— —— (1961). The influence of hydrocortisone on the action excess of vitamin A on limb bone rudiments in culture. *J. exp. Med.* **114**, 343–62.

—— —— and PELC, S. R. (1956). Influence of excess vitamin A on the sulphate metabolism of bone rudiments grown *in vitro*. *J. Physiol., Lond.* **134**, 179–88.

FISCHMAN, D. A. and HAY, E. D. (1962). Origin of osteoclasts from mononuclear leucocytes in generating newt limbs. *Anat. Rec.* **143**, 329–38.

FITTON JACKSON, S. (1969). Unpublished results.

FLEISCH, H. and FELIX, R. (1979). Diphosphonates. *Calcif. Tiss. Int.* **27**, 91–4.

—— and NEUMAN, W. F. (1961). Mechanism of calcification: role of collagen, poly-phosphates and phosphatase. *Am. J. Physiol.* **200**, 1296–1300.

FLETCHER, W., LOUTIT, J. F., and PAPWORTH, D. G. (1966). Interpretation of levels of strontium 90 in human bone. *Br. med. J.* **2**, 1225–30.

FOSTER, G. V. (1968). Magnesium metabolism. In *Recent advances in clinical pathology* (ed. S. C. Dyke) pp. 131–45. Churchill, London.

—— BYFIELD, P. G. H., and GUDMUNDSSON, T. V. (1972). Calcitonin. *Clin. Endocr. Met.* **1**, 93–124.

—— MACINTYRE, I., and PEARSE, A. G. E. (1964). Calcitonin production and the mito-chondrion rich cells of the dog thyroid. *Nature, Lond.* **203**, 1029–30.

—— DOYLE, F. H., BORDIER, P., and MATRAJT, H. (1966). Effect of thyrocalcitonin on bone. *Lancet* **ii**, 1428–31.

—— JOPLIN, G. F., MACINTYRE, I., MELVIN, K. E. W., and SLACK, E. (1966). Effect of thyrocalcitonin in man. *Lancet* **i**, 107–9.

—— BAGHDIANTZ, A., KUMAR, M. A., SLACK, E., SOLIMAN, H. A., and MACINTYRE, I. (1964). Thyroid origin of calcitonin. *Nature, Lond.* **202**, 1303–5.

FOURMAN, P. and ROYER, P. (1968). *Calcium metabolism and the bone.* (2nd edn). Blackwell, Oxford.

FRAME, B., JACKSON, C. E., REYNOLDS, W. A., and UMPHREY, J. E. (1974). Hypercal-caemia and skeletal effects in chronic hypervitaminosis A. *Ann. Intern. Med.* **80**, 44–8.

FRANKLIN, R., COSTELLO, L. C., STACEY, R. and STEPHENS, R. (1973). Calcitonin effects on plasma and urinary citrate levels in rats. *Am. J. Phys.* **225**, 1178–80.

FRANZ, J., ROSENTHALER, J., ZEHNDER, K., DOEPFNER, W., HUGUERIN, R., and GUTT-MAN, ST. (1968). Isolierung, Aminosaunezusammensetung und tryptischer Abbau von Thyrocalcitonin aus Schweinesachilddrusen. *Helv. chim. Acta* **51**, 218–20.

FRASER, D. and KODICEK, E. (1970). Unique biosynthesis by kidney of a biological active vitamin D metabolite. *Nature, Lond.* **228**, 764–6.

FRASER, D. R. and KODICEK, E. K. (1973). Regulation of 25-hydroxycholecalciferol-1-hydroxylase activity in the kidney by parathyroid hormone. *Nature, New Biol.* **241**, 163–6.

FRASER, D., KOOH, S. W., and SCRIVER, C. R. (1967). Hyperparathyroidism as the cause of hyperaminoaciduria and phosphaturia in human vitamin D deficiency. *Pediatr. Res.* **1**, 425–35.

FRIEDENSTEIN, A. J. (1968). Induction of bone tissue by transitional epithelium. *Clin. Orth. and Rel. Res.* **59**, 21–35.

—— (1973). Determined and inducable osteogenic precursor cells. In *Hard tissue growth, repair and remineralization* pp. 169–85. Ciba Foundation Symposium II (NS), Elsevier–Excerpta Medica–North Holland–Associated Science Publishers, Amster-dam.

—— (1976). Precursor cells of mechanocytes. *Int. Rev. Cytol.* **47**, 327–59.

—— CHAILAKHJIAN, R. K., and LALYKINA, K. S. (1970). The development of fibroblast colonies in monolayer cultures of guinea-pig bone marrow and spleen cells. *Cell Tissue Kinet.* **3**, 393–403.

—— —— LATZINIK, N. V., PANASYUK, A. F., and KEILISS-BOROK, I. V. (1974). Stromal cells responsible for transferring the microenvironment of the hemopoietic tissues. *Transplantation* **17**, 331.

—— DERIGLASOVA, U. F., KULAGINA, N. N., PANASUK, A. F., RUDAKOWA, S. F., LURIA, E. A., and RUDAKOW, I. A. (1974). Precursors for fibroblasts in different populations of hematopoietic cells. *Exp. Hemat. (Copenhagen)* **2**, 83–92.

—— LALYKINA, K. S. and TOLMACHEVA, A. A. (1967). Osteogenic activity of peritoneal fluid cells induced by transitional epithelium. *Acta Anat.* **68**, 532–49.

—— PIATETSKY-SHAPIRO, I. I., and PETRAKOVA, K. V. (1966). Osteogenesis in transplants of bone marrow cells. *J. Embryol. exp. Morph.* **16**, 381–90.

—— PETRAKOVA, K. V., KUROLESOVA, A. I., and FROLOVA, G. P. (1968). Heterotopic transplants of bone marrow. Analysis of precursor cells for osteogenic and haematopoietic tissues. *Transplantation* **6**, 230–47.

FRIEDMAN, J. and RAISZ, L. G. (1965). Thyrocalcitonin: inhibitor of bone resorption in tissue culture. *Science, N.Y.* **150**, 1465–7.

FRIEDMAN, J., AU, W. Y. W., and RAISZ, L. G. (1968). Response of fetal rat bone to thyrocalcitonin in tissue culture. *Endocrinology* **82**, 149–56.

FRIJLINK, W. B., BIJVOET, O. L. M., TE-VELDE, J., and HEYNEN, G. (1979). Treatment of Paget's disease with (3-amino-1-hydroxypropylidene)-1,1-biphosphonate (A.P.D.). *Lancet* **i**, 799–803.

FROST, H. M. (1967). The dynamics of osteoid tissue. In *L'Osteomalacia Tours* 1965 (ed. D. J. Hioco) pp. 3–18. Masson et Cie, Paris.

FUJII, K., and TANZER, M. L. (1977). Osteogenesis imperfecta: biochemical studies of bone collagen. *Clin. Orthop.* **124**, 271–7.

GAILLARD, P. J., WASSENAAR, A. M., and WIJKE-WHEELER, M. E. VAN. (1977). *Proc. K. ned. Akad. Wet. Amsterdam* **80**, 267–79.

GALLAGHER, J. C., RIGGS, B. L., FISMAN, J., ARNAUD, S., and DELUCA, H. F. (1976). Impaired intestinal calcium absorption in post menopausal osteoporosis: possible role of vitamin D metabolites and PTH. *Clin. Res.* **24**, 360A.

—— —— JOHNSON, K. A., and DELUCA, H. F. (1979). Treatment of osteoporosis with synthetic, 1,25-dihydroxy vitamin D. *Calcif. Tiss. Int.* **27**, Suppl. No. 51, p. A13.

—— AARON, J., HORSEMAN, A., WILKINSON, R., and NORDIN, B. E. C. (1973). Corticosteroid osteoporosis. *Clin. Endocr. Met.* **2**, 355–68.

—— RIGGS, B. L., EISMAN, J., HAMSTRA, A., ARNAUD, S. B., and DELUCA, H. F. (1979). Intestinal calcium absorption and serum vitamin D metabolites in normal subjects and osteoporotic patients: effect of age and dietary calcium. *J. clin. Invest.* **64**, 729–36.

GARABEDIAN, M., TANAKA, Y., HOLLICK, M. F., and DELUCA, H. F. (1974). Response of intestinal calcium transport and bone calcium mobilization to 1,25-dihydroxy-vitamin D_3 in thyroparathyroidectomized rats. *Endocrinology* **94**, 1022–7.

GLICK, S. M., ROTH, J., YALLOW, R. S., and BERSON, S. A. (1965). The regulation of growth hormone secretion. *Recent Prog. Horm. Res.* **21**, 241–83.

GLIMCHER, M. J. (1976). Composition, structure and organization of bone and other mineralized tissues and the mechanism of calcification. *Handbook of Physiology, Endocrinology VII*, Chapter 3, pp. 25–116. Williams and Wilkins Co., Baltimore.

GODARD, C. and ZAHND, G. R. (1971). Growth hormone and insulin in severe infantile malnutrition. II. Plasma insulin and growth hormone during intravenous glucose tolerance test. *Helv. paed. Acta* **26**, 276–85.

GONICK, H. C. and BROWN, M. (1970). Critique of compartmental analysis of calcium kinetics in man based on study of 27 cases. *Metabolism* **19**, 919–33.

GOSS, R. J. (1970). Problems of antlerogenesis. *Clin. Orthop.* **69**, 227–38.

GOTHLIN, G. and ERICSSON, J. L. E. (1976). The osteoclast. *Clin. Orthop.* **120**, 201–31.

GOULD, B. S. (1960). Ascorbic acid and collagen fibre formation. *Vitam. Horm.* **18**, 89–120.

—— (1968). The role of certain vitamins in collagen formation. In *Treatise on collagen* (ed. B. S. Gould) Vol. 2A, pp. 323–65. Academic Press, London.

—— (1970). Possible folate-ascorbic interaction in collagen formation. In *Chemistry and molecular biology of the intercellular matrix* (ed. E. A. Balazs) Vol. 1, pp. 431–7. Academic Press, London.

GOYER, R. A. (1973). Pathological effects of lead. *Int. Rev. exp. Pathol.* **12**, 1–77.

GRAHAM, R. F., PREECE, M. A., and O'RIORDAN, J. L. H. (1977). A highly sensitive competitive-protein binding assay for 24,25- and 25,26- dihydroxycholecalciferols. *Calc. Tiss. Res.* **22**, Suppl. 416–21.

GRANT, M. E. and PROCKOP, D. J. (1972). The biosynthesis of collagen. *New Engl. J. Med.* **286**, 194–9.

GREENBERG, A. H., NAJJAR, S., and BLIZZARD, R. M. (1974). Effects of thyroid hormone on growth differentiation and development. In *Handbook of physiology, section 7, endocrinology* **3**, *thyroid* (ed. M. A. Greer and D. H. Solomon) pp. 377–89.

GRIFFITHS, G. C., NICHOLS, G., ASHER, J. D., and FLANAGAN, B. (1965). Heparin osteoporosis. *J. Am. med. Ass.* **193**, 91–4.

GROSS, J. and LAPIERE, C. M. (1962). Collagenolytic activity in amphibian tissues: A tissue culture assay. *Proc. natn Acad. Sci. USA* **48**, 1014–22.

HAAS, H. G., DAMBACHER, M. A., LAUFFENBURGER, TH, LAMMLE, B., and OLAM, J. (1979). Efficiency of 1,25-$(OH)_2D_3$ in post menopausal osteoporosis. *Calcif. Tiss. Int.* **27**, Suppl. 55, P. A14.

HABENER, J. F. and POTTS, J. T. Jr. (1976). Chemistry biosynthesis, secretion and metabolism of parathyroid hormone. *Handbook of physiology, Vol. 7, Section 7*, pp. 313–42.

—— —— (1979*a*). Cleavage-associated enhancement of an antigenic site in the biologically active NH_2-terminal region of parathyroid hormone. *Endocrinology* **105**, 115–19.

—— —— (1979*b*). Subcellular distribution of parathyroid hormone, hormonal precursors and parathyroid secretory function. *Endocrinology* **104**, 265–75.

HADDAD, J. G., MIN, C., WALGATE, J., and HAHN, T. (1976). Competition by 24,25-hydroxycholecalciferol in the competitive protein binding assay of 25-hydroxycalciferol. *J. clin. Endocr. Metab.* **43**, 712–15.

—— —— MENDELSOHN, M., SLATOPOLSKY, E., and HAHN, T. (1977). Competitive protein binding radioassay of 24,25-dihydroxy vitamin D in sera from normal and anephric patients. *Arch. Biochem. Biophys.* **182**, 390–5.

HAJEK, A. S. and SOLURSH, M. (1977). The effect of ascorbic acid on growth and synthesis of matrix components by cultured chick embryo chondrocytes. *J. exp. Zool.* **200**, 377–88.

HALEY, J. E., TJIO, J. H., SMITH, W. W., and BRECHER, G. (1975). Haematopoietic differentiative properties of murine spleen implanted in the omenta of irradiated and non irradiated hosts. *Exp. Haem.* **3**, 187–96.

HALL, B. K. (1978). *Developmental and cellular skeletal biology*. Academic Press, New York.

HALSE, J. (1979). Parathyroid function in acromegaly. *Calcif. Tiss. Int.* **27**, Suppl. 58.

—— and GORDELADZE, J. O. (1978). Urinary hydroxyproline excretion in acromegaly. *Acta endocr.* **89**, 483–91.

HAM, A. W. (1974). *Histology* (7th edn) p. 394. Pitman, London.

—— and CORMACK, D. H. (1979). *Histology* (8th edn) Chapters 14, 15, 16, pp. 367–485. J. B. Lippincott Co., Philadelphia.

HANCOX, N. H. (1972). The osteoclast. In *The biochemistry and physiology of bone* (ed. G. H. Bourne) (2nd edn) pp. 45–67. Academic Press, New York.

—— and BOOTHROYD, B. (1966). Electron microscope observations of osteogenesis. In *The Fourth Symposium on Calcified Tissue* (ed. P. J. Gaillard, A. van den Hooff, and

R. Steendijk) pp. 42–3. International Congress Series No. 120. Excerpta Medica, Amsterdam.

HANNA, S. and MACINTYRE, I. (1960). Influence of aldosterone on metabolism of magnesium. *Lancet* **ii**, 348–50.

HARDINGHAM, T. E. and MUIR, H. (1972). The specific interaction of hyaluronic acid with cartilage proteoglycans. *Biochim. biophys. Acta* **279**, 401–5.

HARLAND, B. F., SPIVEY FOX, M. R., and FRY, B. E. Jr. (1975). Protection against zinc deficiency by prior excess dietary zinc in young Japanese quail. *J. Nutr.* **105**, 1509–18.

HARPER, R. A. and POSNER, A. S. (1966). Measurement of non-crystalline calcium phosphate in bone mineral. *Proc. Soc. exp. Biol. Med.* **122**, 137–42.

HARRIS, E. D. and CARTWRIGHT, E. C. (1977). Mammalian collagenases, In *Proteinases in mammalian cells and tissues* (ed. A. J. Barrett) pp. 249–91. North-Holland Publishing Co., Amsterdam.

HARRIS, M. J. and SCHLENKER, R. A. (1977–8). *Quantitative histology of human paranasal sinus and mastoid air cell epithelia.* ANL 78–65, part II, pp. 55–69.

HARRIS, S. S. (1977). Effect of vitamin A deficiency on calcium and glycosaminoglycan metabolism in guinea pig bone. *J. Nutr.* **107**, 2198–2205.

HARRIS, W. H. and HEANEY, R. P. (1969). Skeletal renewal and metabolic bone disease. *N. Engl J. Med.* **280**, 193–202.

HARRISON, G. E. (1980). Whole body retention of the alkaline earths in adult man. *Hlth Phys.* (In press.)

—— CARR, T. E. F., and SUTTON, A. (1967). Distribution of radioactive calcium, strontium, barium and radium following intravenous injection into a healthy man. *Int. J. radiat. Biol.* **13**, 235–47.

—— —— —— and RUNDO, J. (1966). Plasma concentration and excretion of calcium 47, strontium 85, barium 133 and radium 223 following successive intravenous doses to a healthy man. *Nature, Lond.* **209**, 526–7.

—— HOWELLS, G. R., and POLLARD, J. (1967). Comparative uptake and elution of ^{45}Ca, ^{85}Sr, ^{133}Ba, and ^{223}Ra in bone powder. *Calc. Tiss. Res.* **1**, 105–13.

HASTINGS, A. B. and HUGGINS, C. B. (1933). Experimental hypocalcaemia. *Proc. Soc. exp. Biol. Med.* **30**, 458–9.

HAUSCHKA, P. V. and GALLOP, P. M. (1977). Purification and calcium-binding properties of osteocalcin, the γ-carboxyglutamate-containing protein of bone. In *Calcium binding proteins and calcium function* (ed. R. H. Wasserman, R. A. Corradino, E. Carafoli, R. H. Kretsinger, D. H. Maclennan, and F. L. Siegel) pp. 338–47. North Holland, New York.

—— and REID, M. L. (1978). Vitamin K dependence of a calcium-binding protein containing γ carboxyglutamic acid in chicken bone. *J. biol. Chem.* **253**, 9063–8.

—— LIAN, J. B., and GALLOP, P. M. (1975). Direct identification of the calcium-binding amino acid, γ-carboxyglutamate, in mineralized tissue. *Proc. Natn Acad. Sci. USA* **72**, 3925–9.

—— —— —— (1978). Vitamin K and mineralization. *Trends in Biochem. Sci.* **3**, 75–8.

HAUSSLER, M. R., BOYCE, D. W., LITTLEDIKE, E. T., and RASMUSSEN, H. (1971). A rapidly acting metabolite of vitamin D_3. *Proc. natn. Acad. Sci. USA* **68**, 177–81.

—— HUGHES, M., BAYLINK, B., LITTLEDIKE, E. T., CORK, D., and PITT, M. (1977). Influence of phosphate depletion on the biosynthesis and circulating level of 1-25-dihydroxy vitamin D. *Adv. exp. Med. Biol.* **81**, 233–50.

HEANEY, R. P. (1963). Evaluation and interpretation of calcium kinetic data in man. *Clin. Orthop.* **31**, 153–83.

—— (1976a). Calcium kinetics in plasma: as they apply to the measurements of bone formation and resorption rates. In *The biochemistry and physiology of bone* (ed. G. H. Bourne) (2nd edn) Vol. 4, pp. 105–33. Academic Press, New York.

—— (1976*b*). Oestrogens and post menopausal osteoporosis. *Clin. Obstet. Gynaec.* **19,** 791–802.

—— and WHEDON, G. D. (1958). Radiocalcium studies of bone formation rate in human metabolic bone disease. *J. clin. Endocr. Metab.* **18,** 1246–67.

HEERSCHE, J. N. M. (1978). Mechanism of osteoclastic bone resorption: A new hypothesis. *Calc. Tiss. Res.* **26,** 81–4.

—— MARCUS, R., and AURBACH, G. D. (1974). Calcitonin and the formation of 3'5'-Amp in bone and kidney. *Endocrinology* **94,** 241–7.

HENNEMAN, D., PAK, C. V. C., BARTTER, F. C., LIFSCHITZ, M. D., and SANZENBACHER, L. (1972). The solubility and synthetic rate of bone collagen in idiopathic osteoporosis. *Clin. Orthop.* **88,** 275–82.

HENRY, H. L. and NORMAN, A. W. (1975). Studies on the mechanism of action of calciferol. VII. Localization of 1,25-dihydroxyvitamin D_3 in chick parathyroid glands. *Biochem. Biophys. Res. Commun.* **62,** 781–8.

HERRING, G. M. (1964). Mucosubstances of cortical bone. In *Bone and tooth symposium* (ed. H. J. J. Blackwood) pp. 263–8. Pergamon Press, Oxford.

—— (1968). The chemical structure of tendon cartilage, dentin and bone matrix. *Clin. Orthop.* **60,** 261–99.

—— (1969). Comparison of carbohydrate-containing macromolecules in tendon and bone matrix. In *Biochemistry and physiology of connective tissue* (ed. M. Adam, Z. Deyl, and J. Rosmus) pp. 195–6. Geoindustria, Prague.

—— (1972). The organic matrix of bone. In *The biochemistry and physiology of bone* (ed. G. H. Bourne) (2nd edn) Vol. 1, pp. 127–89. Academic Press, New York.

—— (1976). A comparison of bone matrix and tendon with particular reference to glycoprotein content. *Biochem. J.* **159,** 749–55.

—— (1977). Methods for the study of the glycoproteins and proteoglycans of bone using bacterial collagenase. *Calc. Tiss. Res.* **24,** 29–36.

—— (1979). Bone glycoproteins. In *Biochemie des tissus conjonctifs normaux et pathologiques No. 287,* pp. 209–13. Colloques int. CNRS.

—— and OLDROYD, D. (1968). Unpublished observations.

HERRMAN-ERLEE, M. P. M., GAILLARD, P. J., and NIJWEIDE, P. J. (1979). Studies on the interrelation between the effects of PTE, PGE, and 1,25-$(OH)_2D_3$ on embryonic bone in vitro. *Calcif. Tiss. Int.* **27,** suppl. 63, p. A16.

HEYNEN, G., KANIS, J. A., OLIVER, D., LEDINGHAM, J. G. G., and RUSSELL, R. G. G. (1976). Evidence that endogenous calcitonin protects against renal bone disease. *Lancet* **ii,** 1322–6.

HILLYARD, C. J., STEVENSON, J. C., and MACINTYRE, I. (1978). Relative deficiency of plasma calcitonin in normal women. *Lancet* **i,** 961–2.

—— COOKE, T. J. C., COOMBES, R. C., EVANS, I. M. A., and MACINTYRE, I. (1977). Normal planned calcitonin, circadian variation and response to stimuli. *Clin. Endocr.* **6,** 291–8.

HIOCO, D., BORDIER, P. H., MIRAVET, L., DENYS, H., and TUN CHOT, S. (1970). Prolonged administration of calcitonin in man; biological, isotopic and morphological effects. In *Calcitonin 1969, Proceedings of the Second International Symposium* (ed. S. Taylor and G. V. Foster) pp. 514–22. Heinemann Medical Books Ltd., London.

HIRSCH, P. F., GAUTHIER, G. F., and MUNSON, P. L. (1963). Thyroid hypocalcaemic principle and recurrent laryngeal nerve injury as factors affecting the response to parathyroidectomy in rats. *Endocrinology* **73,** 244–52.

HJERTQUIST, S. (1964*a*). Microchemical analyses of glycosaminoglycans (mucopolysaccharides) in normal and rachitic epiphyseal cartilage. *Acta Soc. Med. upsal.* **69,** 22–40.

—— (1964*b*). The glycosaminoglycans (mucopolysaccharides) of the epiphyseal plates in normal and rachitic dogs. Studies using a column procedure with cetylpyridinium chloride. *Acta Soc. Med. upsal.* **69,** 83–104.

HÖHLING, H. J., KREILOS, R., NEUBAUER, G., and BOYDE, A. (1971). Electron microscopy and electron microscopical measurements of collagen mineralization in hard tissue. *Z. Zellforsch. Mikrosk. Anat.* **122,** 36–52.

HOLICK, M. F. and DELUCA, H. F. (1978). Metabolism of vitamin D. In *Vitamin D* (ed. D. E. M. Lawson) pp. 51–91. Academic Press, London.

—— GARABEDIAN, M., and DELUCA, H. F. (1972). 1,25-dihydroxycholecalciferol: Metabolite of vitamin D_3 active on bone in anephric rats. *Science, N.Y.* **176,** 1146–7.

—— SCHNOES, H. K., and DELUCA, H. F. (1971). Identification of 1,25-dihydroxy-cholecalciferol a form of vitamin D_3 metabolically active in the intestine. *Proc. natn Acad. Sci. USA* **68,** 803–4.

—— MCNEILL, S. C., CLARK, M. B., HOLICK, S. A., and POTTS, J. T. (1979). The skin: A unique endocrine organ responsible for the photobiosynthesis of vitamin D_3. *Calcif. Tiss. Int.* **28,** abs. 174.

—— KLEINER-BOSSALER, A., SCHNOES, H. K., KASTEN, P. M., BOYLE, I. T., and DELUCA, H. F. (1973). 1,24,25-trihydroxyvitamin D_3. *J. biol. Chem.* **248,** 6691–6.

HOLTROP, M. E. and RAISZ, L. G. (1979). Comparison of the effects of 1,25-dihydroxy-cholecalciferol, prostaglandin E_2 and osteoclast activating factor with parathyroid hormone on the ultrastructure of osteoclasts in cultured long bones of foetal rats. *Calc. Tiss. Res.* **29,** 201–5.

—— and WEINGER, J. M. (1971). Ultrastructural evidence for a transport system in bone. In *Parathyroid hormone and the calcitonins* (ed. R. V. Talmage and P. L. Munson) pp. 365–74. International Congress Series No. 243, Excerpta Medica, Amsterdam.

—— RAISZ, L. G., and SIMMONS, H. A. (1974). The effects of parathyroid hormone, colchicine or calcitonin on the ultrastructure and the activity of osteoclasts in organ culture. *J. Cell Biol.* **60,** 346–55.

HOLTROP, M. E. and KING, G. J. (1977). The ultrastructure of the osteoclast. *Clin. Orthop.* **123,** 177–96.

—— KING, G. T., COX, K. A., and REIT, B. (1979). Time related changes in the ultra-structure of osteoclasts after injection of parathyroid hormone in young rats. *Calcif. Tiss. Int.* **27,** 129–35.

—— COX, K., CLARK, M., HOLICK, M., and ANAST, C. (1979). The effect of 1,25-dihydroxy cholecalciferol on the ultrastructure of osteoclasts in young rats. *Calcif. Tiss. Int.* **28,** abs. p. 175.

HORTON, J. E., RAISZ, L. G., SIMMONS, H. A., OPPENHEIM, J. J., and MERGENHAGEN, S. E. (1972). Bone resorbing activity in supernatant fluid from cultured human peripheral blood leukocytes. *Science, Wash.* **177,** 793–5.

HOSKING, D. J., VAN AKEN, J., BIJVOET, O. L. M., and WILL, E. J. (1976). Paget's bone disease treated with diphosphonate and calcitonin. *Lancet* **i,** 615–16.

HOWARD, J. E. (1956). Present knowledge of parathyroid function, with special emphasis upon its limitations. In *Bone structure and metabolism* (ed. G. E. W. Wolstenholme and C. M. O'Connor) pp. 206–38. Little Brown, Boston.

HOWELL, D. S. (1971). Current concepts of calcification. *J. Bone Jt Surg.* **53A,** 250–8.

—— and CARLSON, L. (1965). The effect of papain on mineral deposition in the healing of rachitic epiphysis. *Exp. Cell Res.* **37,** 582–96.

—— and PITA, J. C. (1976). Calcification of growth plate cartilage with special reference to studies on micropunctual fluids. *Clin. Orthop.* **118,** 208–29.

———— MARQUEZ, J. F., and GATTER, R. A. (1969). Demonstration of macro-molecular inhibitor(s) of calcification and nucleational factor(s) in fluids from calcifying sites in cartilage. *J. clin. Invest.* **48**, 630–41.

HUGGINS, C. B. (1930). Influence of urinary tract mucosa on the experimental formation of bone. *Proc. Soc. exp. Biol. Med.* **27**, 349–51.

HUNT, B. J. and BÉLANGER, L. F. (1972). Localized, multiform subperiosteal hyperplasia and generalized osteomyelosclerosis in magnesium deficient rats. *Calc. Tiss. Res.* **9**, 17–27.

HURLEY, L. S. and SWENERTON, H. (1971). Lack of mobilization of bone and liver zinc under teratogenic conditions of zinc deficiency in rats. *J. Nutr.* **101**, 597–603.

HUTCHINSON, T. A., POLANSKY, S. M., and FEINSTEIN, A. R. (1979). Post menopausal oestrogens protect against fractures of hip and distal radius. A case control study. *Lancet* **i**, 705–9.

IRVING, J. T. (1965). Bone matrix lipids and calcification. In *Calcified tissues* (ed. L. J. Richelle and M. J. Dallemagne). Proceedings of the Second European Symposium, pp. 313–24. Collection des Colloques de L'Université de Liège.

—— and WUTHIER, R. E. (1968). Histochemistry and biochemistry of calcification with special reference to the role of lipids. *Clin. Orthop.* **56**, 237–60.

JANDE, S. S. and BÉLANGER, L. F. (1971). Electron microscopy of osteocytes and the pericellular matrix in rat trabecular bone. *Calc. Tiss. Rec.* **6**, 280–9.

—— —— (1973). The life cycle of the osteocyte. *Clin. Orthop.* **94**, 281–305.

JASIN, H. E., FINK, C. W., WISE, W., and ZIFF, M. (1962). Relationship between urinary hydroxyproline and growth. *J. clin. Invest.* **41**, 1928–35.

JEE, W. S. S. and NOLAN, P. D. (1963). Origin of osteoclasts from the fusion of phagocytes. *Nature, Lond.* **200**, 225–6.

—— PARK, H. Z., ROBERTS, W. E., BLACKWOOD, E. L., and KENNER, G. H. (1970). Corticosteroid and bones. In *Research in Radiobiology, Annual Report of Work in Progress in the Internal Irradiation Programme*, COO.119.942, pp. 312–53.

JONGEBLOED, W. L., VAN DEN BERG, P. J., and ARENDS, J. (1974). The dissolution of single crystals of hydroxyapatite in citric acid and lactic acid. *Calc. Tiss. Res.* **15**, 1–9.

JOTEREAU, F. V. and LE DOUARIN, N. W. (1978). The developmental relationship between osteocytes and osteoclasts. A study using the quail-chick nuclear marker in endochondral ossification. *Dev. Biol.* **63**, 253–65.

JOWSEY, J. (1963). Microradiography of bone resorption. In *Mechanisms of hard tissue destruction* (ed. R. F. Sognnaes) pp. 447–69, Publication No. 75. American Association for the Advancement of Science, Washington DC.

—— (1969). Effect of long-term administration of porcine calcitonin in the development of dietary osteoporosis in cats. *Endocrinology* **85**, 1196–1201.

JULLIENNE, C., CALMETTES, C., RAULAIS, D., MILHAUD, G., and MOUKHTAR, M. S. (1978). Immunochemical characterization of calcitonin in human disorders. In *Endocrinology of calcium metabolism* (ed. D. H. Copp and R. V. Talmage) pp. 55–63. Excerpta Medica, Amsterdam.

JUNG, A., BARTHOLDI, P., MERMILLOD, B., REEVE, J., and NEER, R. (1978). Critical analysis of methods for analysing human calcium kinetics. *J. theor. Biol.* **73**, 131–57.

—— BISAZ, S., and FLEISCH, H. (1973). The binding of pyrophosphate and two diphosphonates by hydroxyapatite crystals. *Calc. Tiss. Res.* **11**, 269–80.

KAHN, A. J. and SIMMONS, D. J. (1975). Investigation of cell lineage in bone using a chimaera of chick and quail embryonic tissue. *Nature, Lond.* **258**, 325–7.

—— STEWART, C. C., and TEITELBAUM, S. L. (1978). Contact-mediated bone resorption by human monocytes in vivo. *Science, N.Y.* **199**, 988–90.

KAHNT, F. W., RINIKER, B., MacINTYRE, I., and NEHER, R. (1968). Thyrocalcitonin.

I. Isolierung und Characterisierung wirksamer Peptide aus Schweineschilddrusen. *Helv. chim. Acta* **51**, 214–17.

KALU, D. N., HILLYARD, C., and FOSTER, G. V. (1972). Effect of glucagon on bone collagen metabolism in the rat. *J. Endocr.* **55**, 245–52.

—— DOYLE, F. H., PENNOCK, J., and FOSTER, G. V. (1970). Parathyroid hormone and experimental osteosclerosis. *Lancet* **i**, 1363–6.

KANG, A. H. and TRELSTAD, R. L. (1973). A collagen defect in homocystinuria. *J. clin. Invest.* **52**, 2571–8.

KANIS, J. A., HEYNEN, G., RUSSELL, R. G. G., SMITH, R., WALTON, R. J., and WARNER, G. T. (1977). In *Vitamin D*, Proc. Third Workshop (ed. A. W. Norman) pp. 793–5. De Gruyter, Berlin.

KAPLAN, S. L., ABRAMS, C. A. L., BELL, J. J., CONTE, F. A., and GRUMBACH, M. M. (1968). Growth and growth hormone. *Pediat. Res.* **2**, 43–63.

KEELER, R., WALKER, V., and COPP, D. H. (1970). Natriuretic and diuretic effects of salmon calcitonin in rats. *Can. J. Physiol. Pharmacol.* **48**, 838–41.

KEMBER, N. F. (1960). Cell division in endochondral ossification. *J. Bone Jt Surg.* **42B**, 824–39.

—— (1971). Cell population kinetics of bone growth: The first ten years of autoradiographic studies with tritiated thymidine. *Clin. Orthop.* **76**, 213–30.

KENNEDY, A. L., SHERIDAN, B., and MONTGOMERY, D. A. D. (1978). ACTH and cortisol response to bromocriptine and results of long-term therapy in Cushing's disease. *Acta Endocr.* **89**, 461–8.

KENT, P. W., JOWSEY, J., STEDDON, L. M., OLIVER, R., and VAUGHAN, J. (1956). Deposition of ^{35}S in cortical bone. *Biochem. J.* **62**, 470–6.

KIMMEL, D. B. and JEE, W. S. S. (1977). Quantitative histology of trabecular bone surfaces in young adult beagles. In *Research in Radiobiology, Annual Report of Work in Progress in the Internal Irradiation Program* pp. 152–61. Radiobiology Laboratory, University of Utah College of Medicine COO.119.252.

—— —— (1978a). Study of skeletal kinetics of young adult beagles. *Research in Radiobiology. Annual Report of Work in Progress in the Internal Irradiation Program* pp. 234–6. Radiobiology Laboratory, University of Utah College of Medicine. COO.119.253.

—— —— (1978b). Comparison of biologic activity of young adult human and beagle trabecular bone. In *Research in Radiobiology, Annual Report of Work in Progress in the Internal Irradiation Program* pp. 237–42. Radiobiology Laboratory, University of Utah College of Medicine. COO.119.253.

KISTLER, A. (1978). Inhibition of vitamin A action in rat bone cultures by inhibitors of RNA and protein synthesis. *Experientia* **34**, 1159–61.

KLEIN, D. C. and RAISZ, L. G. (1970). Prostaglandins and bone resorption. *Endocrinology* **86**, 1436–40.

KOCHHAR, D. M. (1977). Cellular basis of congenital limb deformity induced in mice by vitamin A. *Birth Defects* **13**, 111–54.

KODICEK, E. (1965). The effect of ascorbic acid on biosynthesis of components of connective tissue. In *Structure and function of connective and skeletal tissue* pp. 307–19, (NATO Scientific Affairs Division). Butterworth, London.

KRANE, S. M., BROWNELL, G. L., STANBURY, J. B., and CORRIGAN, H. (1956). The effect of thyroid disease on calcium metabolism in man. *J. clin. Invest.* **35**, 874–87.

KREAM, B. E., JOSE, M., YAMADA, S., and DELUCA, H. F. (1977). A specific high affinity binding macromolecule for 1,25-dihydroxyvitamin D in foetal bone. *Science, N.Y.* **197**, 1086–8.

KREMPIN, B., FRIEDRICH, E., and RITZ, E. (1978). Effect of PTH on osteocyte ultra-structure. *Adv. exp. Med. Biol.* **103,** 437–50.

KSHIRSAGAR, S. G., LLOYD, E., and VAUGHAN, J. (1966). Discrimination between strontium and calcium in bone and the transfer from blood to bone in the rabbit. *Br. J. Radiol.* **39,** 131–40.

—— VAUGHAN, J., and WILLIAMSON, M. (1965). The occurrence of squamous carcinoma and osteosarcoma in young rabbits injected with ^{90}Sr (50–100 µc/kg). *Br. J. Cancer* **19,** 777–86.

LACROIX, P. (1971). The internal remodeling of bone. In *The biochemistry and physiology of bone* (ed. G. H. Bourne) (2nd edn) Vol. 3, pp. 119–44. Academic Press, New York.

LAI, C. C., SINGER, L., and ARMSTRONG, W. D. (1975). Bone composition and phosphatase activity in magnesium deficiency in rats. *J. Bone Jt Surg.* **57A,** 516–22.

LAPRESLE, C. (1971). Rabbit cathepsin D and E. In *The tissue proteinases. Proceedings of the Royal Society Wates Symposium, Cambridge 1970* (ed. A. J. Barrett and J. T. Dingle) pp. 135–55. North Holland, Amsterdam.

LAWRENCE, A. M., GOLDFINE, I. D., and KIRSTEINS, L. (1970). Growth hormone dynamics in acromegaly. *J. clin. Endocr. Metab.* **31,** 239–47.

LAWSON, D. E. M. (1978). Biochemical responses of the intestine to vitamin D. In *Vitamin D* (ed. D. E. M. Lawson) pp. 167–200. Academic Press, London.

LAZARUS, G. S. (1973). Studies on the degradation of collagen by collagenases. In *Lysosomes in biology and pathology* (ed. J. T. Dingle) Vol. 3, pp. 338–64. North Holland, Amsterdam.

LEA, L. and VAUGHAN, J. (1957). The uptake of ^{35}S in cortical bone. *Q. Jl microsc. Sci.* **98,** 369–75.

LEAVER, A. G. and SHUTTLEWORTH, C. A. (1966). The isolation from human dentine and ox bone of phosphate containing peptides. *Archs oral Biol.* **11,** 1209–11.

—— —— (1968). Studies on the peptides, free amino acids and certain related compounds isolated from ox bone. *Archs oral Biol.* **13,** 509–25.

—— PRICE, R., and SMITH, A. J. (1975). The insoluble fraction isolated after digestion of the demineralized human dentine matrix with collagenase. *Archs oral Biol.* **23,** 511–13.

—— —— and TRIFFITT, J. T. (1965). The separation of citric acid from other bone constituents by a series of chromatographic procedures. *J. Dent. Res.* **44,** 1177–8.

—— TRIFFITT, J. T., and HOLBROOK, I. B. (1975). Newer knowledge of non-collagenous protein in dentin and cortical bone matrix. *Clin. Orthop.* **11,** 269–92.

LEBLOND, C. P. and WEINSTOCK, M. (1971). Radioautographic studies of bone formation. In *The biochemistry and physiology of bone* (ed. G. H. Bourne) (2nd edn) Vol. 3, pp. 181–200. Academic Press, New York.

LEE, J. and LAYCOCK, J. (1978). *Essential endocrinology.* Oxford University Press.

LEHMANN, J., LITZOW, J. R., and LENNON, E. J. (1966). The effects of chronic acid loads in normal man: further evidence for the participation of bone mineral in the defence against chronic metabolic acidosis. *J. clin. Invest.* **45,** 1608–14.

LEHNINGER, A. L., REYNAFARJE, B., VERCESI, A., and TEW, W. P. (1978). Transport and accumulation of calcium in mitochondria. *Ann. N.Y. Acad. Sci.* **307,** 248–9.

LEMKES, H. H. P., REITSMA, P. H., FRIJLINK, W., VERLINDEN-OOMS, H., and BIJVOET, L. M. (1978). A new diphosphonate: Dissociation between effects on cells and mineral in rats and a preliminary trial in Paget's disease. *Adv. exp. Med. Biol.* **103,** 459–69.

LEVENE, C. I. and BATES, C. J. (1976). The effect of hypoxia on collagen synthesis in cultured 3T6 fibroblasts and its relationship to the mode of action of ascorbate. *Biochim. biophys. Acta* **444,** 446–52.

—— OCKLEFORD, C. D., and BARBER, C. L. (1977). Scurvy: a comparison between ultrastructural and biochemical changes observed in cultured fibroblasts and the collagen they synthesize. *Virchows Archiv (cell pathology)* **23**, 325–38.

LIEBERHERR, M., VREVEN, J. and VAES, G. (1973). The acid and alkaline phosphatases, inorganic pyrophosphatases and phosphoprotein phosphatase of bone. *Biochim. biophys. Acta* **293**, 160–9.

LIKINS, R. C., McCANN, H. G., POSNER, A. S., and SCOTT, D. B. (1960). Comparative fixation of calcium and strontium by synthetic hydroxyapatite. *J. biol. Chem.* **235**, 2152–6.

LINCOLN, G. A., YOUNGSON, R. W., and SHORT, R. V. (1970). The social and sexual behaviour of the red deer stag. *J. Repro. Fert. Suppl.* **11**, 71–103.

LINDGREN, J. U. and LINDHOLM, T. S. (1979). Effect of 1-alpha-hydroxy vitamin D on osteoporosis in rats induced by oophorestomy. *Calcif. Tiss. Int.* **27**, 161–4.

LINDHOLM, T. S., SEVASTIKOGLO, J. A., and LINDGREN, U. (1978). Short term effects of varying doses of 1-α-hydroxyvitamin D_3 on blood and urine chemistry and calcium absorption of osteoporotic patients. *Clin. Orthop.* **135**, 226–31.

—— —— —— (1978). Interim report on treatment of osteoporotic patients with 1-hydroxyvitamin D_3 and calcium. *Clin. Orthop.* **135**, 232–40.

LIPP, W. (1967). Blood serum protein and the mineralization of bone ground substance. *Histochemie* **9**, 339–53.

LITTMAN, M. S., KIRSH, I. E., and KEANE, A. T. (1977–8). Radium induced malignant tumours of the mastoid and paranasal sinuses, pp. 5–6. Radiological and Environmental Research Division Annual Report. Centre for Human Radiobiology. Argonne National Laboratory ANL.78.65.

LLOYD, E. (1968). Relative binding of strontium and calcium in protein and non-protein fractions of serum in the rabbit. *Nature, Lond.* **217**, 355–6.

—— and HODGES, D. (1971). Quantitative characterization of bone. A computer analysis of microradiographs. *Clin. Orthop.* **78**, 230–50.

LLOYD, E. L. and HENNING, C. B. (1978–9). ANL Progress Report 1978–9, ANL-79-65, Part II.

—— —— and GEMMELL, M. A. (1977–8). The geometry of flattened cells on endosteal surfaces of human bone. Implications for the induction of osteosarcoma and the shape of the dose–response relationship. *Radiological and Environmental Research Division, Annual Report, Centre for Human Radiobiology, Argonne National Laboratory* ANL.78.65. pp. 9–19.

LOUTIT, J. F. (1979). Personal communication.

—— and NISBET, N. W. (1979). Resorption of bone. *Lancet* **ii**, 26–8.

—— and SANSOM, J. M. (1976). Osteopetrosis of micro-opthalmic mice. A defect of the haematopoietic stem cell. *Calc. Tiss. Res.* **20**, 251–9.

LOWE, C. E., BIRD, E. D., and THOMAS, W. C. (1962). Hypercalcaemia in myxoedema. *J. clin. Endocr.* **22**, 261–7.

LUCY, J. A., DINGLE, J. T., and FELL, H. B. (1961). Studies on the mode of action of excess of vitamin A. 2. A possible role of intracellular proteases in the degradation of cartilage matrix. *Biochem. J.* **79**, 500–8.

LUSCOMBE, M. and PHELPS, C. F. (1967). Action of degradative enzymes on the light fraction of bovine septa protein polysaccharide. *Biochem. J.* **103**, 103–9.

McCARTY, Jr., D. J., HOGAN, J. M., GATTER, R. A., and GROSSMAN, M. (1966). Studies on pathological calcification in human cartilage. *J. Bone Jt Surg.* **48A**, 309–25.

McCONAGHY, P. (1972). The production of 'sulphation factor' by rat liver. *J. Endocr.* **52**, 1–9.

MacCALLUM, W. G. and VOEGTLIN, C. (1909). On the relation of tetany to the parathyroid glands and to calcium metabolism. *J. exp. Med.* **11**, 118–51.

MacIntyre, I. (1978). Discussion: Hormonal regulation of bone formation. *Recent Prog. Horm. Res.* **34**, 350.

—— Parsons, J. A., and Robinson, C. J. (1967). The effect of thyrocalcitonin on the blood-bone calcium equilibrium in the perfused tibia of the cat. *J. Physiol.* **191**, 393–405.

Mack, P. B., Lachance, P. A., Vose, G. P., and Vogt, F. B. (1967). Bone demineralization of foot and hand of Gemini-Titan IV, V and VII astronauts during orbital flight. *Am. J. Roentgen.* **100**, 503–11.

McLean, F. C. (1957). The parathyroid hormone and bone. *Clin. Orthop.* **9**, 46–60.

—— and Urist, M. R. (1968). *Fundamentals of the physiology of skeletal tissue* (3rd edn) p. 12. University of Chicago Press, Chicago.

Majerson, H. S. (1964). The physiologic importance of lymph. In *Handbook of physiology, Section 2, Circulation* **11**, 1035–73.

Majeska, R. J., Holwerda, D. L., and Wuthier, R. E. (1979). Localization of phosphatidylserine in isolated chick epiphyseal cartilage matrix vesicles with trinitrobenzenesulphonate. *Calcif. Tiss. Int.* **27**, 41–6.

Maletkos, C. J., Keane, A. T., Telles, N. C., and Evans, R. D. (1966). The metabolism of intravenously administered radium and thorium in simulated radium dial paints. Radioactivity Centre, Mass. Inst. of Technology Annual Report, MIT-952-3, pp. 202–317.

Manolagas, S. C., Anderson, D. C., and Lindsay, R. (1979). Adrenal steroids and the development of osteoporosis in oophorectomized women. *Lancet* **ii**, 597–60.

Marinelli, L. D. (1958). Radioactivity and the human skeleton. *Am. J. Roentgen.* **80**, 729–39.

Marks, S. C. and Walker, D. G. (1976). Mammalian osteopetrosis and bone resorption. In *The biochemistry and physiology of bone* (ed. G. H. Bourne) (2nd edn), Vol. IV, pp. 227–301. Academic Press, New York.

Maroudas, A. (1970). Distribution and diffusion of solutes in articular cartilage. *Biophys. J.* **10**, 305–79.

Marshall, J. H. (1964). Theory of alkaline earth metabolism. *J. theor. Biol.* **6**, 386–412.

—— (1969). Measurements and models of skeletal metabolism. In *Mineral Metabolism* III (ed. C. L. Comar and F. Bronner) pp. 1–122. Academic Press, New York.

—— Lloyd, E. L., Rundo, J., Liniecki, J., Marotti, I., Mays, C. W., Sissons, H. A., and Snyder, W. S. (1972). *Alkaline earth metabolism in adult man.* ICRP Publication 20, Pergamon Press, Oxford. [Also published *Hlth Phys.* (1973), **29**, 125.]

Marshall, J. H. and Onkelinx, C. (1968). Radial diffusion and power function retention of alkaline earth radioisotopes in adult bone. *Nature, Lond.* **217**, 742–3.

Marshall, W. A. (1978). Puberty. In *Human growth* (ed. F. Falkner and J. M. Tanner) Vol. 2, pp. 141–81. Baillière Tindal, London.

Martin, J. H. and Matthews, J. L. (1970). Mitochondrial granules in chondrocytes, osteoblasts and osteocytes. *Clin. Orthop.* **68**, 273–8.

Martin, T. J., Robinson, C. J., and MacIntyre, I. (1966). The mode of action of thyrocalcitonin. *Lancet* **i**, 900–2.

Massin, J. P., Vallee, G., and Savoie, J. C. (1974). Compartmental analysis of calcium kinetics in man's application of a four-compartmental model. *Metabolism* **23**, 399–415.

Massry, S. G. (1977). Pharmacology of magnesium. *Ann. Rev. Pharmacol. Toxicol.* **17**, 67–82.

Matrajt, H., Tun Chot, Bordier, P., and Hioco, D. (1971). Effect of calcitonin on vitamin A induced changes in bone in the rat. *Endocrinology* **88**, 129–37.

Matthews, J. L. and Martin, J. H. (1971). Intracellular transport of calcium and its relationship to homeostasis and mineralization. *Am. J. Med.* **50**, 589–97.

—— —— KENNEDY, 3rd, J. W., and COLLINS, E. J. (1973). An ultrastructural study of calcium and phosphate deposition and exchange in tissues. In *Hard tissue growth, repair and remineralization* pp. 187–211. Ciba Foundation Symposium No. 11 (NS). Elsevier–Excerpta Medica–North Holland–Associated Science Publishers, Amsterdam.

MATTHEWS, J. L., VANDER WIEL, C., and TALMAGE, R. V. (1978). Bone lining cells and the bone fluid compartment, an ultrastructural study. *Adv. exp. Med. Biol.* **103**, 451–8.

MAWER, E. B., BACKHOUSE, J., DAVIES, M., HILL, L. F., and TAYLOR, C. M. (1976). Metabolic fate of administered 1,25-hydroxycholecalciferol in controls and in patients with hypoparathyroidism. *Lancet* **i**, 1203–6.

MAYBERRY, H. E., VAN DER BRANDE, J. L., VAN WYK, J. J., and WADELL, W. J. (1971). Early localization of ^{125}I-labelled human growth hormone in adrenals and other organs of immature hypophysectomized rats. *Endocrinology* **88**, 1307–9.

MAYS, C. W. (1964). Personal communication to J. H. Marshall.

—— LLOYD, R. D., CHRISTENSEN, W. R., ATHERTON, D. R., and PITCHFORD, G. S. (1963). Radium metabolism in a man. *Radiat. Res.* **19**, 210 (plus data from C. W. Mays 1968).

MEDICAL RESEARCH COUNCIL. *Monitoring report* No. 19. (1973). HMSO, London.

MELLANBY, E. (1919). An experimental investigation on rickets. *Lancet* **i**, 407–12.

—— (1944–5). Nutrition in relation to bone growth and the nervous system. *Proc. R. Soc.* **B132**, 28–46.

MELSON, G. L., CHASE, L. R., and AURBACH, G. D. (1970). Parathyroid hormone sensitive adenyl cyclase in isolated renal tubules. *Endocrinology* **86**, 511–18.

MENCZEL, J., POSNER, A. S., and HARPER, R. A. (1965). Age changes in the crystallinity of rat bone apatite. *Israel J. med. Sci.* **1**, 251–2.

MERIMÉE, T. J., LILLICRAP, D. A., and RABINOWITZ, D. (1965). Effect of arginine on serum-levels of human growth hormone. *Lancet* **ii**, 668–70.

—— HALL, J., RABINOWITZ, D., McKUSICK, V. A., and RIMOIN, D. L. (1968). An unusual variety of endocrine dwarfism: subresponsiveness to growth hormone in a sexually mature dwarf. *Lancet* **ii**, 191–3.

—— RIMOIN, D. L., CAVALLI-SFORZA, L. C., RABINOWITZ, D., and McKUSICK, V. A. (1968). Metabolic effects of human growth hormone in the African pygmy. *Lancet* **ii**, 194–5.

MESSER, H. H. and COPP, D. H. (1974). Changes in response to calcitonin following prolonged administration to intact rats. *Proc. Soc. exp. Biol. Med.* **146**, 643–7.

METCALF, D. (1972). The colony stimulating factor (CSF). *Aust. J. exp. Biol. med. Sci.* **50**, 547–57.

—— and MOORE, M. A. S. (1971). *Haematopoietic cells, Frontiers of Biol.* **24**, North Holland, Amsterdam.

MEUNIER, P. J., ALEXANDRE, C., EDOUARD, C., MATHIEU, L., CHAPUY, M. C., BRESSOT, C., VIGNON, E., and TRECHSEL, U. (1979). Effects of disodium dichloromethylene diphosphonate on Paget's disease of bone. *Lancet* **ii**, 489–92.

MILHAUD, G. and JOB, J. C. (1966). Thyrocalcitonin effect on idiopathic hypercalcaemia. *Science, N.Y.* **154**, 794–6.

—— and LABAT, M-L. (1978). Thymus and osteopetrosis. *Clin. Orthop.* **135**, 260–71.

—— —— (1979). Osteopetrosis reconsidered as a curable immune disorder. *Biomedicine* **30**, 71–5.

—— MOUKHTAR, M. S., BOURICHON, J., and PERAULT, A. M. (1965). Existence et activité de la thyrocalcitonine chez l'homme. *C.R. Acad. Sci. (Paris)* **261**, 4513–16.

—— CALMETTES, C., JULLIENNE, A., THARAUD, D., BLOCH-MICHEL, H., CAVAILLON,

J. P., COLIN, R., and MOUKHTAR, M. S. (1972). A new chapter in human pathology; Calcitonin disorders and therapeutic use. In *Calcium, parathyroid hormone and the calcitonins* (ed. R. V. Talmage and P. L. Munson) pp. 56–70. Excerpta Medica, Amsterdam.

MILLER, C. E. and FINKEL, A. J. (1964/5). An examination of retention patterns in patients who received radium by multiple injection 33 years earlier. *Radiological and Environmental Research Division. Annual Report* pp. 7–90. Argonne National Laboratory ANL 2717.7.

MILLER, E. J. (1976). Biochemical characteristics and biological significance of the genetically-distinct collagens. *Mol. Cell Biochem.* **13**, 165–92.

MILLER, S. C. and JEE, W. S. S. (1973). The effects of disodium ethane-1-hydroxy-1 diphosphonate (EHDP) and disodium dichloromethanane diphosphonate (Cl_2MDP) on bone of the proximal tibia of the growing rat. *Research in Radiobiology, Annual Report of Work in progress in the Internal Irradiation Programme* pp. 274–487. University of Utah College of Medicine. COO.119.248.

―― ―― (1975). Ethane-1-hydroxy-1, 1-diphosphonate (EHDP). Effects on growth and modelling of the rat tibia. *Calc. Tiss. Res.* **18**, 215–31.

―― ―― KIMMEL, D. B., and WOODBURY, L. (1977). Ethane-1-hydroxy-1, 1-diphosphonate (EHDP). Effects on incorporation and accumulation of osteoclast nuclei. *Calc. Tiss. Res.* **22**, 243–52.

MINAIRE, P., MEUNIER, P., EDOUARD, C., BERNARD, J., COURPRON, P., and BOURRET, J. (1974). Quantitative histological data on disuse osteoporosis―comparison with biological data. *Calc. Tiss. Res.* **17**, 57–73.

MOORE, L. A., HUFFMAN, C. F., and DUNCAN, C. W. (1935). Blindness in cattle associated with constriction of optic nerve and probably of nutritional origin. *J. Nutr.* **9**, 533–51.

MOORE, M. A. S. and METCALF, D. (1970). Ontogeny of the haemopoietic system: yolk sac origin of *in vivo* and *in vitro* colony forming cells in the developing mouse embryo. *Br. J. Haemat.* **18**, 279–96.

MORGAN, B. (1973). Aging and osteoporosis in particular spinal osteoporosis. *Clin. Endocr. Met.* **2**, 187–201.

MORRIS, A., DAY, J. B., BASSINGTHWAITE, J. B., AN, K., and KELLY, P. J. (1979). Potassium and fluid spaces of canine cortical bone. *Calcif. Tiss. Int.* **28**, abs. p. 163.

MORRISON, R. I. S. (1970). The breakdown of proteoglycans by lysosomal enzymes and its specific inhibition by an antiserum to cathepsin D. In *Chemistry and molecular biology of the intercellular matrix* (ed. E. A. Balazs) Vol. 3, pp. 1638–1706. Academic Press, New York.

MOSS, M. L. (1966). Bone. In *Histology* (ed. R. O. Greep) (2nd edn) pp. 155–73. McGraw-Hill, New York.

MUIR, H. (1978). Proteoglycans of cartilage. *J. clin. Path.* (Suppl.) **12**, 67–81.

―― BULLOUGH, P., and MAROUDAS, A. (1970). The distribution of collagen in human articular cartilage with some of its physiological implications. *J. Bone Jt Surg.* **52B**, 554–63.

MÜLLER, P. K., RAISCH, K., and MATZEN, K. (1977). Presence of type III collagen in bone from a patient with osteogenesis imperfecta. *Eur. J. Pediatr.* **125**, 29–37.

MUNDY, G. R. (1979). Personal communication.

―― and RAISZ, L. G. (1974). Drugs for disorders of bone: pharmacological and clinical considerations. *Drugs* **8**, 250–89.

—— RAISZ, L. G., COOPER, R. A., SCHECHTER, G. P., and SALMON, S. E. (1974). Evidence for the secretion of an osteoclast stimulating factor in myeloma. *New Engl. J. Med.* **291**, 1041–6.

—— —— and SHAPIRO, J. L. (1977). Big and little forms of osteoclast activating factor. *J. clin. Invest.* **60**, 122–37.

—— SHAPIRO, J. L., BANDELIN, J. G., CANALIS, E. M., and RAISZ, L. G. (1976). Direct stimulation of bone resorption by thyroid hormone. *J. clin. Invest.* **58**, 529–34.

—— ALTMAN, A. J., GONDEK, M. D., and BANDELIN, J. G. (1977). Direct resorption of bone by human monocytes. *Science, N. Y.* **196**, 1109–11.

—— VARANI, J., ORR, W., GONDEK, M. D., and WARD, P. A. (1978). Resorbing bone is chemotactic for monocytes. *Nature, Lond.* **275**, 132–5.

MURAD, F., BREWER, Jr. H. B., and VAUGHAN, M. (1970). Effect of thyrocalcitonin on adenosine 3′:5′ cyclic phosphate formation by rat kidney and bone. *Proc. natn Acad. Sci. USA* **65**, 446–53.

MUROTA, S. I., ENDO, H., and TAMAOKI, B. I. (1967). Identification of metabolites of cortisol in culture bone and their effects upon bone formation. *Biochim. biophys. Acta* **136**, 379–85.

—— SHIKITA, M., and TAMAOKI, B. I. (1966). Conversion of cortisol to tetrahydrocortisol by cultured chick embryo femora. *Biochim. biophys. Acta* **117**, 424–32.

MURPHY, G., REYNOLDS, J. J., BRETZ, U., and BAGGIOLINI, M. (1977). Collagenase is a component of the specific granules of human neutrophil leucocytes. *Biochem. J.* **162**, 195–7.

NACHTIGALL, L. E., NACHTIGALL, R. H., NACHTIGALL, R. D., and BECKMAN, E. M. (1979). Oestrogen replacement therapy 1. A 10-year prospective study in the relationship to osteoporosis. *Obstet. and Gynec.* **53**, 277–81.

NEER, R., BERMAN, M., FISHER, L., and ROSENBERG, L. E. (1967). Multicompartmental analysis of calcium kinetics in normal adult males. *J. clin. Invest.* **46**, 1364.

—— PARSONS, J. M., KRANE, S. M., DEFTOS, L. J., SHIELDS, C. G., COPP, D. H., and POTTS, J. T. (1969). Pharmacology of calcitonin: Human studies. In *Calcitonin 1969. Proceedings of the Second International Symposium* (ed. S. Taylor and G. V. Foster) pp. 547–54. Heinemann Medical Books Ltd., London.

NEUMAN, M. W., NEUMAN, W. F. and LANE, K. (1979). Formation and serum disappearance of parathyroid hormone in the infused dog. *Calcif. Tissue Int.* **28**, 79–81.

NEUMAN, W. F. (1969). The milieu interieur of bone: Claude Bernard revisited. *Fed Proc.* **28**, 1846–50.

—— BROMMAGE, R., and MYERS, C. R. (1977). The measurement of Ca^{2+} effluxes from bone. *Calcif. Tiss. Res.* **24**, 113–17.

—— and RAMP, W. K. (1971). The concept of bone membrane. In *Cellular mechanisms for calcium transfer and homeostasis* (ed. G. Nichols and R. H. Wasserman) pp. 197–209. Academic Press, New York.

—— and NEUMAN, M. W. (1958). *The chemical dynamics of bone mineral.* University of Chicago Press, Chicago.

—— —— and MYERS, C. R. (1979a). The linkage between cell energetics and Ca^{2+} fluxes in calvaria. *Calcif. Tissue Int. Suppl.*, Vol. 27, No. 120, p. A30.

—— —— —— (1979b). Blood:bone disequilibrium. iii. Linkage between cell energetics and Ca fluxes. *Am. J. Physiol.* **236**, C 244–8.

—— —— SAMMON, P. J., SIMON, W., and LANE, K. (1975). The metabolism of labelled parathyroid hormone. iii. Studies in rats. *Calc. Tiss. Res.* **18**, 251–61.

NEWTON, D., RUNDO, J., and HARRISON, G. E. (1977). The retention of alkaline earth elements in man with special reference to barium. *Hlth Phys.* **33**, 45–53.

NEWTON-JOHN, H. F. and MORGAN, D. B. (1968). Osteoporosis: disease on senescence. *Lancet* **i**, 232–3.

—— —— (1970). The loss of bone with age, osteoporosis and fractures. *Clin. Orthop.* **71**, 229–52.

NIALL, H. D., HOGAN, M. L., TREGEAR, G. W., SEGRE, G. V., HWANG, P., and FRIESEN, H. (1973). The chemistry of growth hormone and the lactogenic hormones. *Recent Prog. Horm. Res.* **29**, 387–404.

NICOLAYSEN, R. (1937). Studies upon the mode of action of vitamin D. ii. The influence of vitamin D on the faecal output of endogenous calcium and phosphorus in the rat. *Biochem. J.* **31**, 107–21.

NILSSON, A. (1973). Influence of oestrogenic hormones on carcinogenesis and toxicity of radiostrontium. *Acta Radiol. Ther. Phys. Biol.* **12**, 209–28.

NISSENSON, R. A. and ARNAUD, C. D. (1979). Properties of the parathyroid hormone receptor-adenylate cyclase system in chicken renal plasma membrane. *J. biol. Chem.* **254**, 1469–75.

NORDIN, B. E. C., PEACOCK, M., and WILKINSON, R. (1972). Hypercalciuria and calcium stone disease. *Clin. Endocr. Metab.* **1**, 169–83.

—— WILKINSON, R., MARSHALL, D. H., GALLAGHER, J. C., WILLIAMS, A. and PEACOCK, M. (1976). Calcium absorption in the elderly. 11th European Symposium on Calcified Tissues. *Calc. Tiss. Res.* **21**, Suppl. 422–51.

NORIMATSU, H., VANDER WIEL, C. J., and TALMAGE, R. V. (1979). Electron microscopic study of the effects of calcitonin on bone cells and their extracellular milieu. *Clin. Orthop.* **139**, 250–8.

NORMAN, A. W. (1978). Calcium and phosphorus absorption. In *Vitamin D* (ed. D. E. M. Lawson) pp. 93–132. Academic Press, London.

—— and DELUCA, H. F. (1963). The preparation of 3H vitamin D_2 and D_3: their localization in the rat. *Biochemistry* **2**, 1160–8.

NORRIS, W. P., SPECKMAN, T. W., and GUSTAFSON, P. F. (1955). Studies of the metabolism of radium in man. *Am. J. Roentgenol.* **73**, 785–802.

OMDAHL, J. L. and DELUCA, H. F. (1973). Regulation of vitamin D metabolism and function. *Phys. Rev.* **53**, 327–72.

OPPENHEIMER, J. H. (1973). Interaction of drugs with thyroid hormone binding sites. *Ann. N.Y. Acad. Sci.* **226**, 330–40.

ORNOY, A., GOODWIN, D., NOFF, D., and EDELSTEIN, S. (1978). 24,25-dihydroxyvitamin D is a metabolite of vitamin D essential for bone formation. *Nature, Lond.* **276**, 517–19.

ORR, W. L., HOLT, L. E. Jr., WILKINS, L., and BOONE, F. H. (1923). The calcium and phosphorus metabolism in rickets, with special reference to ultraviolet ray therapy. *Am. J. Dis. Childn* **26**, 362–72.

OWEN, M. (1963). Cell population kinetics of an osteogenic tissue. 1. *J. Cell Biol.* **19**, 19–32.

—— (1967). Uptake of ^{3}H-uridine into precursor pools and RNA in osteogenic cells. *J. Cell Sci.* **2**, 39–56.

—— (1970). The origin of bone cells. *Int. Rev. Cytol.* **28**, 213–38.

—— (1971). Cellular dynamics of bone. In *The physiology and biochemistry of bone* (ed. G. H. Bourne), (2nd edn) Vol. 3, pp. 271–98. Academic Press, New York.

—— (1978). Histogenesis of bone cells. *Calc. Tiss. Res.* **25**, 205–7.

—— and MACPHERSON, S. (1963). Cell population kinetics of an osteogenic tissue II. *J. cell Biol.* **19**, 33–44.

—— and SHETLAR, M. R. (1968). Uptake of ^{3}H glucosamine by osteoclasts. *Nature, Lond.* **220**, 1335–6.

—— and TRIFFITT, J. T. (1972). Plasma glycoproteins and bone. In *Calcium, parathyroid hormone and the calcitonins* (ed. R. V. Talmage and P. L. Munsen) pp. 316–26. Excerpta Medica, Amsterdam.

—— —— (1976). Extravascular albumin in bone tissue. *J. Phys.* **257**, 293–307.

—— and VAUGHAN, J. (1959*a*). Dose rate measurements in the rabbit tibia following uptake of ^{90}Sr. *Br. J. Radiol.* **32**, 714–24.

—— —— (1959*b*). Radiation dose and its relation to damage in the rabbit tibia following a single injection and daily feeding of ^{90}Sr. *Br. J. Cancer* **13**, 424–38.

—— HOWLETT, C. R., and TRIFFITT, J. T. (1977). Movement of ^{125}I albumin and ^{125}I polyvinylpyrrolidone through bone tissue fluid. *Calc. Tiss. Res.* **23**, 103–12.

—— —— and MELICK, R. A. (1973). Albumin in bone. In *Hard tissue growth, repair and remineralization*, pp. 263–93. Ciba Foundation Symposium No. 11 (NS). Elsevier–Excerpta Medica–North Holland–Associated Science Publishers, Amsterdam.

PAPWORTH, D. and VENNART, J. (1973). Retention of ^{90}Sr in human bone at different ages and the resulting radiation doses. *Physics Med. Biol.* **18**, 169–86.

PARFITT, A. M. (1976*a*). The actions of parathyroid hormone on bone. Part I. *Metabolism* **25**, 809–44.

—— (1976*b*). The actions of parathyroid hormone on bone. Part II. *Metabolism* **25**, 909–55.

—— and DENT, C. E. (1970). Hyperthyroidism and hypercalcaemia. *Q. Jl Med.* **39**, 171–87.

PARSONS, J. A. (1976). Parathyroid physiology and the skeleton. In *Biochemistry and physiology of bone* (ed. G. H. Bourne), Vol. IV, pp. 159–225. Academic Press, New York.

—— (1978). Functional interactions between vitamin D metabolism and other calcium regulating hormones. In *Vitamin D* (ed. D. E. M. Lawson) pp. 387–415. Academic Press, London.

—— DARLY, A. J., and REIT, B. (1973). Anabolic effect of parathyroid hormone on bone demonstrated by chronic infusion to dogs. *Endocrinology 1973, Proceedings of the Fourth International Symposium, London* (ed. S. Taylor). Heinemann Medical Books Ltd.

—— MEUNIER, P., NEER, R. M., and REEVE, J. (1979). Clinical responses of the skeleton to the synthetic amino terminal fragment of human parathyroid hormone. *Calcif. Tiss. Int.* **28**, 103–5.

PARTHEMORE, J. G. and DEFTOS, L. J. (1978). Calcitonin secretion in normal human subjects. *J. clin. Endocr. Metab.* **47**, 184–8.

PARTRIDGE, S. M. (1968). Trace metals and the cross linking system of the protein fibres of connective tissue. In *Proc. 7th Symp. Group European Nutritionists, Cambridge.* Biblthca nutr. dieta. **13**, 99–110.

PASTERNAK, C. A. (1968). Metabolic aspects of vitamin A deficiency in rats and cultured tumour cells. In *Proc. 7th Symp. Group European Nutritionists, Cambridge.* Biblthca nutr. dieta. **13**, 159–61.

PATERSON, C. R., WOODS, C. G., and MORGAN, D. B. (1968). Osteoid in metabolic bone disease. *J. Path. Bact.* **95**, 449–56.

PATT, H. M. (1976). Bone marrow interactions. In *The health effects of plutonium and radium* (ed. W. S. S. Jee) pp. 609–16. J. W. Press, Salt Lake City, Utah.

—— and MALONEY, M. A. (1975). Marrow regeneration after local injury. A review. *Exp. Haem.* **3**, 135–48.

PATT, H. M. and MALONY, M. A. (1976). Regulation of stem cells after local bone marrow injury. The role of the osseous environment. In *Stem cells* (ed. A. B. Cairne, P. K. Lala, and D. G. Osmond). Academic Press, New York.

PAYNE, R. B., CARVER, M. E., and MORGAN, D. B. (1979). Interpretation of serum total calcium: effects of adjustment for albumin concentration on frequency of abnormal values and on detection of change in the individual. *J. clin. Path.* **32,** 56–60.

PEACOCK, M. and NORDIN, B. E. C. (1973). Plasma calcium homeostasis. In *Hard tissue growth, repair and remineralization*, pp. 409–38. Ciba Foundation Symposium No. 11 (NS). Elsevier–Excerpta Medica–North Holland–Associated Science Publishers, Amsterdam.

—— GALLAGHER, J., and NORDIN, B. (1974). Action of 1-hydroxyvitamin D_3 on calcium absorption and bone resorption in man. *Lancet* **i,** 385–9.

PEARSE, A. G. E. (1968). Common cytochemical and ultrastructural characteristics of cells producing polypeptide hormones (the APUD series) and their relevance to thyroid and ultimobranchial C cells and calcitonin. *Proc. R. Soc.* **B170,** 71–80.

—— and POLAK, J. M. (1972). The neural crest origin of the endocrine polypeptide cells of the APUD series. In *Endocrinology 1971* (ed. S. Taylor) pp. 145–52. Heinemann Medical Books Ltd., London.

PERESS, N. A., ANDERSON, H. C., and SAYDERA, S. W. (1974). The lipids of matrix vesicles from bovine foetal epiphyseal cartilage. *Calc. Tiss. Res.* **14,** 275–81.

PETERS, T. J. and SMILLIE, I. S. (1971). Studies on chemical composition of menisci from the human knee joint. *Proc. R. Soc. Med.* **64,** 261–2.

PHILLIPS, L. S. and VASSIPOULOU-SELLIN, R. (1980). Somatomedins. *N. Engl. J. Med.* **302,** 371–80, 438–46.

PIMSTONE, B. L., BECKER, D. J., and HANSON, J. D. L. (1971). The effect of malnutrition on human growth hormone secretion. In *Second International Symposium on growth hormone*, pp. 17–18. Abstr. 30. International Congress Series No. 236, Excerpta Medica, Amsterdam.

PINCUS, G., DORFMAN, R. I., ROMANOFF, L. P., RUBIN, B., BLOCK, E., CARLO, J., and FREEMAN, H. (1955). Steroid metabolism in aging men and women. *Recent Prog. Horm. Res.* **11,** 307–34.

POOLE, A. R., BARRATT, M. G., and FELL, H. B. (1973). The role of soft connective tissue in the breakdown of pig articular cartilage cultivated in the presence of complement-sufficient antiserum to pig erythrocytes. II. Distribution of immunoglobulin G. *Int. Archs Allergy appl. Immun.* **44,** 469–88.

POSNER, A. S. (1978a). The chemistry of bone mineral. *Bull. Hosp. Joint Dis.* **39,** 126–44.

—— (1978b). Intra mitochondrial storage of stable amorphous calcium phosphate. *Ann. N.Y. Acad. Sci.* **307,** 248–9.

—— BETTS, F., and BLUMENTHAL, N. C. (1976–7). Role of ATP and Mg in the stabilization of biological and synthetic amorphous calcium phosphate. *Calc. Tiss. Res. Suppl.* **22,** 208–12.

—— EAVES, E. D., HARPER, R. A., and ZIPKIN, I. (1963). X-ray diffraction analysis of fluoride on human bone apatite. *Archs oral Biol.* **8,** 549–56.

POTTS, J. T., BUCKLE, R. M., SHERWOOD, L. M., RAMBERG, C. F., MAYER, C. P., KRONFELD, D. S., DEFTOS, L. J., CARE, A. D., and AURBACH, G. D. (1968). Control of secretion of parathyroid hormone. In *Parathyroid hormone and thyrocalcitonin (calcitonin)* (ed. R. V. Talmage and L. F. Belanger) pp. 407–16. International Congress Series No. 159. Excerpta Medica, Amsterdam.

POTTS, J. T. Jr and DEFTOS, L. J. (1974). Parathyroid hormone, calcitonin, vitamin D and bone mineral metabolism. In *Duncan's disease of metabolism* (ed. P. K. Bondy and L. E. Rosenberg) (7th edn) pp. 1225–1430. Saunders, Philadelphia.

Prader, A., Tanner, J. M., and Harnack, G. H. A. von. (1963). Catch-up growth following illness or starvation. *J. Pediat.* **62,** 646–59.

Preece, M. A. (1976). The effect of administered corticosteroids on the growth of children. *Postgrad. med. J.* **52,** 625–30.

—— and Tanner, J. M. (1977). Results of intermittent treatment of growth hormone deficiency with human growth hormone. *J. clin. Endocr. Metab.* **45,** 169–70.

Price, C. H., Moore, M., and Jones, D. B. (1972). FBJ virus induced tumours in mice. A histopathological study of FBJ virus tumours and their relevance to murine and human osteosarcoma arising in bone. *Br. J. Cancer* **26,** 15–27.

Price, P. A., Otsaka, A. S., and Posner, J. W. (1977). Comparison of γ-carboxyglutamic acid-containing proteins from bovine and sword fish bone. Primary structure and Ca^{++} binding. In *Calcium binding proteins and calcium function* (ed. R. H. Wasserman, R. A. Corradino, E. Carafoli, R. H. Kretsinger, D. H. Maclennan, and F. L. Siegel) pp. 333–7. North Holland, New York.

—— —— Poser, J. W., Kristaponis, J., and Ramon, N. (1976). Characterization of a γ-carboxyglutamic acid-containing protein from bone. *Proc. natn. Acad. Sci. USA* **73,** 1447–51.

Pritchard, J. J. (1972). The osteoblast. In *The Biochemistry and physiology of bone* (ed. G. H. Bourne) (2nd edn) Vol. 1, pp. 21–43. Academic Press, New York.

Prockop, D. J., Kivirikko, K. I., Tuderman, L., and Guzman, N. A. (1979). The biosynthesis of collagen and its disorders. *New Engl. J. Med.* **301,** 13–23, 77–85.

Pugliarello, M. C., Vittur, F., de Bernard, B., Bonucci, E., and Ascenzi, A. (1973). Analysis of bone composition at the microscopic level. *Calc. Tiss. Res.* **12,** 209–16.

Puschett, J. B., Fernandez, P. C., Boyle, I. T., Gray, R. W., Amdahl, J. L., and DeLuca, H. F. (1972). The acute renal tubular effects of 1,25-dihydroxycholecalciferol. *Proc. Soc. exp. Biol. Med.* **141,** 379–84.

Pyke, R. E., Mack, P. B., Hoffman, R. A., Gilchrist, W. W., Hood, W. N., and George, C. P. (1968). Physiologic and metabolic changes in Macaca Nemestrina on two types of diet during restraint and non restraint. iii. Excretion of calcium and phosphorus. *Aerospace Med.* **39,** 704–8.

Rabinovitch, A. L. and Anderson, H. C. (1976). Biogenesis of matrix vesicles in cartilage growth plates. *Fedn Proc.* **35,** 112–16.

Radfar, N., Ansusingha, K., and Kenny, F. M. (1976). Circulating bound and free estradiol and esterone during normal growth and development and in premature thelarche and isosexual precosity. *J. Pediatr.* **89,** 719–23.

Raisz, L. G. (1965). Inhibition by Actinomycin D of bone resorption induced by parathyroid hormone or Vitamin A. *Proc. Soc. exp. Biol. Med.* **119,** 614–17.

—— and Niemann, U. (1969). Effect of phosphate, calcium and magnesium on bone resorption and hormonal response in tissue culture. *Endocrinology* **85,** 446–52.

—— Au, W. Y. W., and Tepperman, J. (1961). Effect of changes in parathyroid activity on bone metabolism in vitro. *Endocrinology* **68,** 446–52.

—— Au, W. Y. W., Friedman, J., and Nieman, I. (1967). Thyrocalcitonin and bone resorption. *Am. J. Med.* **43,** 684–90.

—— Trummel, C. L., Holick, M. F., and DeLuca, H. F. (1972). 1,25 dihydroxycholecalciferol: a potent stimulator of bone resorption in tissue culture. *Science, N.Y.* **175,** 768–9.

—— Trummel, C. L., Wener, J. A., and Simmons, H. A. (1972). Effect of glucocorticoids on bone resorption in tissue culture. *Endocrinology* **90,** 961–7.

—— Canalis, E. M., Dietrich, J. W., Kream, B. E., and Gworek, S. C. (1978). Hormonal regulation of bone formation. *Recent Prog. Horm. Res.* **34,** 335–48.

—— Maina, D. M., Gworek, S. C., Dietrich, J. W., and Canalis, E. M. (1978).

Hormonal control of bone collagen synthesis *in vitro*: inhibitory effect of 1-hydroxylated vitamin D metabolites. *Endocrinology* **102,** 731–5.

—— DIETRICH, J. W., SIMMONS, H. A., SEYBERTH, H. W., HUBBARD, W., OATES, J. A. (1977). Effect of prostaglandin endoperoxides and metabolites on bone resorption *in vitro*. *Nature, Lond.* **267,** 532–4.

—— LUBEN, R. A., MUNDY, G. R., DIETRICH, J. W., HORTON, J. E., and TRUMMEL, C. L. (1975). Effect of osteoclast activating factor from human leucocytes on bone metabolism. *J. clin. Invest.* **56,** 408–13.

RAJAN, K. T. (1969). The cultivation in vitro of post foetal mammalian cartilage and its response to hypervitaminosis. A. *Exp. Cell Res.* **55,** 419–22.

—— and HOPKINS, A. M. (1970). Human digits in organ culture. *Nature, Lond.* **227,** 621–2.

RAO, L. E., HEERSCHE, J. N. N., STURTRIDGE, W. C., and MARCHUK, L. L. (1979). Immunohistochemical localization of calcitonin receptors in bone and kidney. *Calcif. Tiss. Int.* **28,** 154.

RAO, V. H. and BOSE, S. M. (1971). Effect of certain vitamins on the formation of cross-links in the collagen of lathyritic rats. *J. Vitam.* **17,** 19–23.

RASMUSSEN, H. (1968). The parathyroids. In *Textbook of endocrinology* (ed. R. H. Williams) (4th edn) pp. 847–965. Saunders, Philadelphia.

—— (1972). The cellular basis of mammalian calcium homeostasis. *Clin. Endocr. Metab.* **1,** 3–20.

—— and BORDIER, P. (1974). The physiological and cellular basis of metabolic bone disease, pp. 43–7. Williams and Wilkins Co., New York.

—— and GOODMAN, D. B. P. (1977). Calcium and cyclic nucleotides. *Physiol. Rev.* **57,** 421–509.

REDDY, S. and SUTTIE, J. W. (1979). Possible physiological role of the Vitamin K dependent bone proteins. In *Vitamin K Metabolism and Vitamin K-dependent proteins* (ed. J. W. Suttie) pp. 255–8. University Park Press, Baltimore.

REEVE, J. (1978). The turnover time of calcium in the exchangeable pools of bone in man and the long term effect of a parathyroid hormone fragment. *Clin. Endocr.* **8,** 445–55.

—— and HESP, R. (1976). A model-independent comparison of the rate of uptake and short time retention of ^{47}Ca and ^{85}Sr. by the skeleton. *Calc. Tiss. Res.* **22,** 183–9.

—— —— and WOOTTON, R. (1976). A new tracer method for the calculation of rates of bone formation and breakdown in osteoporosis and other generalized skeletal disorders. *Calc. Tiss. Res.* **22,** 191–206.

—— VEALL, N., and WOOTTON, R. (1978). Problems in the analysis of dynamic tracer studies. *Clin. Sci. mol. Med.* **55,** 225–30.

REEVE, J., WOOTTON, R., and HESP, R. (1976). A new method for calculating the accretion rate of bone calcium and some observations on the suitability of ^{85}Sr as a tracer for bone calcium. *Calc. Tiss. Res.* **20,** 121–35.

REEVES, J. D., AUGUST, C. S., HUMBERT, J. R., and WESTON, W. L. (1979). Host defence in infantile osteopetrosis. *Pediatrics* **64,** 202–6.

REITSMA, P. H., BIJVOET, O. L. M., FRIJLINK, W. B., VISMANS, F. J. F. E., and VAN BREUKELEN, F. J. M. (1980). Pharmacology of disodium (3-amino-1-hydroxy-propylidene)-1-Bis-Phosphonate. To be published.

REYNOLDS, J. J. (1967). The synthesis of collagen by chick bone rudiments in vitro. *Exp. Cell Res.* **47,** 42–8.

—— (1968). Inhibition by calcitonin of bone resorption induced in vitro by vitamin A. *Proc. R. Soc.* **B170,** 61–9.

—— (1972). Skeletal tissue in culture. In *The biochemistry and physiology of bone* (ed. G. H. Bourne) Vol. 1, pp. 69–126. Academic Press, New York.

—— (1973). Bone remodelling: *in vitro* studies on vitamin D metabolites. In *Hard tissue, growth, repair and remineralization*, pp. 315–30. Ciba Foundation Symposium No. 11 (NS). Elsevier–Excerpta Medica–North Holland–Associated Science Publishers, Amsterdam.

—— (1974). *The role of 1,25-dihydroxycholecalciferol in bone metabolism*. Biochemical Society Special Publication No. 3, pp. 91–102.

—— and DINGLE, J. T. (1970). A sensitive *in vitro* method for studying the induction and inhibition of bone resorption. *Calc. Tiss. Res.* **4**, 339–49.

—— PAVLOVITCH, H., and BALSAN, S. (1976). 1,25-dihydroxycholecalciferol increases bone resorption in thyroparathyroidectomized mice. *Calc. Tiss. Res.* **21**, 207–12.

—— MURPHY, G., SELLERS, A., and CARTWRIGHT, E. (1977). A new factor that may control collagen resorption. *Lancet* **ii**, 333–5.

RHINELANDER, F. W. (1972). Circulation of bone. In *The physiology and biochemistry of bone* (ed. G. H. Bourne) (2nd edn) Vol. 2, pp. 1–76.

RIGGS, B. L., JOWSEY, J., KELLY, P. J., HOFFMAN, D. L., and ARNAUD, C. D. (1973). Studies on pathogenesis and treatment in post menopausal and senile osteoporosis. *Clin. Endocr. Metab.* **2**, 317–32.

—— RYAN, R. J., WAHNER, H. W., JIANG, N. S., and MATTOX, V. R. (1973). Serum concentrations of oestrogen, testosterone and gonadotrophins in osteoporotic and non osteoporotic post-menopausal women. *J. clin. Endocr. Met.* **36**, 1097–9.

ROBERTSON, W. G. (1976). Measurement of ionized calcium in body fluids. *Ann. clin. Biochem.* **13**, 540–8.

ROBINSON, D. R., TASHJIAN, A. H. Jr, and LEVINE, L. (1975). Prostaglandin E induced bone resorption by rheumatoid synovia. A model for bone destruction in rheumatoid arthritis. *Arthritis Rheum.* **18**, 422.

ROBINSON, R. A. and WATSON, M. L. (1955). Crystal collagen relationships in bone as observed in the electron microscope. III. Crystal and collagen morphology as a function of age. *Ann. N.Y. Acad. Sci.* **60**, 596–628.

ROBISON, G. A., BUTCHER, R. W., and SUTHERLAND, E. W. (1971). *Cyclic AMP*, pp. 363–73. Academic Press, New York.

ROBISON, R. (1923). The possible significance of hexosophosphoric esters in ossification. ix. Calcification *in vitro*. *Biochem. J.* **24**, 1927–41.

RONA, R. J. and TANNER, J. M. (1977). Aetiology of idiopathic growth hormone deficiency in England and Wales. *Arch. Dis. Childh.* **52**, 197–208.

ROOT, A. W., ROSENFIELD, R. L., BANGIOVANNI, A. M., and EVERLEIN, W. R. (1967). The plasma growth hormone response to insulin induced hypoglycaemia in children with retardation of growth. *Pediatrics* **39**, 844–52.

—— SNYDER, P. J., REZVANI, I., DIGEORGE, A. M., and UTIGER, R. D. (1973). Inhibition of thyrotropin-releasing hormone-mediated secretion of thyrotropin by human growth hormone. *J. clin. Endocrinol.* **36**, 103–7.

ROSENBERG, L. (1973). Cartilage proteoglycans. *Fedn Proc. Fedn Am. Soc. exp. Biol.* **32**, 1467–73.

ROSENBLATT, M., SEGRE, G. V., TREGEAR, G. W., SHEPHARD, G. L., TYLER, G. A., and POTTS, J. T. Jr. (1978). Human parathyroid hormone, synthesis and chemical, biological and immunological evaluation of the carboxyl terminal region. *Endocrinology* **103**, 978–84.

ROUGET, C. (1873). Mémoire sur le dévelopement de la tunique contractile des vaisseaux. *C. r. hebd Séanc. Acad. Sci., Paris* **79**, 559.

ROWLAND, R. E. (1966). Exchangeable bone calcium. *Clin. Orthop.* **49**, 233–48.

—— and MARSHALL, J. H. (1959). Radium in human bone: the dose in microscopic volumes of bone. *Radiat*. **11**, 299–313.

ROYER, P. and MATHIEU, H. (1962). Métabolisme du calcium dans l'insuffisance thyroidienne humaine et experimentale. *Path. Biol*. **10**, 1035–45.

RUNDO, J. (1968). The retention of barium 133 in man. *Int. J. Radiat. Biol*. **13**, 301–2.

RUSSELL, J. E., TERMINE, J. D., and AVIOLI, L. V. (1973). Abnormal bone mineral maturation in the chronic uraemic state. *J. clin. Invest*. **52**, 2848–52.

RUSSELL, R. G. G. (1976). Regulation of calcium metabolism. *Ann. clin. Biochem*. **13**, 518–39.

—— and FLEISCH, H. (1976). Pyrophosphate and diphosphonates. In *The biochemistry and physiology of bone* (ed. G. H. Bourne) (2nd edn) Vol. IV, pp. 61–104. Academic Press, New York.

—— and SMITH, R. (1973). Diphosphonates: experimental and clinical aspects. *J. Bone Jt Surg*. **55B**, 66–86.

—— CASEY, P. A., and FLEISCH, H. (1968). Stimulation of phosphate excretion by the renal arterial infusion of 3′5′ AMP (cyclic AMP), a possible mechanism of action of parathyroid hormone. *Calcif. tissue Res*. Suppl. 54–54a.

—— SMITH, R., WALTON, R. J., PRESTON, C., BASSON, R., HENDERSON, R. G., and NORMAN, A. W. (1974). 1,25-dihydroxycholecalciferol and 1-α-hydroxycholecalciferol on hypoparathyroidism. *Lancet* **ii**, 14–17.

SAKAMOTO, S., GOLDHABER, P., and GLIMCHER, M. J. (1973). The effect of heparin on the amount of enzyme released in tissue culture and on the activity of the enzyme. *Calc. Tiss. Res*. **12**, 247–58.

SALMON, W. D. and DAUGHADAY, W. H. (1957). A hormonally controlled serum factor which stimulates sulphate incorporation by cartilage in vitro. *J. Lab. clin. Med*. **49**, 825–36.

SAVILLE, P. D. (1970). Observations on 80 women with osteoporotic spine fractures. In *Osteoporosis* (ed. U. S. Barzel) pp. 38–46. Grune and Stratton, New York.

—— (1973). The syndrome of spinal osteoporosis. *Clin. Endocr. Metab*. **2**, 177–85.

SCARPACE, P. J. and NEUMAN, W. F. (1976a). The blood:bone disequilibrium. (1) The active accumulation of K^+ into bone extracellular fluid. *Calc. Tiss. Res*. **20**, 137–49.

—— —— (1976b). The blood: bone equilibrium. (ii) Evidence against the active accumulation of calcium or phosphate into the bone extracellular fluid. *Calc. Tiss. Res*. **20**, 151–8.

SCHACHTER, D., FINKELSTEIN, J. D., and KOWARSKI, S. (1964). Metabolism of vitamin D. Preparation of radioactive vitamin D and its intestinal absorption in the rat. *J. clin. Invest*. **43**, 787–96.

SCHENK, R., MERZ, W. A., FLEISCH, H., MUHLBAUER, R. C., and RUSSELL, R. G. G. (1973). Effect of ethane-1-hydroxy-1, 1-diphosphonate (EHDP) and dichloromethylene diphosphate U_2MDF on the calcification and resorption of cartilage and bone in the tibial epiphysis and metaphysis of rats. *Calc. Tiss. Res*. **11**, 196–214.

SCHERFT, J. P. (1972). The lamina limitans of the organic matrix of calcified cartilage and bone. *J. Ultrastruct. Res*. **38**, 318–31.

—— (1978). The lamina limitans of the organic bone matrix: Formation in vitro. *J. Ultrastruct. Res*. **64**, 173–81.

SCHLUNDT, H., NERANCY, J. T., and MORRIS, J. P. (1933). The detection and estimation of radium in living persons. IV. The retention of soluble radium salts administered intravenously. *Am. J. Roentgenol. Radiat. Therapy* **30**, 515–22.

SCHMIDT, J. (1962). Osteopetrosis myxoedematosa with nephrolethiasis. *Z. Kinderheilk*. **86**, 602–18.

SCHWARTZ, E. R. and ADAMY, L. (1977). Effect of ascorbic acid on aryl sulphatase activities and sulphated proteoglycan metabolism in chondrocyte cultures. *J. clin. Invest.* **60**, 96–106.

SCHWARTZ, R. and REDDI, A. H. (1979). Influence of magnesium depletion on matrix induced endochondral bone formation. *Calcif. Tiss. Int.* **29**, 15–20.

SEGRÉ, G. V., HABENER, J. F., POWELL, D., TREGEAR, G. W., and POTTS, J. T. Jr. (1972). Parathyroid hormone in human plasma. Immunochemical characterization and biological implications. *J. clin. Invest.* **51**, 3163–72.

—— ROSENBLATT, M., REINER, B. L., MAHAFFY, J. E., and POTTS, J. T. (1979). Characterization of parathyroid hormone receptors in canine renal cortical plasma membrane using a radioiodinated sulphur free hormone analogue. *J. biol. Chem.* **254**, 6980–6.

—— TULLY, G., ROSENBLATT, M., LAUGHARN, J., REIT, B., and POTTS, J. T. (1979). Evaluation of an *in vitro* parathyroid hormone (bPTH) antagonist in intact dogs. *Calcif. Tiss. Int.* **28**, abs. 171.

SELIGER, W. G. (1970). Tissue fluid movement in compact bone. *Anat. Rec.* **166**, 247–55.

SELLERS, A. and REYNOLDS, J. R. (1977). Identification and partial characterization of an inhibitor of collagenase from rabbit bone. *Biochem. J.* **167**, 353–60.

—— —— and MEIKLE, M. C. (1978). Neutral metallo-proteinases of rabbit bone. *Biochem. J.* **171**, 493–6.

SERAFINI-FRACASSINE, A. and SMITH, J. W. (1974). *The structure and biochemistry of cartilage.* Churchill Livingston, Edinburgh.

SEYBERTH, H. W., RAISZ, L. G., and OATES, J. A. (1978). Prostaglandins and hypercalcaemic states. *Ann. Rev. Med.* **29**, 23–9.

SHAPIRO, I. M. (1970). The phospholipids of mineralized tissue. *Calc. Tiss. Res.* **5**, 21–9.

—— (1971). The neutral lipids of bovine bone. *Archs oral Biol.* **16**, 411–21.

SHETLAR, M. R., SHURLEY, H., and HERN, D. (1972). The effects of parathyroid extract upon incorporation of $1,^{14}C$ glucosamine into bone. *Proc. Soc. exp. Biol. Med.* **139**, 340–4.

SHIM, S. S. and PATTERSON, F. P. (1967). A direct method of qualitative study of bone blood circulation. *Surgery Gynec. Obstet.* **125**, 261–8.

SHORT, R. V. (1976). The evolution of human reproduction. *Proceedings of the Royal Society London* **B195**, pp. 3–24.

—— (1980). The hormonal control of growth at puberty. In *Growth in animals*, (ed. T. L. J. Lawrence) pp. 25–45. Butterworth & Co., London.

SIEGEL, R. C., PINNILL, S. R., and MARTIN, G. R. (1970). Cross-linking of collagen and elastin. Properties of lysyl oxidase. *Biochemistry* **9**, 4486–92.

SILBERBERG, M. and SILBERBERG, R. (1971). Steroid hormones and bone. In *The Biochemistry and physiology of bone* (ed. G. H. Bourne) Vol. 3, pp. 401–84. Academic Press, New York.

SILVERMAN, F. N. and CURRARINO, G. (1960). Roentgen manifestations of hereditary metabolic diseases in childhood. *Metabolism* **9**, 248–81.

SINGER, F. R. and HABENER, J. F. (1974). Multiple immuno reactive form of calcitonin in human plasma. *Biochem. Biophys. Res. Commun.* **61**, 710–16.

SISSONS, H. A. (1970). Dimensions of cells covering bone surfaces. Medical Research Council (London) Subcommittee on Permissible Levels. PIRC/PL/70/4.

—— (1971). The growth of bone. In *The physiology and biochemistry of bone* (ed. G. H. Bourne) Vol. III, pp. 145–80. Academic Press, New York.

—— HOLLEY, K. J., and HEIGHWAY, J. (1967). Normal bone structure in relation to osteomalacia, Tours 1965 (ed. D. J. Hioco), pp. 19–37. Maison et Cie, Paris.

SLAVKIN, H. C., CROISSANT, R., and BRINGES, P. Jr. (1972). Epithelialmesenchymal interactions during odontogenesis. III. A simple method for the isolation of matrix vesicles. *J. Cell Biol.* **53,** 841–9.

—— BRINGES, P. Jr., CROISSANT, R., and BAVETTA, J. A. (1972). Epithelial-mesenchymal interaction during odontogenesis. II. Intercellular matrix vesicles. *Mech. Age Devol.* **1,** 1–13.

SMITH, A. J. and LEAVER, A. G. (1978). The effect of periodate degradation and collagenase digestion on the organic matrix of human dentin. *Archs oral Biol.* **23,** 535–42.

SMITH, B. S. W. and NISBET, D. L. (1968). Biochemical and pathological studies on magnesium deficiency in the rat. *J. comp. Path.* **78,** 149–59.

SMITH, D. A., FRASER, S. A., and WILSON, G. M. (1973). Hyperthyroidism and calcium metabolism. *Clin. Endocr. Metab.* **2,** 333–54.

SMITH, W. G., DAVIS, R. H., and FOURMAN, P. (1960). Calcium deprivation in hypoparathyroidism. A method of diagnosis using sodium phytate. *Lancet* **ii,** 510–13.

SNEID, D. S., JACOBS, L. S., WELDON, V. V., TRIVEDI, B. L., and DAUGHADAY, W. H. (1975). Radio receptor-inactive growth hormone associated with stimulated secretion in normal subjects. *J. clin. Endocr. Metab.* **41,** 471–4.

SORGENTE, N., KUETTNER, K. E., SOBLE, L. B., and EISENSTEIN, R. (1975). The resistance of certain tissues to invasion. ii. Evidence for extractable factors in cartilage which inhibit invasion by vascularized mesenchyme. *Lab. Invest.* **32,** 217–22.

SPENCER, H., WARREN, J. M., KRAMER, L., and SAMACHSON, J. (1973). Passage of calcium and strontium across the intestine in man. *Clin. Orthop.* **91,** 225–34.

—— KRAMER, L., SAMACHSON, J., HARDY, E. P., and RIVERA, J. (1973). Strontium 90 calcium interrelationships in man. *Hlth Phys.* **24,** 525–33.

STANBURY, S. W., HILL, L. F., and MAWER, E. B. (1973). Renal and skeletal interaction: The role of vitamin D. In *Hard tissue growth, repair and mineralization* pp. 391–408. Ciba Foundation Symposium No. 11 (NS). Elsevier–Excerpta Medica–North Holland–Associated Scientific Publishers, Amsterdam.

STARKEY, P. M. and BARRETT, A. J. (1977). Macroglobulin, a physiological regulation of proteinase activity. In *Proteinases in mammalian cells and tissues* (ed. A. J. Barrett) pp. 663–96. North Holland Publishing Co., Amsterdam.

STAUB, B. B., HAMBURGER, R. J., and GOLDBERG, M. (1972). Tracer micro-injection study of renal tubular phosphate resorption in the rat. *J. clin. Invest.* **51,** 2271–6.

STEELE, T., ENGLE, J., TANAKA, Y., LORENC, R., DUDGEON, K., and DELUCA, H. (1975). Phosphatemic acid of 1,25-dihydroxyvitamin D_3. *Am. J. Physiol.* **229,** 489–95.

STEIN, A. H. Jr, MORGAN, H. L., and PORRAS, R. F. (1958). The effect of presser and depresser drugs on intramedullary bone marrow pressure. *J. Bone Jt Surg.* **40A,** 1103–10.

STEVENSON, J. C., HILLYARD, C. J., MACINTYRE, I., COOPER, H., and WHITEHEAD, M. I. (1979). A physiological role for calcitonin: protection of the maternal skeleton. *Lancet* **ii,** 769–71.

STOCKWELL, R. A. (1978). Chondrocytes. *J. clin. Path. Suppl.* **12,** 7–13.

—— (1979). *Biology of cartilage cells.* Cambridge University Press, London.

STRUMPF, M., KOWALSKI, A., and MUNDY, G. R. (1978). Effect of glucocorticoids on osteoclast stimulating factor. *J. Lab. clin. Med.* **92,** 772–8.

STYNE, D. M. and GRUMBACH, M. M. (1978). Puberty in the male and female: its physiology and disorders. In *Reproductive endocrinology* (ed. S. S. C. Yen and R. R. Jaffe) pp. 189–240. W. B. Saunders Co., Philadelphia.

SUNDAR RAJ, C. V., CHURCH, R. L., KLOBUTCHER, L. A., and RUDDLE, F. H. (1977). Genetics of the connective tissue proteins: assignment of the gene for human type 1 procollagen to chromosome 17 by analysis of cell hybrids and microcell hybrids. *Proc. natn. Acad. Sci. USA* **74,** 4444–8.

SUTHERLAND, E. W., ØYE, I., and BUTCHER, R. W. (1965). The action of epinephrine and the role of adenyl cyclase system in hormone action. *Recent Prog. Horm. Res.* **21**, 623–42.

SUTTIE, J. W. (1979). *Vitamin K metabolism and vitamin K-dependent proteins*. University Park Press, Baltimore.

SUTTON, A., HARRISON, G. E., CARR, T. E. F., and BARLTROP, D. (1971). Reduction in the absorption of dietary strontium in children by an alginate derivative. *Int. J. Radiat. Biol.* **19**, 79–85.

SUTTON, R. A. L., HARRIS, C. A., WONG, N. L. M., and DIRKS, J. (1977). The effects of vitamin D on renal tubular calcium transport. In *Vitamin D: biochemical, chemical and clinical aspects related to calcium metabolism* (ed. A. W. Norman, J. V. Schaefer, H. F. Coburn, H. F. DeLuca, D. Fraser, H. G. Grigoleit, V. Grigoleit, and D. Herrath) pp. 451–3. Walter de Gruyter, Berlin.

SYKES, B. and SOLOMON, E. (1978). Assignment of a type 1 collagen structural gene to human chromosome 7. *Nature, Lond.* **272**, 548–9.

TALMAGE, R. V. (1969). Calcium homeostasis — calcium transport — parathyroid action: the effects of parathyroid hormone on the movement of calcium between bone and fluid. *Clin. Orthop.* **67**, 211–24.

—— (1970). Morphological and physiological considerations in a new concept of calcium transport in bone. *Am. J. Anat.* **129**, 467–76.

—— and GRUBB, S. A. (1977). A laboratory model demonstrating osteocyte–osteoblast control of plasma calcium concentrations. Table model for plasma calcium control. *Clin. Orthop.* **122**, 299–306.

—— and VANDER WIEL, C. J. (1979). The influence of calcitonin on the plasma and urine phosphate and ^{32}P changes produced by parathyroid. *Calcif. Tiss. Int.* **28**, ab. p. 155.

—— DOPPETT, S. H., and COOPER, C. W. (1975). Relationship of blood concentration of calcium phosphate, gastrin and calcitonin to the onset of feeding in the rat. *Proc. Soc. exp. Biol. Med.* **149**, 855–9.

TANAKA, Y. and DELUCA, H. F. (1973). The control of 25-hydroxy vitamin-D metabolism by inorganic phosphorus. *Archs Biochem. Biophys.* **154**, 566–74.

—— CASTILLO, L., and DELUCA, H. F. (1976). Control of the renal vitamin D hydroxy-lases in birds by the sex hormones. *Proc. natn. Acad. Sci. USA* **73**, 2701–5.

TANNER, J. M. (1972). Human growth hormone. *Nature, Lond.* **237**, 433–9.

—— WHITEHOUSE, R. H., HUGHES, P. C. R., and CARTER, B. S. (1976). Relative importance of growth hormone and sex steroids for the growth at puberty of trunk length, limb length and muscle width in growth-hormone-deficient children. *J. Pediat.* **89**, 1000–8.

—— —— MARUBINI, E., and RESELE, L. F. (1976). The adolescent growth spurt of boys and girls of the Harpenden growth study. *Ann. hum. Biol.* **3**, 109–26.

TASHJIAN, A. H. Jr., VOELKEL, E. F., LEVINE, L., and GOLDHABER, P. (1972). Evidence that the bone resorption-stimulating factor produced by mouse fibrosarcoma cells is prostaglandin E_2. A new model for the hypercalcaemia of cancer. *J. exp. Med.* **136**, 1329–43.

—— WRIGHT, D. R., IVEY, J. L., and PONT, A. (1978). Calcitonin binding sites in bone: relationship to biological response and 'escape'. *Recent Prog. Horm. Res.* **34**, 285–334.

TAVASSOLI, M., RATZAN, R. J., and CROSBY, W. H. (1973). Studies on regeneration of heterotopic splenic autotransplants. *Blood* **41**, 701–9.

TAYLOR, A. N. (1974). In vitro phosphate transport in chick ilium: Effect of chole-calciferol, calcium, sodium and metabolic inhibitors. *J. Nutr.* **104**, 489–94.

TAYLOR, C. M., DE SILVA, P., and HUGHES, S. E. (1977). Competitive protein-binding assay for 24,25 dihydroxycholecalciferol. *Calc. Tiss. Res.* **22,** Suppl. 40–4.

TAYLOR, T. G. (1960). The nature of bone citrate. *Biochim. biophys. Acta* **39,** 148–9.

TEITELBAUM, S. L., STEWART, C. C., and KAHN, A. J. (1979). Rodent peritoneal macrophages as bone resorbing cells. *Calcif. Tiss. Int.* **27,** 255–61.

TEOTIA, S. P. S. and TEOTIA, M. (1973). Secondary hyperparathyroidism in patients with endemic skeletal fluorosis. *Br. med. J.* **i,** 637–40.

TERMINE, J. D. and POSNER, A. S. (1967). Amorphous/crystalline interrelationships in bone mineral. *Calc. Tiss. Res.* **1,** 8–23.

THOMAS, L. (1956). Reversible collapse of rabbit ears after intravenous papain and prevention of recovery by cortisone. *J. exp. Med.* **104,** 245–52.

THYBERG, J. (1972). Ultrastructural localization of aryl sulphatase activity in the epiphyseal plate. *J. ultrastruct. Res.* **38,** 332–42.

—— (1975). Electron microscopic studies on the uptake of particles by different cell types in the guinea pig metaphysis. *Cell. Tiss. Res.* **156,** 301–15.

—— and FRIBERG, U. (1972). Electron microscopic enzyme histochemical studies on the cellular genesis of matrix vesicles in the epiphyseal plate. *J. ultrastruct. Res.* **41,** 43–59.

—— NILSSON, S., and FRIBERG, U. (1975). Electron microscopic and enzyme cytochemical studies on the guinea pig metaphysis with special reference to the lysosomal systems of different cell types. *Cell Tiss. Res.* **156,** 273–99.

TIPTON, I. H. and COOK, M. J. (1963). Trace elements in human tissue. Part II. Adult subjects from the United States. *Hlth Phys.* **9,** 103–45.

—— and SHAFER, J. J. (1964). *Trace elements in human tissue, rib and vertebra.* Oak Ridge National Laboratory 3697, Excerpt 179.

—— SCHROEDER, H. A., PERRY, H. M. Jr, and COOK, M. J. (1965). Trace elements in human tissue. Part III. Subjects from Africa, the Near and Far East and Europe. *Hlth Phys.* **11,** 403–51.

TONNA, E. A. (1960). Osteoclasts and the aging skeleton: a cytological, cytochemical and autoradiographic study. *Anat. Rec.* **137,** 251–69.

—— (1961). The cellular complement of the skeletal system studied autoradiographically with tritiated thymidine during growth and aging. *J. Biophys. Biochem. Cytol.* **9,** 813–24.

—— (1966). A study of osteocyte formation and distribution in aging mice complemented with 3H proline autoradiography. *J. Geront.* **21,** 124–30.

—— (1972). An electron microscopical study of osteocyte release during osteoclasis in mice at different ages. *Clin. Orthop.* **87,** 311–17.

TOSHIYOKI, Y. and MUNDY, G. R. (1979). Regulation of osteoclast activating factor (OAF) production by prostaglandin (PG) is mediated by cyclic AMP. *Calcif. Tiss. Int.* **28,** ab. p. 152.

TOVERUD, S. U. and MUNSON, P. L. (1976). *Abstr. 58, Ann. Meet. Am. Endocr. Soc.*, p. 104 quoted Cooper *et al.* 1978.

TRELSTAD, R. L., RUBIN, D., and GROSS, J. (1977). Osteogenesis imperfecta congenita: Evidence for a generalized molecular disorder of collagen. *Lab. Invest.* **36,** 501–8.

TRIFFITT, J. T. (1976). Haemopoietic inductive microenvironments. In *Stem cells* (ed. A. B. Cairnie, P. K. Lala, and D. G. Osmond) pp. 255–61. Academic Press, New York.

—— and OWEN, M. (1973). Studies on bone matrix glycoproteins. *Biochem. J.* **136,** 125–34.

—— and OWEN, M. (1977a). Preliminary studies on the binding of plasma albumin to bone tissue. *Calc. Tiss. Res.* **23,** 303–5.

—— and OWEN, M. E. (1977b). Plasma macromolecules in bone interstitial fluid. *Calc. Tiss. Res.* **24,** Suppl. p. R 24, No. 95.

—— Jones, R. O., and Patrick, G. (1972). Uptake of ^{45}Ca and ^{85}Sr by bone in tissue culture. *Calc. Tiss. Res.* **8**, 211–16.

—— Terepka, A. R., and Neuman, W. F. (1968). A comparative study of the exchange *in vivo* of major constituents of bone mineral. *Calc. Tiss. Res.* **2**, 165–76.

—— Owen, M. E., Ashton, B. A., and Wilson, J. M. (1978). Plasma disappearance of rabbit α_2HS-glycoprotein and its uptake by bone tissue. *Calc. Tiss. Res.* **26**, 155–61.

Triffitt, J. T., Gebauer, U., Ashton, B. A., Owen, M. E., and Reynolds, J. J. (1976). Origin of plasma α-HS-glycoprotein and its accumulation in bone. *Nature, Lond.* **262**, 226–7.

Trummel, C. L., Raisz, L. G., Blunt, J. W., and DeLuca, H. F. (1969). 25-hydroxy-cholecalciferol stimulation of bone resorption in tissue culture. *Science, N.Y.* **163**, 1450–1.

Turner, R. C., Radley, J. M., and Mayneord, W. V. (1958). Alpha ray activities of humans and their environment. *Nature, Lond.* **181**, 518–21.

Urist, M. R. (1973). Enzymes in bone morphogenesis. In *Hard tissue growth, repair and mineralization* pp. 143–67. Ciba Foundation Symposium No. 11 (NS), Elsevier–Excerpta Medica–North Holland–Associated Science Publishers, Amsterdam.

—— (1976). Biochemistry of calcification. In *The biochemistry and physiology of bone* (ed. G. H. Bourne) (2nd edn) Vol. 4, pp. 2–53. Academic Press, New York.

—— and Iwata, H. (1973). Preservation and biodegradation of the morphogenetic property of bone matrix. *J. theor. Biol.* **38**, 155–67.

—— Nogami, H., and Terashima, Y. (1975). A substratum of bone matrix gelatin for chondrogenesis in tissue culture and *in vivo*. In *Extracellular matrix influences on gene expression* (ed. H. C. Slavkin and R. C. Greulich) pp. 609–18. Academic Press, London.

—— Mikulski, A. J., Nakagawa, M., and Yen, K. (1977). A bone matrix calcification-initiator non collagenous protein. *Am. J. Phys.* **232**, C 115–27.

Vaes, G. (1968*a*). The role of lysosomes and of their enzymes in the development of bone resorption induced by parathyroid hormone. In *Parathyroid hormone and thyrocalcitonin (calcitonin)* (ed. R. V. Talmage and L. F. Bélanger) pp. 318–28. International Congress Series No. 159. Excerpta Medica, Amsterdam.

—— (1968*b*). On the mechanism of bone resorption. *J. Cell Biol.* **39**, 676–97.

—— (1969). Lysosomes and cellular physiology of bone resorption. In *Lysosomes in biology and pathology* (ed. J. T. Dingle and H. B. Fell) Vol. 1, pp. 217–53. North Holland, Amsterdam.

—— (1973). Digestive capacity of lysosomes. In *Lysosomes and storage diseases* (ed. H. G. Hers and F. van Hoot) pp. 43–77. Academic Press, New York.

Van Breukelin, F. J. M., Bijvoet, O. L. M., and Van Oosterom, A. T. (1979). Inhibition of osteolytic bone lesions by (3-amino-1-hydroxypropylidene)-1,1-Bis phosphonate (A.P.D.). *Lancet* **i**, 803–5.

Vander Wiel, C. J., Grubb, S. A., and Talmage, R. V. (1978). The presence of lining cells on surfaces of human trabecular bone. *Clin. Orthop.* **134**, 350–5.

Van Furth, R. (1975). Modulation of monocyte production. In *Mononuclear phagocytes in immunity, infection and pathology* (ed. R. Van Furth) pp. 161–72. Blackwell, Oxford.

—— and Cohn, Z. A. (1968). The origin and kinetics of mononuclear phagocytes. *J. exp. Med.* **128**, 415–25.

—— Langevoort, H. L., and Schaberg, A. (1975). Mononuclear phagocytes in pathology. In *Mononuclear phagocytes in immunity, infection and pathology* (ed. R. Van Furth) pp. 1–10. Blackwell, Oxford.

—— Cohn, Z. A., Hirsch, J. G., Humphrey, J. H., Spector, W., and Langevoort,

H. C. (1972). The mononuclear phagocyte system: a new classification. *Bull. Wld Hlth Org.* **46**, 845–52.

VAN OSS, C. J., GILLMAN, C. F., BRONSON, P. M., and BORDER, J. R. (1974). Opsonic properties of human serum α2 HS glycoprotein. *Immun. Commun.* **3**, 329–35.

VAN WYK, J. J., UNDERWOOD, L. E., BASEMAN, J. B., HINTZ, R. L., CLEMMONS, D. R., and MARSHALL, R. N. (1975). Exploration of the insulin-like and growth-promoting properties of somatomedin by membrane receptor assays. *Adv. Metab. Disord.* **8**, 127–50.

VAUGHAN, J. (1970). Note on the character of cells on trabecular bone surfaces in adult human vertebrae. Medical Research Council (London), Subcommittee on Protection against Ionizing Radiation. PIRC/PL/70/1.

—— (1972). Bone surfaces: what are they? In *Radiobiology of plutonium* (ed. B. J. Stover and W. S. S. Jee) pp. 323–31. J. W. Press, Utah.

—— (1973). Skeletal tumours induced by internal radiation. In *Bone: certain aspects of neoplasia* (ed. G. H. C. Price and F. G. M. Ross) pp. 337–89. Butterworth and Co., London.

—— and WILLIAMSON, M. (1967). Variation in 'turnover rates' in different parts of the skeleton in relation to tumour incidence due to strontium-90 deposition. In *Strontium metabolism, Proceedings of the International Symposium on some aspects of strontium metabolism held at Chapelcross, Glasgow and Strontian, 5–7 May, 1966* (ed J. M. A. Lenihan, J. F. Loutit, and J. H. Martin). Academic Press, London.

—— —— (1969). ^{90}Sr in the rabbit: the relative risks of osteosarcoma and squamous cell carcinoma. In *Sun Valley Symposium on delayed effects of bone-seeking radionuclides* (ed. C. W. Mays, W. S. Jee, R. D. Lloyd, B. J. Stover, J. H. Dougherty, and G. N. Taylor) pp. 337–55. University of Utah Press.

VEIS, A. and BHATNAGER, R. S. (1970). The microfibrillar structure of collagen and the placement of intermolecular covalent cross linkages in 'Chemistry and Molecular Biology of the Intercellular Matrix, Vol. 1, ed. E. A. Balazs. Academic Press, London.

VILLANUEVA, A., FROST, H. M., ILNICKI, L., FRAME, B., SMITH, R., and ARNSTEIN, R. (1966). Cortical bone dynamics measured by means of tetracycline labelling in 21 cases of osteoporosis. *J. Lab. clin. Med.* **68**, 599– .

VITTUR, F., PUGLIARELLO, M. C., and BERNARD, B. DE. (1971). Chemical modifications of cartilage matrix during endochondral calcification. *Experientia* **27**, 126–7.

—— —— —— (1972). The calcium-binding properties of a glycoprotein isolated from pre-osseous cartilage. *Biochem. biophys. Res. Commun.* **48**, 143–52.

VOLKMAN, A. and GOWANS, J. L. (1965). The origin of macrophages from bone marrow in the rat. *Br. J. exp. Path.* **46**, 62–70.

VON DER MARK, K. and CONRAD, G. (1979). Cartilage cell differentiation. *Clin. Orthop.* **139**, 185–205.

VREVEN, J., LIEBERHERR, M., and VAES, G. (1973). The acid and alkaline phosphatases, inorganic pyrophosphatases and phosphoprotein phosphatase of bone. II. Distribution in subcellular fractions of bone tissue homogenates and structure linked latency. *Biochim. biophys. Acta* **293**, 170–7.

WACKER, W. E. C. and PARISI, A. F. (1968). Magnesium metabolism. *New Engl. J. Med.* **278**, 658–63, 712–17, 772–6.

WAHL, L. M., WAHL, S. M., MERGENHAGEN, S. E., and MARTIN, G. R. (1975). Collagenase production by lymphokine—activated macrophages. *Science, N.Y.* **187**, 261–3.

WALKER, D. G. (1973). Osteopetrosis in mice cured by temporary parabiosis. *Science, N.Y.* **180**, 875.

—— (1975a). Bone resorption in osteopetrotic mice by transplants of normal bone marrow and spleen cells. *Science, N.Y.* **190**, 784–5.

—— (1975b). Bone resorption restored in osteopetrotic mice by transplants of normal bone marrow and spleen cells. *Science, N.Y.* **190**, 785–7.

WASS, J. A. S., THORNER, M. O., MORRIS, D. V., REES, L. H., and MASON, A. S. (1977). Long term treatment of acromegaly with bromocriptine. *Br. med. J.* **i**, 875–8.

WASSERMAN, R. H. and COMAR, C. L. (1961). The parathyroids and the intestinal absorption of calcium strontium and phosphate ions in the rat. *Endocrinology* **69**, 1074–9.

—— and TAYLOR, A. N. (1966). Vitamin D_3 induced calcium binding protein in chick intestinal homogenates. *Nature, Lond.* **198**, 30–2.

—— —— (1973). Intestinal absorption of phosphate in the chick : Effect of vitamin D_3 and other parameters. *J. Nutr.* **103**, 586–99.

WASSERMAN, F. and YAEGER, J. A. (1965). Fine structure of the osteocyte capsule and of the wall of the lacunae in bone. *Z. Zellforsch. Mikrosk. Anat.* **67**, 636–52.

—— FULLMER, C. S., and TAYLOR, A. N. (1978). The vitamin D dependent calcium binding proteins. In *Vitamin D* (ed. D. E. M. Lawson) pp. 133–66. Academic Press, London.

—— CORRADINO, R. A., CARAFOLI, E., KRETSINGER, R. H., MACLENNAN, D. H., and SIEGEL, F. L. (ed.) (1977). *Calcium binding proteins and calcium function.* North Holland, New York.

WEBER, J. C., PONS, V., and KODICEK, E. (1971). The localization of the 1,25-dihydroxy-cholecalciferol in bone cell nuclei of rachitic chicks. *Biochem. J.* **125**, 147–53.

WEBLING, D. D'A. and HOLDSWORTH, E. S. (1966). Bile salts and calcium absorption. *Biochem. J.* **100**, 652–60.

WEINGER, J. M. and HOLTROP, M. E. (1974). An ultrastructural study of bone cells. The occurrence of microtubules, microfilaments and tight junctions. *Calc. Tiss. Res.* **14**, 15–29.

WEISS, L. (1973). Histology of bone marrow. In *Histology* (ed. R. O. Greep and L. Weiss) pp.393. McGraw Hill Book Company, New York.

—— (1976). The haemopoietic microenvironment of the bone marrow: An ultrastructural study of the stroma in rats. *Anat. Rec.* **186**, 161–84.

WEISS, R. A. and ROOT, W. S. (1959). Innervation of the vessels of the marrow cavity of certain bones. *Am. J. Physiol.* **197**, 1255–7.

WELLS, H. and LLOYD, W. (1968). Possible involvement of cyclic AMP in the actions of thyrocalcitonin and parathyroid hormone. In *Parathyroid hormone and thyro-calcitonin (calcitonin)* (ed. R. V. Talmage and L. F. Bélanger) pp. 332–3. International Congress Series No. 159. Excerpta Medica, Amsterdam.

WERB, A. and BURLEIGH, M. C. (1974). A specific collagenase from rabbit fibroblasts in monolayer culture. *Biochem. J.* **137**, 373–85.

WERB, Z. and REYNOLDS, J. J. (1975). Rabbit collagenase. Immunological identity of the enzyme released from cells and tissues in normal and pathological conditions. *Biochem. J.* **151**, 665–9.

WEST, T. E. T., JOFFE, M., SINCLAIR, L., and O'RIORDAN, J. L. (1971). Treatment of hypercalcaemia with calcitonin. *Lancet* **i**, 675–8.

WESTEN, H. and BAINTON, D. F. (1979). Association of alkaline phosphatase positive cells in bone marrow with granulocytic precursors. *J. exp. Med.* **150**, 919–37.

WESTON, P. D. (1969). A specific antiserum to lysosomal cathepsin D. *Immunology* **17**, 421–8.

—— BARRETT, A. J., and DINGLE, J. T. (1969). Specific inhibition of cartilage breakdown. *Nature, Lond.* **222**, 285–6.

WEZEMAN, F. H. (1976). 25-hydroxy vitamin D_3. Autoradiographic evidence of site of action in epiphyseal cartilage and bone. *Science, N.Y.* **194**, 1069–71.

WHALEN, J. P., KROOK, L., NUNEZ, E. A., PENNOCK, J., and DOYLE, F. H. (1973). Calcitonin and remodelling of bones in the growing rat. In *Endocrinology 1973, Proceedings of the Fourth International Symposium, London* (ed. S. Taylor). Heinemann Medical Books Ltd., London.

WHITELAW, D. M. and BATHO, H. F. (1975). Kinetics of monocytes. In *Mononuclear phagocytes in immunity, infection and pathology* (ed. R. Van Furth) pp. 175–85.

WHITESIDE, L. A., SIMMONS, D. J., and LESKER, P. A. (1977). Comparison of regional bone blood flow in areas of differing osteoblastic activity in the rabbit tibia. *Clin. Orthop.* **124**, 267–70.

WIDDOWSON, E. M. and DICKERSON, J. W. T. (1964). *Chemical composition of the body* (ed. C. L. Comar and F. Bronner) Vol. 2A, pp. 1–246. Academic Press, New York.

WIEBKIN, O. W., HARDINGHAM, T. E., and MUIR, H. (1975). The interaction of proteoglycans and hyaluronic acid and the effect of hyaluronic acid on proteoglycan synthesis of adult cartilage. In *Dynamics of connective tissue macromolecules* (ed. P. M. C. Burleigh and A. R. Poole) pp. 81–104. North Holland Publishing, Amsterdam.

WILKINS, L. (1965). *The diagnosis and treatment of endocrine disorders in childhood and adolescence.* (3rd edn). Thomas Springfield, Illinois.

—— and FLEISCHMANN, W. (1941). The diagnosis of hypothyroidism in childhood. *J. Am. med. Ass.* **116**, 2459–65.

WILKINSON, R., ANDERSON, M., and SMART, G. A. (1972). Growth hormone deficiency in lactogenic hypothyroidism. *Br. med. J.* **ii**, 87–8.

WILLIAMS, P. A. and PEACOCKE, A. R. (1967). The binding of calcium and yttrium ions to a glycoprotein from bovine cortical bone. *Biochem. J.* **105**, 1177–85.

WILLIAMSON, M. and VAUGHAN, J. (1967). Histochemistry of the mucosaccharides in the epiphyseal plate of young rabbits. *Nature, Lond.* **215**, 711–14.

WILLS, M. R. (1973). Intestinal absorption of calcium. *Lancet* **i**, 820–3.

WILSON, J. M., ASHTON, B., and TRIFFITT, J. T. (1977). The interaction of a component of bone organic matrix with the mineral phase. *Calc. Tiss. Res.* **22**, Suppl. 458–60.

WILSON, P. W. and LAWSON, D. E. M. (1977). 1,25-dihydroxyvitamin D stimulation of specific membrane proteins in chick intestine. *Biochim. biophys. Acta* **497**, 805–11.

WINTER, J. S. D. (1978). Prepubertal and pubertal endocrinology. In *Human Growth* **2**, 183–213 (ed. F. Falkner and J. M. Tanner). Balliere Tindall, London.

WOESSNER, J. F. Jr. (1973*a*). Purification of cathepsin D from cartilage and uterus and its action on the protein polysaccharide complex of cartilage. *J. biol. Chem.* **248**, 1634–42.

—— (1973*b*). Cartilage cathepsin D and its action on matrix components. *Fedn Proc.* **32**, 1485–8.

WOODARD, H. Q. (1962). The elementary composition of human cortical bone. *Hlth Phys.* **8**, 513–17.

WOODS, C. G. (1973). Discussion. In *Proc. 1st Workshop Bone Histomorphometry* (ed. J. G. Jaworski), p. 201. University of Ottawa Press.

WOODS, C. G., EARNSHAW, M., and KANIS, J. (1977). The relationship between calcification front and osteoblasts. *Calc. Tiss. Res.* **24**, Suppl. R 26, No. 102.

WOOTTON, R. (1974). The single-passage extraction of ^{18}Fe in rabbit bone. *Clin. Sci. Mol. Med.* **47**, 73–7.

—— and REEVE, J. (1979). Difference between Leeds fractures and London fractures. *Br. med. J.* **1**, 1017.

—— —— and VEALL, N. (1976). The clinical measurement of skeletal blood flow. *Clin. Sci. Mol. Med.* **50**, 261–8.

—— —— —— (1977). Skeletal blood flow and calcium kinetics in metabolic bone disease. *Calc. Tiss. Res.* **22**, Suppl. 325–8.

WUTHIER, R. E. (1966). Two-dimensional chromatography on silica gel loaded paper for the microanalysis of polar lipids. *J. Lipid Res.* **7**, 544–50.

—— (1968). Lipids of mineralizing epiphyseal tissues in the bovine foetus. *J. Lipid Res.* **9**, 68–78.

—— (1969). A zonal analysis of inorganic and organic constituents of the epiphysis during endochondral calcification. *Calc. Tiss. Res.* **4**, 20–38.

—— (1971). Zonal analysis of phospholipids in the epiphyseal cartilage and bone of normal and rachitic chickens and pigs. *Calc. Tiss. Res.* **8**, 36–53.

—— (1975). Lipid composition of isolated epiphyseal cartilage cells, membranes and matrix vesicles. *Biochim. biophys. Acta* **409**, 128–43.

—— and GORE, S. T. (1977). Partition of inorganic ions and phospholipids in isolated cell, membrane and matrix vesicle fractions: evidence for Ca-P$_1$-acidic phospholipid complexes. *Calc. Tiss. Res.* **24**, 163–71.

—— and IRVING, J. T. (1964). The lipids in developing calf bone. *J. Dent. Res.* **43**, 814–15.

—— and SHAPIRO, I. M. (1966). Discovery of two unidentified lipids associated with the mineral phase of calcified tissues. *Int. Assoc. Dent. Res. Abstracts*, p. 40.

YONEDA, T. and MUNDY, G. R. (1979). Prostaglandins are necessary for osteoclast-activating production by activated peripheral blood leucocytes. *J. exp. Med.* **149**, 279–83.

YOUNG, R. A. and ELLIOT, J. C. (1966). Atomic scale bases for several properties of apatites. *Archs oral Biol.* **11**, 699–707.

YOUNG, R. W. (1962). Regional differences in cell generation time in growing rat tibiae. *Exp. Cell Res.* **26**, 562–7.

—— (1963). Nucleic acids, protein synthesis and bone. *Clin. Orthop.* **26**, 147–60.

—— (1964). Specialization of bone cells. In *Bone biodynamics* (ed. H. M. Frost) pp. 17–47. Churchill, London.

ZACHMANN, M., FERRANDEZ, M. D., MURSET, G., GNEHM, H. E., and PRADER, A. (1976). Testosterone treatment of excessively tall boys. *J. Pediat.* **88**, 116–23.

ZAMOSCIANYK, H. and VEISS, A. (1966). The isolation and chemical characterization of a phosphate-containing sialoglycoprotein from developing bovine teeth. *Fedn Proc.* **25**, p. 409, abs. 1237.

Index